THE ROLE OF DEMOGRAPHICS IN OCCUPATIONAL STRESS AND WELL BEING

RESEARCH IN OCCUPATIONAL STRESS AND WELL BEING

Series Editors: Pamela L. Perrewé,
Christopher C. Rosen and
Jonathon R. B. Halbesleben

Recent Volumes:

Volume 1: Exploring Theoretical Mechanisms and Perspectives

Volume 2: Historical and Current Perspectives on Stress and Health

Volume 3: Emotional and Physiological Processes and Positive Intervention Strategies

Volume 4: Exploring Interpersonal Dynamics

Volume 5: Employee Health. Coping and Methodologies

Volume 6: Exploring the Work and Non-Work Interface

Volume 7: Current Perspectives on Job-Stress Recovery

Volume 8: New Developments in Theoretical and Conceptual Approaches to Job Stress

Volume 9: The Role of Individual Differences in Occupational Stress and Well Being

Volume 10: The Role of the Economic Crisis on Occupational Stress and Well Being

Volume 11: The Role of Emotion and Emotion Regulation in Job Stress and Well Being

RESEARCH IN OCCUPATIONAL STRESS AND
WELL BEING VOLUME 12

THE ROLE OF DEMOGRAPHICS IN OCCUPATIONAL STRESS AND WELL BEING

EDITED BY

PAMELA L. PERREWÉ
Florida State University, USA

CHRISTOPHER C. ROSEN
University of Arkansas, USA

JONATHON R. B. HALBESLEBEN
University of Alabama, USA

Emerald

United Kingdom – North America – Japan
India – Malaysia – China

Emerald Group Publishing Limited
Howard House, Wagon Lane, Bingley BD16 1WA, UK

First edition 2014

British Library Cataloguing in Publication Data
A catalogue record for this book is available from the British Library

ISBN: 978-1-78350-647-7
ISSN: 1479-3555 (Series)

ISOQAR
REGISTERED
ISOQAR certified Management System, awarded to Emerald for adherence to Environmental standard ISO 14001:2004.

Certificate Number 1985
ISO 14001

INVESTOR IN PEOPLE

CONTENTS

LIST OF CONTRIBUTORS *vii*

EDITORIAL ADVISORY BOARD *ix*

OVERVIEW *xi*

RACE, STRESS, AND WELL-BEING IN ORGANIZATIONS: AN INTEGRATIVE CONCEPTUALIZATION
Gerald R. Ferris, Shanna R. Daniels and Jennifer C. Sexton *1*

A REVIEW OF MINORITY STRESS RELATED TO EMPLOYEES' DEMOGRAPHICS AND THE DEVELOPMENT OF AN INTERSECTIONAL FRAMEWORK FOR THEIR COPING STRATEGIES IN THE WORKPLACE
Thomas Köllen *41*

AGE, OCCUPATIONAL STRAIN, AND WELL-BEING: A PERSON-ENVIRONMENT FIT PERSPECTIVE
Hannes Zacher, Daniel C. Feldman and Heiko Schulz *83*

AGE, RESILIENCE, WELL-BEING, AND POSITIVE WORK OUTCOMES
Rachel King and Steve Jex *113*

RELIGION AND SPIRITUALITY AS FACTORS THAT INFLUENCE OCCUPATIONAL STRESS AND WELL-BEING
Christopher J. L. Cunningham *135*

ANTECEDENTS, OUTCOMES, PREVENTION AND COPING STRATEGIES FOR LESBIAN, GAY, AND BISEXUAL WORKPLACE STRESS
Isaac Sabat, Alex Lindsey and Eden King *173*

OCCUPATIONAL STRESS: CONSIDERING THE COMPLEX INTERPLAY OF SEX, GENDER, AND JOB ROLES
Shannon L. Rawski, Emilija Djurdjevic and Leah D. Sheppard *199*

DEMOGRAPHIC FACTORS AND WORKER WELL-BEING: AN EMPIRICAL REVIEW USING REPRESENTATIVE DATA FROM THE UNITED STATES AND ACROSS THE WORLD
Louis Tay, Vincent Ng, Lauren Kuykendall and Ed Diener *235*

ABOUT THE AUTHORS *285*

LIST OF CONTRIBUTORS

Christopher J. L. Cunningham — Department of Psychology, The University of Tennessee at Chattanooga, Chattanooga, TN, USA

Shanna R. Daniels — Department of Management, Florida State University, Tallahassee, FL, USA

Ed Diener — Department of Psychology, University of Illinois at Urbana-Champaign, Champaign, IL, USA

Emilija Djurdjevic — College of Business Administration, University of Rhode Island, Kingston, RI, USA

Daniel C. Feldman — Terry College of Business, University of Georgia, Athens, GA, USA

Gerald R. Ferris — Department of Management, Florida State University, Tallahassee, FL, USA

Steve Jex — Department of Psychology, Bowling Green State University, Bowling Green, OH, USA

Eden King — Department of Psychology, George Mason University, Fairfax, VA, USA

Rachel King — Department of Psychology, Bowling Green State University, Bowling Green, OH, USA

Thomas Köllen — Department of Management, Vienna University of Economics and Business, Vienna, Austria

Lauren Kuykendall — Department of Psychological Sciences, Purdue University, West Lafayette, IN, USA

Alex Lindsey	Department of Psychology, George Mason University, Fairfax, VA, USA
Vincent Ng	Department of Psychological Sciences, Purdue University, West Lafayette, IN, USA
Shannon L. Rawski	Department of Management, University of Arkansas, Fayetteville, AR, USA
Isaac Sabat	Department of Psychology, George Mason University, Fairfax, VA, USA
Heiko Schulz	Department of Personnel Development, Techniker Krankenkasse, Hamburg, Germany
Jennifer C. Sexton	Department of Management, West Virginia University, Morgantown, WV, USA
Leah D. Sheppard	Sauder School of Business, University of British Columbia, Vancouver, BC, Canada
Louis Tay	Department of Psychological Sciences, Purdue University, West Lafayette, IN, USA
Hannes Zacher	Department of Psychology, University of Groningen, Groningen, The Netherlands

EDITORIAL ADVISORY BOARD

OVERVIEW

In our 12th volume of Research in Occupational Stress and Well Being, we offer eight chapters that examine the role of demographics in occupational stress and well being. The first two chapters consider the influences of minority status on employee stress and well-being, with a focus on developing frameworks that explain how and why minorities experience a unique form of stress in organizations. In our lead chapter, Gerald R. Ferris, Shanna R. Daniels, and Jennifer C. Sexton develop an integrative conceptualization that describes the relationship between race and work stress, with a focus on understanding intermediary processes. In the second chapter, Thomas Köllen develops an integrative model that explains how individuals who are minorities may experience stress due to innate characteristics of organizational processes (e.g., hierarchization, marginalization, and discrimination).

The next section of volume 12 focuses on the relationship between employee age and work stress. The third chapter, by Hannes Zacher, Daniel C. Feldman, and Heiko Schulz, draws from person-environment fit theory to develop a model that explains the relationship between age and employee stress. Specifically, this chapter presents a conceptual model that explains relationships among age, person-environment fit, and occupational strain and well-being. The fourth chapter, by Rachel King and Steve Jex, outlines the importance of considering age in well-being and resilience research. More specifically, the authors draw from the organizational psychological and developmental psychology literatures to develop models that explain how age impacts resilience, well-being, and positive work outcomes.

The final section of this volume focuses on chapters that discuss religion, gender, and sexual orientation. The fifth chapter, by Christopher J. L. Cunningham, explores religion and spirituality as a demographic difference that is relevant to occupational stress and well-being. In this chapter, the author reviews religion and spirituality concepts, integrates these into common occupational stress theories, and identifies directions for future research in this domain. In the sixth chapter, Isaac Sabat, Alex Lindsey, and Eden King identify the mechanisms that explain stress experienced by lesbian, gay, and bisexual (LGB) employees, with a focus on identifying theoretically relevant antecedents, outcomes, and prevention and coping strategies for LGB-workplace stress. The seventh chapter, by Shannon L. Rawski, Emilija Djurdjevic, and Leah D. Sheppard, considers the relationship between biological stress and job stress. In this chapter, the authors develop theory to explain the effects of sex and gender-based role conflict on work stress outcomes (e.g., stress, burnout, and well-being). In the eighth chapter, Louis Tay, Vincent Ng, Lauren Kuykendall, and Ed Diener utilize large, representative samples to examine how age, gender, and race/ethnicity relate to worker well-being. Though many of the observed relationships in this study were complex, and difficult to interpret, the results confirmed that demographic differences influence worker well-being and additional theoretical and empirical work is necessary to understand these relationships.

Together, these chapters offer insight into the role of demographics in occupational stress research. These chapters challenge our traditional thinking and offer several exciting directions for future research. We hope you enjoy volume 12 of Research in Occupational Stress and Well Being.

Pamela L. Perrewé
Christopher C. Rosen
Jonathon R. B. Halbesleben
Editors

RACE, STRESS, AND WELL-BEING IN ORGANIZATIONS: AN INTEGRATIVE CONCEPTUALIZATION

Gerald R. Ferris, Shanna R. Daniels and Jennifer C. Sexton

ABSTRACT

Although employee race has been an actively investigated area of scientific inquiry for decades, a thorough and informed understanding of the role of race in the organizational sciences has eluded us for a number of reasons. The relationship of race and stress in organizations is a prime example of this neglect and deficiency in our knowledge base, as little work has been done in this area. We attempt to address this limitation in the literature by proposing an inductively derived, review-centric framework that attempts to articulate the multiple intermediate linkages that explain the process dynamics taking place in the relationship between employee race and health and well-being in organizations. We argue that socialization processes, social networks, information and resource access, and mentoring contribute to distance and differences between racial minorities and nonminorities concerning control, reputation,

The Role of Demographics in Occupational Stress and Well Being
Research in Occupational Stress and Well Being, Volume 12, 1–39

ISSN: 1479-3555/doi:10.1108/S1479-355520140000012001

performance, and political understanding and skill, which in turn, creates barriers to success, and increased stress and strain for racial minorities. The implications of this framework along with directions for future theory and research are discussed in this chapter.

Keywords: Race; stress; strain reactions; political skill; well-being; social networks

INTRODUCTION

For many years, scholars have noted the importance of the study of race in organizations, and it has been an active area of inquiry (e.g., Cox, 2004; Nkomo, 1992, 2009; Nkomo & Stewart, 2006; Proudford & Nkomo, 2006). Furthermore, with the advent of employment legislation in the 1960s, early research on race focused on equal opportunity and hiring decisions (e.g., Huang, Frideger, & Pearce, 2013; Ilgen & Youtz, 1986; Segrest Purkiss, Perrewé, Gillespie, Mayes, & Ferris, 2006), and the impact of race in organizations has been extensive, affecting important job outcomes like compensation and advancement (e.g., James, 2000; Roberson & Block, 2001). Cox and Nkomo (1990) reported that 71% of the published research in this area reported significant race effects. Also, with the U.S. workforce reflecting an increasing proportion of ethnic and racial minorities (e.g., U.S. Census Bureau, 2004), we clearly need to develop an informed understanding of the role race plays in the organizational sciences because of its theoretical and practical importance (Cox, 2004).

Unfortunately, the degree and extent of this understanding has lagged behind (Cox, 2004; Nkomo, 1992). Indeed, Brief and Hayes (1997) noted that organizational scholars have failed to meet their obligation to more substantially enrich our understanding of race at work. Also, even though complex societal, organizational, and psychological factors may account for race effects, Nkomo (1992) argued that race research to date has provided little insight into such potential dynamics. Additionally, despite the implicit strain consequences of race research in organizations over the years, no efforts to date have been made to explicate the relationship between race and work stress.

In this chapter, we attempt to address this limitation in the literature by proposing a conceptualization of race and work stress, which argues that socialization processes, social networks, information and resource access, and mentoring contribute to differences between racial minorities and nonminorities concerning control, reputation, performance, and political understanding and skill. In turn, these differences create barriers to success, resulting in increased stress and strain for racial minorities. We discuss the implications of this conceptualization, propose some directions for future theory and research, and present a theoretical framework of the relationships discussed going forward.

RACE AND BEHAVIOR IN ORGANIZATIONS

As we noted at the outset of this chapter, much research on race in organizations over the past several decades has focused on the disadvantages that racial minorities experience in hiring/selection, performance evaluation, compensation, and career progress decisions (e.g., Dovidio & Gaertner, 2000; Huang et al., 2013; Ilgen & Youtz, 1986; James, 2000; Roberson & Block, 2001; Segrest Purkiss et al., 2006). A multitude of reasons have been offered for such discrimination effects against racial minorities, including race-differential performance criteria used for decision making, prevalent contextual biased attitudes, lack of accountability of raters/decision makers, and so forth (Dipboye & Halverson, 2004). To move scholarship on race and behavior in organizations forward, researchers need to better understand how employees are affected by, and effectively cope with, discrimination (Colella, McKay, Daniels, & Signal, 2012).

Furthermore, because the ultimate dependent variable in most of this research is the employment-related decision made, with investigations not going further to assess racial minority attitudes and strain consequences, there is much more to learn about the subjective strain-related experiences of discrimination on racial minorities. Extant data suggest that racial-ethnic discrimination has detrimental effects on one's mental health, particularly for African-Americans, Hispanics, and Asians (Colella et al., 2012). These studies show that reports of greater discrimination are linked to lower psychological well-being (Gee, 2002; James, Lovato, & Khoo, 1994; Williams, Yu, Jackson, & Anderson, 1997), lower self-reported health (James et al., 1994; Williams et al., 1997), and a higher number of poor mental health days (Roberts, Swanson, & Murphy, 2004). Although this research has established that there is a relationship between perceived racial discrimination and stress, more scholarship is needed to provide additional explanations for the link.

Therefore, we adopt an alternative perspective in this chapter that moves our understanding of discrimination and its impact on work-related outcomes beyond race-differential performance criteria and prevalent contextually biased attitudes. We propose that getting hired, receiving favorable performance evaluations, being paid well, and winning out in promotion competitions have as much or more to do with distance, positioning, access to contextually relevant information, and development of skill and understanding of politics in organizations than simply being due to racially biased attitudes of white majority managers. Finally, we discuss how these social and political processes can play a role in the stress and strain experienced by racial minorities in the workplace.

The issues related to network distance and positioning, as well as access to information, understanding, and skill building reflect the need for more social and political competencies, and those are areas where racial minorities typically are at a decided disadvantage compared to white majority employees. If racial minorities are not as skilled in social and political influence efforts at work, it may well be reflective of information access and skill deficiency problems. Unfortunately, such lack of savvy, political skill, and failure to understand the way things get done around the organization may result in positioning problems relative to social structure for racial minorities compared to white majority employees, which further compound their social influence effectiveness.

For example, Ferris and King (1992) proposed and tested a distance conceptualization of discrimination in organizations, arguing that distance between supervisors and subordinates correlated significantly and negatively with performance ratings for older compared to younger employees. Ratings of subordinate performance are susceptible to active influence attempts by subordinates, and such influence attempts usually necessitate closer (i.e., rather than more distant) proximity to one another. Ferris and King suggested that older employees were placed at a competitive disadvantage compared to younger employees because the greater distance from their supervisors permitted them less of an opportunity to influence their own performance evaluations. The Ferris and King conceptualization was framed as a model of age discrimination, but just as easily could be applied to race, whereby attitudes drive positioning and distance, which prevents access to opportunity.

So, if management does indeed structure work differently for racial minorities, where they are positioned at greater distance (i.e., physical and psychological) from their bosses, they are at a disadvantage in efforts to influence the performance evaluations their boss gives them. Additionally, this increased physical and psychological distance reduces access to resources, information, opportunities, and so forth that could assist racial minorities with both job performance and career advancement. Thus, their lower resulting performance ratings could become a vicious cycle that hinders racial minorities' upward mobility within the organization.

In a somewhat related manner, Cox and Nkomo (1986) found that raters of job performance in organizations used different criteria to evaluate ratees depending upon the ratees' race. More objective, job-related criteria were used to evaluate same-race ratees, whereas more subjective, social behavior criteria were used to evaluate different-race ratees. Therefore, for example, white raters used subjective, social criteria to evaluate black subordinates, and because performance on these types of criteria are subject to impression management and influence by ratees on the raters, ratees could affect their ratings received if they were skillful in this area of impression management. However, because this typically has been an area of skill deficiency for minorities at work (e.g., Fernandez, 1981), they tend to not fare well in this process, thus being evaluated poorly on performance criteria on which they never should have been evaluated.

Similarly, Hayes (1995) proposed and found support for the notion that network positioning and social capital acquisition mediated the relationship between employee race and advancement progress of racial minorities with respect to managerial advancement in organizations. However, an important question remains: Precisely what factors explain how individuals get well positioned in organizations so that they can take advantage of job and career opportunities, and not experience strain-related consequences from blocked opportunities? We analyze this issue in greater detail in a later section of this chapter, and argue that it might be political understanding and skill that predict such network positioning, distance reduction, and information and resource access that are so critical to both career success and employee stress and well-being.

Similarly, organizational positioning and status is theorized to affect when and why racial minority employees might suppress personal values to conform to the dominant culture or values of the workplace. Hewlin (2003) suggested that facades of conformity, which are "false representations created by employees to appear as if they embrace organizational values" (p. 634), represent a mechanism used by employees to disguise personal values that are different from those held by the organization. Facades may be espoused in various forms, both verbally and nonverbally. However, they also can be a conscious expression of conformity that transpires in the workplace, and in interpersonal exchanges, when there is incongruity between one's personal and organizational values. In many ways, personal values are connected to a person's identity, and are entrenched in one's gender, race, and socioeconomic status.

Although facades of conformity are applicable to all employees, they may function differently depending on individuals' organizational position, status, and race (Hewlin, 2003). Racial minorities, who are not well positioned in the organization, may perceive that they must present outward manifestations of conformity in order to be accepted socially, and to reap the benefits of the dominant group. In essence, racial minority employees who express facades of conformity are in many ways engaging in a form of political behavior. In an empirical test of facades of conformity, Hewlin (2009) found that minority organization positioning is strongly associated with creating facades of conformity, and in turn, emotional exhaustion. The results of this line of research suggest that organization positioning might influence racial minority employees to present false representations of their self, but in so doing, they will incur personal costs that prove detrimental to their well-being.

In a similar vein, research on emotional labor (i.e., which is defined as the effort, planning, and control needed to express organizationally desired emotion during interpersonal transactions; Morris & Feldman, 1996) supports the relationship between facades of conformity and experienced stress. It is likely that employees will experience emotional dissonance when the emotional expression required by their job's display rules conflicts with their inner or "real" feelings. Therefore, it is reasoned that the emotional ambivalence that racial minorities experience as a consequence of creating facades of conformity is likely to lead to stress. The consequence of facades of conformity on racial minorities' well-being can be linked to duality of their self-presentation. This notion is supported by Higgins (1989) who argued that when people experience incongruity between their true self and who they perceive they should be, they experience negative emotions such as fear, anxiety, and stress. In this way, racial minorities are at heightened risk to experience stress which results from underplaying their core values, and pretending they align with those of the organization.

TOWARD AN INDUCTIVELY DERIVED REVIEW-CENTRIC FRAMEWORK OF RACE, STRESS, AND WELL-BEING IN ORGANIZATIONS

We propose a framework to collectively and integratively capture the how and why of the race–stress relationship. Then, in subsequent sections of this chapter, we critically review and discuss the literature related to race and behavior in organizations, with a particular eye toward the implications for the stress, health, and well-being of racial minorities. Also, we discuss how access to information and resources, understanding of politics, and development of political skill through mentoring and sponsorship can pose a partial explanation for both racial discrimination in organizations, and also how and why racial minorities experience stress, strain, and health issues in organizations.

Collectively, then, in presenting our conceptual framework and subsequent review and discussion of critical issues, we seek to propose "novel theoretical insights from reviews of existing theory and research," as suggested recently by LePine and Wilcox-King (2010) as alternative ways to develop new theory in the organizational sciences. Indeed, some previous theory and research on race in organizations has discussed concepts of exclusion and access, mentoring and socialization, social networks and accrued social capital, and political skill and understanding. However, these concepts never have been put together in compelling ways in an attempt to develop a more informed understanding of the race–stress relationship in organizations. That being said, we regard our model as more of a working framework at this point, rather than any type of formal theory. Time and further work will tell whether it can achieve theory status at some point in the future.

Framework Development

The proposed framework is presented in Fig. 1, and it draws from prior theory and research on stress, politics, socialization, mentoring, and social

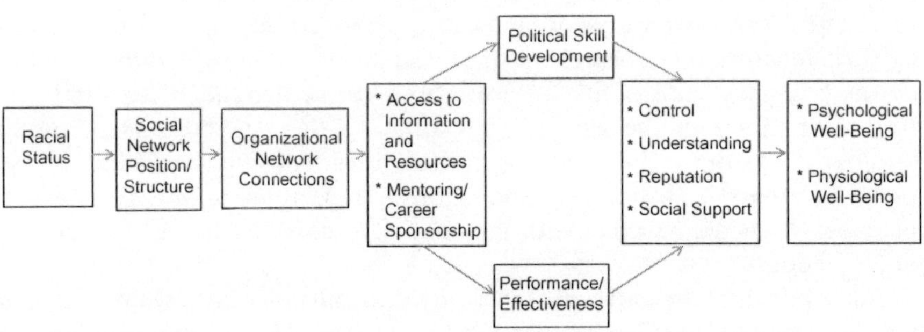

Fig. 1. Framework of Race, Stress, and Well-Being in Organizations.

networks. However, it borrows extensively from the conceptualizations of career progress and social capital by Siebert, Kraimer, and Liden (2001), and also the framework of political skill, health, and well-being by Ferris, Kane, Summers, and Munyon (2011). The implicit message of this framework is that the experience of stress and strain (i.e., vs. health and well-being) in organizations for racial minorities is about relationships and connections, and the information, skills, and visibility that can result from "access" to important people and resources (i.e., vs. exclusion from such preferred pathways, and relegation to outside status). Windows of opportunity seem to be provided for and "opened" for individuals of racial majority status. However, those same windows or points of entry sometimes have to be more cleverly maneuvered so others open them for racial minorities. As such, we believe our framework can shed light on why some racial minorities are closed out and relegated to perpetual "outside" status, whereas other minorities are able to discover the informal organizational road map, which allows them to be successful, happy, and healthy, having achieved "insider" status.

The framework begins by suggesting that individuals' race influences their position in the social network structure. Furthermore, this positioning in the structure leads to individuals being better connected in the organization, both with contacts in other functional areas (i.e., increasing the size and extensiveness of their networks) and contacts with influential others at higher levels in the organization (i.e., increasing the quality and importance of their networks). In turn, such organizational network connections contribute to individuals gaining greater access to critically important information and resources, and also greater legitimacy and visibility one gets from more effective mentoring and career sponsorship.

This is the area described in later sections of the chapter whereby white majority protégés are brought in close by influential white majority mentors. These protégés are promoted and positioned within the organization by their mentors (i.e., increasing their visibility), and educated in the nuances of organizational politics, "how things work around here," and "the ropes" or "rules of the game," thus allowing them to become privileged "insiders." On the other hand, racial minorities typically are excluded from such information, resources, and sponsorship, thus relegating them to unaware "outsider" status, with less ability to compete for effectiveness in organizations.

Such information and skill building contributes to individuals developing their political skill and understanding to higher levels, and also increasing their motivation and performance. Higher performance and political skill will make individuals feel more in control of their work environments. Also, they will develop a more informed understanding of how organizations and politics within them work, which increases their reputations of being perceived by others as more influential and powerful. Such individuals' actual substantive performance will be higher as a result of gaining access to knowledge, information, resources, and mentoring/sponsorship. Additionally, they will increase their reputation and symbolic value as well, which will allow them to compete more effectively for valued rewards in the organization (Ferris & Judge, 1991).

Indeed, Treadway et al. (2013) found that people higher in political skill were able to leverage their performance into greater power in organizations (i.e., as compared to individuals lower in political skill). Also, Siebert et al. (2001, p. 223) argued that information and resources "should increase feelings of both control and competence at work and empowerment." So, the collective impact of social network position, contacts, information, resources, and career sponsorship is that such individuals will realize greater social support. Finally, in addition to enjoying considerable social support and greater reputation, such feelings of control and greater understanding of the organization environment and how it operates, collectively contribute to individuals' high levels of both psychological and physiological well-being, decreased job tension and stress/strain, and increased job and career satisfaction.

A KNOWLEDGE/SKILL ACCESS AND ACQUISITION PERSPECTIVE ON RACE AND STRESS IN ORGANIZATIONS

Organizational scientists have developed a keen interest for years in new employee socialization processes, which reflect the various ways that individuals experience learning, sense making, and understanding about the way things work in organizations. Indeed, socialization has been characterized as the process by which individuals are exposed to and embrace the values, attitudes, and culture of organizations (Bauer, Morrison, & Callister, 1998). Furthermore, one of the principal mechanisms for building savvy and understanding, and transmitting information about how things work in organizations, is mentoring, which has realized increased theory and research interest in recent years (e.g., Noe, Greenberger, & Wang, 2002; Wanberg, Welsh, & Hezlett, 2003). Additionally, socialization research has reported that politics in organizations is one of its most important content areas (Chao, O'Leary-Kelly, Wolf, Klein, & Gardner, 1994), and mentoring has been viewed as the most prevalent mechanism by which individuals learn about organizational politics (Ferris & Judge, 1991), and through which they build political skill (Perrewé, Young, & Blass, 2002).

In the following sections, we present a perspective on race and stress in organizations that complements the framework we just presented. This perspective incorporates theory and research on socialization and mentoring, social networks, information access and exclusion, and contextual knowledge and skill building as a way to better understand the workplace stress and strain of racial minorities in organizations, and how and why they differ from white majority employees. Because much of our thinking has been influenced by theory and research on information availability, access, and social exclusion, we begin with a review of some of this work as a basis for developing the foundations for our ideas.

Race, Social Exclusion, and Stress

There are many socially constructed hierarchies throughout history, one being how racial groups are organized in the United States, and how such hierarchies tend to systematically categorize groups such that some have more power than others. In most instances, majority groups are the primary benefactor of the distribution of power (Graves, 2003; Marger, 2005). The imbalance of power among groups creates situations with in-groups and out-groups, where white majority employees, as in-group members, enjoy much of the power in the United States (Rothenberg, 2005). Consequently, racial minorities fundamentally are placed at a disadvantage, resulting in differential access to opportunities, resources, and support.

Out-group members often experience feelings of vulnerability to those with more power, which can lead to generalized mistreatment in the workplace, resulting in the experience of greater physiological and psychological stress (Ryan & Deci, 2000; Williams, 2007). The effect of in-groups and out-groups can lead to those in the minority/out-group experiencing social isolation in the workplace. Isolation, ostracism, or marginal group membership represent forms of rejection, and in some instances, are viewed as forms of discrimination (Fairhurst & Snavely, 1983; Gerber & Wheeler, 2009; Richman & Leary, 2009; Williams, 2007).

The experience of workplace isolation or exclusion is defined as "the extent to which an individual perceives that he or she is ignored or excluded" at work (Ferris, Brown, Berry, & Lian, 2008, p. 1348). Research on this topic has established that such exclusion is linked to diminished psychological well-being, performance and satisfaction with colleagues (e.g., Baumeister, Twenge, & Nuss, 2002; Hitlan, Cliffton, & DeSoto, 2006), and undesirable behaviors, such as acting rudely, mocking, or arguing with others (Thau, Aquino, & Poortvliet, 2007).

Social exclusion is part of a group of interrelated workplace aggression constructs (e.g., bullying, incivility, social undermining) that are "conceptually distinct, but operationally similar" (Aquino & Thau, 2009; Hershcovis, Reich, Parker, & Bozeman, 2012, p. 2). In many ways, exclusionary acts are similar to workplace incivility or "low-level workplace abuse" (Johnson & Indvik, 2001). Andersson and Pearson (1999) formally defined workplace incivility as "low-intensity deviant behavior with ambiguous intent to harm the target, in violation of workplace norms for mutual respect" (p. 457). According to Pearson, Andersson, and Wegner (2001), these behaviors are considered low-intensity because they involve a "lower magnitude of force" (p. 1401).

Moreover, low-intensity behaviors are not limited to verbal abuse, but also include nonverbal and disrespectful behaviors, such as glaring at, ignoring, or exclusion of a targeted individual. Interestingly, a trend has emerged within this literature which suggests that disrespect and aloofness may at least partially explain why individuals become targets of interpersonal mistreatment and social exclusion (e.g., Anderson & Bushman, 2002; Andersson & Pearson, 1999; Aquino & Thau, 2009). Although research suggests that employees who violate social norms of civility and common courtesy are at risk for being excluded, few studies have explored the roles of race and stress in this relationship.

Cortina's (2008) selective incivility theory is helpful in understanding the interaction of race and incivility. This perspective provides a lens through which researchers can examine interpersonal mistreatment that persists against racial minorities in the workplace. From this standpoint, it is reasoned that individuals holding socially unacceptable beliefs (e.g., sexists or racists) are more likely to instigate workplace incivility. As an identity preservation tactic, individuals with these beliefs behave under the guise of ignorance, and selectively engage in uncivil acts toward out-group members. Such acts are manifestations of their underlying beliefs and motives to undermine members of racial minorities in the workplace.

Cortina (2008) argued that the racial minorities might be most at risk as targets of selective incivility because they are perceived as highly competent and advancing in ways that threaten the dominant white majority. This notion is based on research showing that successful out-groups, such as black professionals and Asians, often are stereotyped as too competent, ambitious, and hardworking, and, at the same time, interpersonally unpleasant and cold (Cortina, 2008). Although these perceptions can trigger admiration to some extent, envy and hostile competition from the dominant white majority also are likely to ensue. To avoid appearances of racism and sexism, the hostility often may take a disguised form, such as "selective incivility" (Cortina, 2008, p. 65).

Although Cortina's (2008) theorizing focused on selective incivility as an outcome, it is also likely that out-groups will experience social exclusion in the same way, and that stress, anxiety, and strain are likely consequences of such experiences. Gottlieb (1997, p. 10) characterized chronic stressors as "persistent demands" that are "woven into the tapestry of life." Many acts of social exclusion would qualify as chronic stress, because exclusion behaviors can create "socially noxious environments" (Gottlieb, 1997, p. 5) for employees, which can trigger mental health problems.

Socialization and Mentoring Processes

The serial approach of the Van Maanen and Schein (1979) taxonomy of socialization tactics often is referred to as "mentoring," because experienced organizational members serve as role models and essentially informally educate newcomers into the ways things get done in organizations. Noe et al. (2002) stated that, "Research needs to investigate the role of mentoring in helping protégés gain political skills" (p. 162). Further, these researchers argued that an important outcome of mentoring is the exposure and visibility of new employees (i.e., protégés), which can result from the increased networking ability that is gained from access to important work and social networks (Siebert et al., 2001).

Learning Content in Mentoring Relationships

Tactics have been an active area of research in socialization for years, but so has the content regarding what the tactics are seeking to impart or transmit (e.g., Fisher, 1986). Based on earlier work, Chao et al. (1994) empirically identified six content categories of organizational socialization (i.e., performance and proficiency, people, politics, language, organizational goals and values, and history). The politics category of socialization content involves: Gaining information regarding power structures, formal and informal work relationships, and learning to handle political behavior. Chao et al. (1994) argued that individuals who are familiar with, and well socialized into, organizational politics may be more promotable than those who achieve greater socialization in the other content areas.

We view the tactics and content perspectives on socialization as fitting well together, and we see tactics as leading to content, which in turn, leads to individual and organizational outcomes. More specifically, we see that mentoring directly contributes to increased understanding of the politics content area, which, in turn, leads to the development of political skill. As such, this perspective incorporates arguments about the content of mentoring experiences suggested by Perrewé et al. (2002) and by Lankau and Scandura (2002). Perrewé et al. argued that the development of political understanding and skill in protégés should be the primary focus of mentoring experiences. Additionally, Lankau and Scandura suggested both work content and interpersonal, social, and political competencies tend to be the focus of the individual learning that goes on in mentoring relationships.

Knowledge and Understanding of Organization Politics through Mentoring

New members in organizations actively seek information to comprehend and make sense of their environments. Furthermore, they usually turn to more experienced and knowledgeable members of the organization for such information (Miller & Jablin, 1991; Morrison, 1993; Ostroff & Kozlowski, 1992, 1993), which is one way that mentoring relationships are initiated (Perrewé et al., 2002). Ferris and his colleagues proposed that protégés can be construed as apprentices who are enlightened about, and educated in "the ways of the game" in organizations (i.e., shown "the ropes"). Thus, they argued that mentoring is at the heart of this learning process. Furthermore, they also suggested that protégé understanding of politics and development of political skill are accomplished through such mentoring relationships (i.e., Ferris, Bhawuk et al., 1996; Ferris, Frink, Bhawuk, Zhou, & Gilmore, 1996; Ferris, Frink, & Galang, 1993). This knowledge and information transmitted from mentors to protégés takes the form of organizational context, which provides the critically important "roadmap for the intricacies, boundaries, and informal rules of the game of politics" (Ferris, Frink, Bhawuk, et al., 1996, p. 31).

Because organizations can be construed as political arenas, the understanding of organization politics and political skill development are essential for effectiveness (e.g., Perrewé & Nelson, 2004). By itself, hard work and good job performance will not lead to sustained, long-term effectiveness if individuals fail to develop a savvy and understanding of opportunity creation and career positioning. Furthermore, the collective knowledge acquisition and skill development will allow employees entering new environments to reduce the associated anxiety and stress by learning "the ropes," and mastering the informal social aspects of their new roles (Van Maanen, 1978; Van Maanen & Schein, 1979).

Mentoring, Understanding Politics, and Political Skill

Organizations have been characterized as political arenas (Mintzberg, 1983; Pfeffer, 1981). Because individuals wish to understand both the content and context of their work environments, they develop "shared meaning," which then serves as the context for their behaviors (Ferris, King, Judge, & Kacmar, 1991). Behaviors that represent individual tactics and strategies, and are reflective of opportunistic values, are commonly referred to as political behaviors (Ferris, Russ, & Fandt, 1989). Thus, the understanding of politics represents an important part of what socialization imparts in organizations, and such learning helps to shape and enhance individuals' political skill as well (Blass, Brouer, Perrewé, & Ferris, 2007).

Political skill is "the ability to effectively understand others at work, and to use such knowledge to influence others to act in ways that enhance one's personal and/or organizational objectives" (Ferris, Treadway, et al., 2005, p. 127). Socialization processes help to build knowledge of politics in organizations, which instills in individuals a more informed understanding of the organization and how it operates. Such knowledge develops in individuals increased interpersonal perceptiveness, which contributes to a greater understanding of their co-workers and the work environment. This allows them to build coalitions, alliances, and networks, become advantageously positioned in networks, and be effective interpersonally, all of which enhances their political skill (cf. Ferris et al., 2007; Munyon, Summers, Thompson, & Ferris, in press).

More specifically, political skill consists of four underlying dimensions: Social astuteness, networking ability, interpersonal influence, and apparent sincerity. The perceptual acuity and attentional focus (i.e., social astuteness), the situational selection and execution of appropriate influence strategies (i.e., interpersonal influence), the genuine and sincere manner or style (i.e., apparent sincerity), and the development of connections, ties, alliances, and building social capital (i.e., networking ability) all are emphasized in mentoring and socialization processes in different ways.

However, it is fair to conclude that the networking ability dimension appears to have the greatest face validity with mentoring processes because of its subject matter relevance to the content of mentoring experiences, which often focuses on the development of connections, alliances, and influential contacts. Furthermore, it is clear that networking ability is built and strengthened through a greater understanding of organizational politics. Networking ability has been defined, not as a trait or possession, but rather as an informational and control asset that stems from access to networks (Burt, 1997). Politically skilled individuals are cognizant of this, and are adept at developing and utilizing social networks (Ferris, Davidson, & Perrewé, 2005; Ferris, Treadway, et al., 2005), often being viewed as adroit negotiators, and as the brokers of compromise.

Being exposed to a greater understanding of politics in organizations through socialization and mentoring transmits information to individuals about "how things are done around here," and which organizational members are most important and influential. As such, this knowledge and information all serve to increase individuals' political skill. Building such a knowledge and information base will allow individuals to identify the people they want to include in their network. However, this information and knowledge helps individuals to build their network in contextually appropriate ways, through knowledge of the organizational power and influence structures, network positioning, and how to effectively navigate the politics taking place around them. The social network perspective focuses on relationship development and resulting network positioning, and suggests that it may be through well-developed political skill that individuals obtain privileged network positions in organizations, which may provide further information and resource access and contextually relevant skill building (e.g., Brass, 1995).

The foregoing arguments indicate that individuals high in political skill should be able to position themselves advantageously in social networks. Supporting this statement is a study by Kelly and Kaplan (1993). They reported that several strategies differentiated top performers from others, and two of those strategies were "organizational savvy" (i.e., including such behaviors as addressing conflict, navigating competing interests, promoting cooperation) and "networking," which relates closely to political skill. Thus, the theory and research to date suggests that mentors instruct protégés on the nuances of organizational politics, which is critical to their long-term effectiveness, and to the development and shaping of their political skill.

Differential Mentoring Experiences by Race

The foregoing discussion implicitly assumes that all protégés are treated the same, and the general feeling is that this is not the case. In fact, the availability and quality of mentoring may divide along racial lines, with racial minorities finding access to mentoring much more difficult than do members of the white majority. Furthermore, this differential access by race might be a function of the different social network positioning in which racial minorities find themselves.

For example, Blake-Beard, Murrell, and Thomas (2007) suggested that access to mentoring may be driven by the social networks and types of relationships that racial minorities develop within organizations, which can create challenges for several reasons. First, it is often difficult for individuals to find same-race mentors in organizations, due to the lack of availability of racial minorities in higher level positions. Additionally, if racial minority individuals seek other-race mentors (i.e., white majority members), this crossing of racial lines in mentoring relationships creates problems of trust building, making it is more difficult to achieve the kind of authentic collaboration in mixed-race mentoring that one typically seeks in same-race mentoring relationships.

Ibarra's (1993) work on personal networks of minorities attempted to go beyond the observation that minorities tend to be excluded totally from, or have limited access to, organizational networks. She attempted to better explain how racial minorities' networks differ from those of the white majority, as well as the factors that cause those differences. Essentially, she has argued that interaction networks are embedded within organizational contexts, and such networks place constraints on racial minorities in ways that result in their networks being different from those of white majority members (i.e., typically white males). Informal interaction networks in organizations provide a variety of instrumental resources critical for employee effectiveness, in addition to important friendship and social support resources (i.e., expressive benefits). The realization that racial minorities typically have limited access to these networks creates serious limitations including knowledge and relationship access.

Additionally, Thomas (1989) investigated potential race effects on the mentoring relationships of managers, and reported some quite interesting results that he believes have their roots in the slavery legacy. He found that black women in the investigation were not interested in developing mentoring relationships with white mentors because of the historical images of African-American women as white slave owner concubines. Thomas referred to such discomfort as "a racial taboo," and he found that senior white male mentors reflected reluctance to engage in such mentoring relationships for similar reasons. These implicit racial taboos prevented the formation of cross-race mentor-protégé relationships, and they most definitely contributed to work-related frustration and stress for racial minorities.

Because politics is a critically important part of what goes on in organizations, it is important to understand how individuals acquire the information to develop the understanding of organization politics, and shaping of political skill that is believed to increase effectiveness in organizations. Ferris et al. (1993) proposed an explanation for these dynamics, and emphasized that political understanding and skill development relies upon access to privileged information that is selectively transmitted only to certain groups, while other groups are kept ignorant of the nature, dynamics, and operation of the politics.

The Ferris et al. (1993) "political skill deficiency" explanation views politics as reflecting the nuances and informal structure of organizational life, and that the set of rules, skills, and context necessary to deal with these politics are passed on selectively. This results in the selected or privileged individuals (i.e., typically white males) being provided with the information access to develop skills and acquire knowledge focused on the operation and nature of politics, while others are prevented access to such information. Those who are closed out of this informal information network (i.e., typically racial minorities) find it virtually impossible to fully appreciate and comprehend the larger context of organization politics, and how it influences important behavioral dynamics and decision making in organizations. Further, those closed out of access to such information have little opportunity to develop political savvy and skill, placing them at a decided disadvantage in performance and career advancement competitions. Thus, Ferris et al. argued that essentially two groups of people are created as a function of this selective transmission of political information; the knowledgeable, skilled, and aware "insiders," and the clueless, unaware "outsiders."

White males typically represent the majority group or dominant coalition in most organizations, so they usually set the tone, agenda, and informal rules for all other groups (Jackall, 1988). As such, it is white male newcomers to organizations who get selected to be mentored by senior members of the dominant coalition and become "insiders" (i.e., the ones privy to the new contextual knowledge of politics, understanding, and skill, and taught to perfect their skills and apply this new knowledge). The "outsiders" represent the other group who are disadvantaged by being excluded from this private and specialized political network, and they tend to be racial minorities, according to Ferris et al. (1993). These "outsiders" typically are refused membership in the "insiders" club, because politics is seen as a "white man's game." This tends to create considerable information asymmetries between white majority and racial minority newcomers, which result in unfair competition between the two groups in internal organizational tournaments.

If the Ferris et al. (1993) theory is accurate, then racial minorities' political skill deficiency places them at a decided disadvantage regarding career advancement and effectiveness both within and across organizations. Some research has reported that career success is a function of confidence, flexibility, adaptability, and political savvy (Rosen & Lovelace, 1991). Additionally, political skill has been identified as a barrier to women's job and career advancement (Rosen, 1982), and that skill building in the political nuances of management was one of the most important training and development needs for racial minority prospective managers (Fernandez, 1981).

In a long-term qualitative investigation of African-American female managers in organizations, Bell and Nkomo (2001) reported that advancement barriers limited access to informal and social networks within organizations for these female minority managers. However, those who were able to circumvent such barriers shared several common experiences and/or observations. First, they were able to gain access to important information, and garner the support of influential others in their organization. Second, these minority women were able to maintain their own identities (i.e., racial identity), while at the same time maneuvering through the political cultures of their organizations through keen observation of social-structural barriers and cultural challenges. Finally, these women reflected an interactive style that was honest, sincere, and forthright, which allowed them to use their voice and influence in such a manner that they were not perceived as offensive (Bell & Nkomo, 2001).

As African-American female managers, these women in the Bell and Nkomo (2001) study were ostensibly "outsiders," relative to the Ferris et al. (1993) classification, due to their demographic dissimilarity to the dominant coalition or "insiders." However, they still were able to develop political skill, use it to circumvent advancement barriers, and achieve success at high levels of their organizations. Their knowledge and understanding of politics, in conjunction with the political skill they shaped and developed, permitted these female minority managers to build and leverage their social capital through effective interpersonal influence, and gain access to the critical information and resources they needed to compete fairly for effectiveness.

In summary, it appears to be the case that the "political skill deficiency hypothesis," proposed by Ferris and his colleagues (Ferris, Frink, Bhawuk, et al., 1996; Ferris et al., 1993) provides a plausible alternative explanation for the differential treatment and outcomes of racial minorities in organizations today, and one that has received some empirical support (i.e., Blass et al., 2007; Ferris, Bhawuk, et al., 1996). It might be the case that individuals' lack of success and ineffectiveness at work might at least partially be due to not being equipped with the necessary knowledge, skills, and understanding to compete with those who are able to develop such skill and knowledge. Furthermore, racial minorities and women who do succeed in the work world, such as those discussed by Bell and Nkomo (2001), probably do so because they were provided access to special information, resources, experiences, and opportunities by "insider" mentors, who then treated them like "insiders."

Although racial minorities tend to experience more challenges to finding quality mentoring relationships in organizations than do white majority group members, it is clearly not the case that they are not getting any mentoring at all. Instead, it might be that minorities receive mentoring experiences by individuals who are not well positioned, and who do not possess the "insider" knowledge to transmit to them, nor the political clout to help position them advantageously (i.e., by those who are not dominant coalition members). As already noted, research has indicated mentors who are members of the dominant coalition, "insider" group might select individuals similar to themselves to mentor, suggesting that the "insider" group (i.e., typically white males) is reasonably consistent in being self-perpetuating. Therefore, this suggests that the dominant white majority group is advantaged in the workplace, relative to racial minorities, by developing an understanding of organizational political processes, and development of political skill through selective mentoring experiences with demographically similar mentors who also are well positioned, influential organization members.

Implications for Strain Reactions by Minorities in Organizations

Politics as a Stressor

As we have seen, the uncertainty and ambiguity inherent in work environments where racial minorities have incomplete information and access to resources can be stressful and anxiety provoking, and knowledge of organizational politics can help reduce such stress. In fact, uncertainty reduction has been the most frequently cited benefit of political behavior (Ferris & Hochwarter, 2011). More directly, "the ability to secure information through political behavior has been shown to minimize much of the ambiguity-generated strain experienced on the job" (Hochwarter, Ferris, Zinko, Arnell, & James, 2007, p. 567). Also, organizational politics perceptions have been characterized as a workplace stressor with associated strain reactions (e.g., Ferris, Frink, Galang, et al., 1996). However, such strain reactions typically are found only for individuals who possess a low understanding of, and/or control over, politics at work.

Relatedly, Charles and Nkomo (2012) developed a conceptualization of what they refer to as "racialized organizational politics (ROPP)," which they defined as "the extent to which individuals believe their racial category or identity is influencing their social interpretations and meanings within organizations, as well as the opportunity to navigate the environment in a way that is favorable and of benefit to them and members of their racial category or identity" (p. 451). Essentially, their model articulates a number of antecedents of ROPP, as well as consequences (i.e., job satisfaction, organizational commitment, extra-role behaviors, performance, turnover, and withdrawal behaviors). Although they do not specifically identify stress or job tension as consequences or outcomes in their model, these certainly are implied.

Furthermore, because ROPP is a type of organizational politics perceptions (POPS) construct, and POPS has been characterized in prior theory and research as a workplace stressor, by implication, ROPP also can be viewed as a stressor in the work environment. However, also included in the Charles and Nkomo model are a group of "personal mitigating resources," or moderators of the relationships between ROPP and consequences or outcomes, and they include political skill, influence tactics and processes, and psychological capital, to name three. Thus, they argue that if individuals possess these "personal mitigating resources," then they should NOT experience the same negative outcomes as those perceiving ROPP who do not possess such personal resources.

Political Skill as a Strain Reduction Mechanism

Organizational scholars have noted that socialization can be a stressful process (Allen, McManus, & Russell, 1999; Berry, 1990; Nelson, 1987; Van Maanen & Schein, 1979). As such, future research might consider examining political skill, as one of Charles and Nkomo's (2012) "personal mitigating resources," which might serve as a useful coping mechanism in moderating the relationship between socialization processes of racial minorities and work stress and strain. Some research has shown that political skill can serve as a problem-solving coping strategy (Perrewé & Zellars, 1999; Perrewé et al., 2004) that neutralizes the dysfunctional effects of role ambiguity and role conflict stressors experienced in the socialization process (also, see Brief, Aldag, Van Sell, & Melone, 1979).

Ferris et al. (2011) addressed the role of political skill in relation to employee psychological and physiological health and well-being. They proposed an organizing framework suggesting that political skill influences internal or what they referred to as "intrapsychic" effects, which include constructs such as adaptability, control, self-esteem, and proactivity. Their framework also showed political skill impacting "interpersonal" processes, which include constructs like affability, humility, authenticity, and trustworthiness. These two categories of variables then were argued to demonstrate direct effects on physiological and psychological health and well-being, as well as exhibiting indirect effects on those outcomes through the development of networks, coalitions, and work relationships.

Functionally Differentiated Networks

In order to circumvent potential barriers to advancement in organizations, racial minorities have sometimes adopted a network strategy characterized by functional differentiation, which seeks to maximize the career and support benefits that can be obtained by tapping into more than one social circle or network. Typically, this strategy involves inclusion in a group of same-race (i.e., "homophilous") relationships, which provide benefits of social support and advice, as well as ties to the majority group or dominant coalition (i.e., typically white managers), who can be tapped into for access to critical organizational information and other resources (Fernandez, 1981; Ibarra, 1993).

Although the potential benefits of functionally differentiated networks for minority employees can be considerable, an unfortunate consequence is that the two groups or networks sought for inclusion often have little overlap for racial minorities, causing difficulties in effectively integrating themselves into both simultaneously in advantageous ways. Attempting to effectively manage such a differentiated social network structure can be very time consuming and stressful, frequently leading to feelings of alienation from one or the other group, guilt, and loss of resources or support from one of or both groups (Davis & Watson, 1982; Dickens & Dickens, 1982; Kanter, 1977). The sometimes conflicting information and advice regarding career decision and job performance considerations received from the different groups also can produce stress.

Similarly, with respect to sources of stress on racial minority employees, Bell and Nkomo (2001) reported that African-American women experience "biculturality," which refers to the movement from one cultural context to another, thus forcing these women to shape some aspects of their careers in one context (i.e., the white world), and at the same time directing other aspects of their life in another context (i.e., the black community). Thus, bicultural individuals see themselves as navigating two different and distinct cultural worlds. Living in these two worlds can be taxing and complex which can lead to emotional distress. This bicultural stress is a resulting feature of the identity suppression or diminishment process in one context in order to survive in their other incompatible contexts.

Therefore, due to biculturality, black women professionals experience very complicated and challenging lives, characterized by large areas of obligation and responsibility, often without the benefit of adequate social support (Bell, 1990). Consequently, as a result of dealing with the many and conflicting role expectations placed upon them in their lives, which create both role conflict and role overload stressors, these racial minority professional women simply become psychologically and physically exhausted. The emotional exhaustion experienced by bicultural individuals is a result of the ambivalence associated with the inherent duality of their cultural identity. This ambivalence oftentimes has a negative effect on their well-being because of the emotional labor required to effectively manage their complex worlds.

RACE, EXECUTIVE BEHAVIOR, STRESS, AND HEALTH

In the preceding sections, we argued that networking position and distance, access to information, and social and political skill affect racial and nonracial minorities differently. Although this is supported in the literature for those in mid-level positions, it is reasonable to expect that these effects hold for racial minorities as they climb the corporate ladder. Consequently, although there is limited scholarship examining race within organizations at lower hierarchical levels, there are even fewer studies that have examined these effects at the executive level. Although women and racial minorities are now represented in executive positions in greater numbers than before, both parties find themselves underrepresented in the most influential board of director positions (Alliance for Board Diversity, 2010;

Bilimoria & Piderit, 1994; Kesner, 1988; McDonald & Westphal, 2013; Peterson & Philpot, 2006).

Of additional concern, increases in the number of initial board of director appointments for women and racial minorities have not led to subsequent additional appointments. Women and racial minorities are not well represented among board members who hold more than one corporate board seat. Individuals who hold multiple directorships may have a disproportionate influence over the firms where they serve as a director; these directors also are more likely to be selected to powerful advisory boards and regulatory agencies (Domhoff, 2002; Geletkanycz & Hambrick, 1997; Westphal & Stern, 2006).

In their study of directors of U.S. public companies between 1999 and 2006, McDonald and Westphal (2013) found that although racial minorities comprised 22% of board members, only 5% of these minority directors held multiple seats, indicating that racial minorities have substantially less influence than white males over the strategic actions of large firms. The absence of women and racial minorities from both powerful board committees and chair positions, coupled with their lack of multiple board seats, indicates their exclusion from the corporate elite. Additionally, increased representation in the boardroom has not necessarily translated into "C-level" positions; women and racial minorities continue to remain underrepresented in the upper echelons at large corporations (McDonald & Westphal, 2013).

Studies have shown that large corporations are acquiescing to external stakeholder pressure by appointing female or racial minority individuals to their boards of directors (Daily, Certo, & Dalton, 1999; Hillman, Cannella, & Harris, 2002; Hillman, Shropshire, & Cannella, 2007). Research has shown that a greater presence of women and racial minorities on a firm's board may have some positive effects on board effectiveness and functioning. For example, Adams and Ferreira (2009) found that racial minority directors may be more conscientious in executing their director roles, and may be more independent from management. However, research also has shown that women and racial minorities at the executive level may affect overall firm reputation and corporate social performance, suggesting a more symbolic role and justification for their presence at the executive level that goes beyond their human capital. In their study of mediators that explain the relationship between board diversity and firm performance, Miller and del Carmen Triana (2009) found a positive relationship between board racial diversity and firm reputation.

Race has been linked to disadvantages in performance evaluation and career progress decisions, but what happens after racial minorities overcome these initial barriers and achieve a position of executive leadership remains to be understood by management scholars. What little we know is that the disadvantages of race do not disappear once an employee is promoted to the executive level, and racial minority executives may suffer even more so than their lower-level counterparts. This section provides an overview of the ramifications of race faced by racial minority executives, and how these demands can contribute to stress.

Race and Work Stress at the Executive Level in Organizations

Executive job demands vary in difficulty (Hambrick, Finkelstein, & Mooney, 2005; Munyon, Summers, Buckley, Ranft, & Ferris, 2010), and such variations arise from three sets of factors. Task challenges and performance challenges represent contextual factors. For example, a firm's resource limitations and complexity can add to the task challenges faced by an executive. Performance challenges result from pressure to achieve a certain threshold of performance demanded by owners, stakeholders, customers, and employees (Hambrick et al., 2005). Both of these factors are generalized to a specific organization regardless of the executive. The third set of factors resides within individual executives. As such, these factors are idiosyncratic and unique to executives and can impact their performance. Hambrick et al. (2005) identified executive aspirations as an important factor that impacts the demands experienced by executives.

Executives differ in their motivations and aspirations, and consequently, the drive and motivation to achieve high levels of performance actually differs from individual to individual. Strongly motivated executives may place more demands on themselves than contextual conditions alone present. These motivations can come from a variety of sources, such as personality factors (e.g., need for achievement, internal locus of control). Tenure may also impact an executive's motivation. Hambrick and Fukutomi (1991) suggested that younger executives or executives in their early career stages may feel more pressure to prove themselves and establish a reputation of success than more senior executives. Executives also may be motivated to enhance firm performance because of an alignment between company performance and their own salaries in the form of stock options and other performance-based pay plans (Alchian & Demsetz, 1972).

Executive job demands may be even higher for gender and racial minorities. At first glance, the contextual factors faced by these executives appear to be the same as those of their white male counterparts. However, the promotion of females and racial minorities to highly visible top leadership positions garners much attention due to the novelty of such occurrences. Increased scrutiny by investors and other key stakeholders may add to racial minority executives' already large demands. In their study of "She-E-Os," Lee and James (2007) found that investors' reactions to the announcements of female CEOs were significantly more negative than those of their male counterparts. As such, gender and racial minorities in leadership positions also may feel increased pressure to achieve higher levels of performance (Hambrick et al., 2005), or increased expectations of accountability (Munyon et al., 2010). Increased levels of scrutiny coupled with higher intrinsic motivation to succeed can contribute to these executives experiencing higher levels of stress than their white male counterparts.

Race, Social Exclusion, and Stress at the Executive Level in Organizations

Racial minorities in executive leadership positions, especially those that represent the sole minority at the executive level, may find themselves increasingly isolated. Isolation can lead to feelings of vulnerability, subsequently leading to higher levels of physiological and psychological stress (Ryan & Deci, 2000; Williams, 2007). At the executive level, gender and racial minorities are likely to face tokenism (Kanter, 1977; Terjesen, Sealy, & Singh, 2009). The dominant group (i.e., white male executives) will see these racial minority members as representatives of their specific minority instead of as individuals. This loss of individuality for racial minority executives makes it difficult for their ideas to be heard and considered seriously. Research has shown that higher numbers of racial minorities present on boards of directors can mitigate these effects. Erkut, Kramer, and Konrad (2008) found that three or more women members on the board of directors represented a critical mass that allowed for more positive, balanced interactions between female and male directors and normalized their presence. McDonald and Westphal (2013) also found that the presence of incumbent racial minorities on the board of directors mitigated the disadvantage experienced by first-time minority directors.

Isolation of minorities at the executive level also can lead to the creation of in-groups and out-groups. The "corporate elite," or those board members who held multiple directorships, is one such example of an in-group. Racial minority executives may be perceived as highly competent, and advancing in ways that threaten the established upper echelons of the organization. Envy and hostile competition may arise in the form of "selective incivility." Stress, anxiety, and strain may result from this type of social exclusion (Cortina, 2008).

Racial minorities at the executive level also may feel isolated from their lower-level counterparts. Racial minority employees may conform in order to improve their organizational position and status. Conformity may represent a way to mitigate the perceived negative stereotypes associated with their particular racial minority group (Hewlin, 2003). Racial minorities at the executive level within the organization may have increased levels of conformity, or may be more effective at producing a façade that coincides with the wants of the dominant coalition of the organization. As such, these racial minority executives may be excluded from the general population of their minority group. Hewlin (2009) found that minority organizational position is associated with creating facades of conformity. These behaviors can lead to emotional exhaustion. Racial minorities at the executive level also may lack a support system of peers who can provide emotional and social support during times of stress.

Due to their status, racial minorities may feel obligated to signal conformity in order to gain acceptance from and enjoy the benefits of majority group members. Research suggests that racial minorities (i.e., especially a "token" executive) often experience widespread publicity of their employment activities. Thus, their success and failure receive heightened attention compared to their nonminority counterparts (Kanter, 1977). As a result, racial minorities are likely to present a facade of conformity as a strategy to evade negative attention that may result from expressing unacceptable values.

Racial minority executives also may choose to segregate themselves from their minority group. For example, Ashford, Rothbard, Piderit, and Dutton (1998) found evidence that although women at lower levels in firms hope that female directors will advocate for women's issues, senior women often are reluctant to pursue a feminist agenda. The authors suggest that women executives may better understand the political ramifications if their advocacy were to fail. Women directors may see their priorities as the same as their male counterparts, that is, protecting shareholder value. Thus, a change agenda or issues pertaining to women do not fall under their responsibility.

Race, Mentoring, and Stress at the Executive Level in Organizations

Racial minorities in executive leadership positions have difficulty in discovering and fostering relationships with mentors. One consequence of underrepresentation of racial minorities within the corporate elite is the lack of role models and mentors for women and racial minorities (Hillman et al., 2007). In their study of large U.S. corporations, McDonald and Westphal (2013) found that female and racial minority first-time directors received comparatively less mentoring from their incumbent colleagues regarding prevailing norms and the process of board deliberations. A consequence of receiving less mentoring manifested itself in subsequently fewer additional board appointments, creating a vicious circle that makes it difficult to find experienced racial minority mentors. Interestingly, female and racial minority first-time directors were found to be less disadvantaged when the board had a woman or racial minority incumbent member (McDonald & Westphal, 2013). In addition to lacking a mentor, racial minority executives may feel intense pressure to mentor lower-level employees in order to promote racial diversity. This pressure, which can manifest in both formal and informal means, can add to a minority executive's job demands and responsibilities (Hambrick et al., 2005).

DISCUSSION

Implications for Theory and Research

In this chapter, we conducted a critical analysis of theory and research on race and stress, combined with the articulation of a framework that attempts to delineate the organizational phenomena that account for the stress, strain, and well-being that racial minorities experience in organizations. The framework we developed is an inductively derived, review-centric attempt to propose "novel theoretical insights from reviews of existing theory and research," as suggested recently by LePine and Wilcox-King (2010) regarding the development of new theory in the organizational sciences.

The proposed framework draws upon literature in the areas of social network and social capital, information and resource access and exclusion, organization politics and political skill, and socialization and mentoring. Furthermore, it depicts racial minorities typically as the excluded outsiders who are prevented access to organizationally relevant information and resources and mentoring by insiders, which deprives them of control, understanding, visibility, and positioning that is associated with greater levels of stress and strain at work. As such, we believe our perspective and framework has a number of implications for theory and research which we note below.

Future work in this area might consider trying to build in an established stress theory that can be integrated with the work we have already proposed above. For example, much of the material discussed in this chapter seems to fit easily within a job demands control framework (e.g., Karasek, 1979, 1998), which could be incorporated in future efforts to refine the theory in this area. Much of the discussion in this chapter addresses adverse behavior demonstrated toward racial minorities that appear to represent unique job demands that potentially could drain coping resources. In particular, it seems that the stress experienced by minorities is due to either heightened demands placed on them to overcome obstacles to their success, or limited control (i.e., actual or perceived) that result from not having access to high-quality network connections, information, and so forth. This might be an issue for future work to address.

Socialization and Mentoring Processes

Our review and the proposed framework make reference to both mentoring and sponsorship, and they tend to be used interchangeably. However, there are likely important differences between which information is transmitted, or which activities are involved, in the mentoring process based on its intent. Clearly, there is at least a "learning function" to mentoring as well as a sponsorship function, where the former focuses on imparting new context-relevant knowledge, whereas the latter focuses on exposure and visibility (e.g., Noe et al., 2002; Siebert et al., 2001; Wanberg et al., 2003). It might be the case that racial minorities tend to be closed out of both functions, or perhaps they acquire the contextual knowledge, but are never actively promoted and given the exposure that is so important. The two different functions of mentoring need to be clearly sorted out and clarified regarding the way racial minorities are dealt with in organizations at different points in the socialization, mentoring, and career development processes.

A related notion concerns the expectations we have of mentors, relative to what all we think they should provide. On the one hand, we might view mentorship rather simplistically, and assume that a single mentor can possess sufficient knowledge, expertise, and motivation to provide protégé development in virtually all areas. Such talented individuals might exist out there in organizations, but we would suspect they are in short supply (so hold on to them if you find them!). It might be more realistic to expect to have more than one mentor, and that you get different things from different mentors.

Indeed, this is what Siebert et al. (2001) found in their research on social capital and career success. They reported that greater career benefits were realized by individuals who had multiple mentors than those who had only one mentor. This prompted them to call for research on "mentoring networks," whereby you would seek out different mentors to provide different information, knowledge, or support. Indeed, Siebert et al. (p. 233) argued that: "One mentor might provide emotional support and spiritual guidance. Another mentor might help the protégé with task and technical advice. Yet another mentor might assist the protégé in coping with organizational politics." This actually might prove to be a point of differentiation between white majority employees and racial minorities, whereby minorities do not receive multiple mentoring, but instead are fortunate to find a single mentor.

Network Groups

One particular area of work has been proposed to alleviate the workplace stresses and strains on minority employees, and promote well-being, and it is referred to as "employee network groups" (Friedman, 1996; Friedman, Kane, & Cornfield, 1998). Friedman argued that network groups essentially reconfigure social networks of racial minorities in ways that allow for greater information and influential contact access, as well as greater social support. Interestingly, employee network groups create greater racial minority advancement and well-being through the seemingly incompatible processes of assimilation and separation. As such, network groups intend to reduce group categorization barriers by capitalizing on within-group political, social, and career support.

Furthermore, network groups are perceived to ameliorate the anxiety-provoking experiences of the employee socialization process for racial minorities (Van Maanen & Schein, 1979) in general, and the stresses of being "solo" (i.e., the extreme case of an individual who is the only one of that type in a group or organization) in workplace settings in particular (Pettigrew & Martin, 1987). Indeed, Van Maanen and Schein acknowledged the stressful nature of socialization processes for all newcomers, but such stress is intensified for individuals who are of racial minority status, because they most like are being carefully scrutinized, and judgments about such individuals are likely extrapolated to the entire racial minority group.

Therefore, racial minority group members in such new environments need to learn more, and more is at stake for their performance and work behavior. Additionally, much more emotional energy is required to deal with all this, which intensifies the socialization stresses for racial minorities. They accomplish such stress-strain reduction through greater access to information and influential contacts through the extensive exercise of voice

(Hirschman, 1970), and the "comfort effect" of realizing greater peer and social support (Friedman, 1996). Friedman et al. (1998) found that network groups demonstrated positive effects on career optimism (i.e., primarily through mentoring) of racial minorities, after controlling for job level, education, and age.

Directions for Future Research

Empirical Tests of the Framework

An obvious initial direction for future research is to empirically investigate the linkages specified in our framework in organizational settings. We suggest that scholars pursue empirical research here in at least a couple of ways. Because psychometrically sound measures of most of the key constructs in the model are available in the literature, quantitative studies could be pursued to conduct tests of the model, or portions of it. Additionally, the very nature of the subject matter we are examining suggests that this area begs for good qualitative research investigations that can try to develop more detailed and insightful descriptions of the phenomena than can be obtained from typical quantitative survey research efforts.

Indeed, such qualitative investigations are much more time-and labor-intensive, regarding data collection, analysis, and write up. However, the yield from such investigations can be quite valuable. Bell and Nkomo (2001) conducted an eight-year, combination-survey approach and "life history methodology" to uncover the experiences of African-American and white female professional managers in organizations. This was a huge time and resource investment for these two scholars, which they readily admit, but they also believe it was worth the investment. However, such an undertaking is probably not for untenured assistant professors, although qualitative scholars like John Van Maanen and Norm Denzin may well disagree with us on that point.

Consideration of Stressors and Strain Reactions

The proposed framework made explicit reference to organizational politics as a workplace stressor that can differentially impact racial minorities because often they tend to be excluded from knowledge, understanding, and skill building regarding politics. Additionally, implicit reference was made to accountability as a source of stress for racial minorities, particularly because in some cases they are held accountable for different performance criteria (Cox & Nkomo, 1986). In other cases, racial minorities are held accountable for the same performance criteria as white majority group members, but because minorities often do not possess the knowledge and skill to understand the "rules of the game," they can see such accountabilities also as stressful. These specific variables reflect the psycho-social category of stressors, yet there may be other as yet to be identified stressors. Future research should consider whether there might be other work environment stressors that play a particularly important role in the stress and strain experiences of racial minorities in organizations.

Future research needs to carefully consider the operationalization and measurement of the stress, health, and well-being outcome variables in the model. Numerous measures of stress and strain exist, but the appropriate ones to select for examination in the present context is important, as well as the degree to which the measures selected are compatible. Because of the often low correlations demonstrated across psychological and physiological stress, and behavioral health and well-being measures, sometimes reflecting measurement and methodological difficulties, the selection of which measures to collect is critical (e.g., Fried, Rowland, & Ferris, 1984; Jex & Beehr, 1991). Therefore, studies should probably collect several different measures and examine the degree of convergence across those measures.

Difference/Comparability across Racial Minority Categories

Much less seems to be known about the experiences, stress, and health of members of other racial minorities in organizations, than is known about African-Americans (e.g., Cox & Nkomo, 1990). However, Ferdman and Cortes (1992) reported that Hispanic and Asian managers also experienced negative stereotyping, but appear to be less likely than are African-Americans to be excluded from informal networks (Fernandez, 1981). Future research should investigate the stress and strain issues raised in this chapter and conceptualization for other racial minority groups besides African-Americans.

CONCLUSION

This volume of the *Research in Occupational Stress and Well Being* focuses on demographic differences in stress and well-being, with a number of different demographic classifications being examined. When accepting the invitation from the series editors to contribute a chapter about race and stress, although we jumped at the opportunity, we knew this would be no easy task, because there is very little material published in this area. However, we took it as a challenge to find and critically review what we could, but then create new knowledge by building a collective and integrative understanding of the stress, strain, health, and well-being experiences of racial minorities in organizations. In perhaps some small way, we hope this chapter stimulates increased research interest in this much needed area of inquiry.

REFERENCES

Adams, R. B., & Ferreira, D. (2009). Women in the boardroom and their impact on governance and performance. *Journal of Financial Economics*, *94*, 291–309.

Alchian, A. A., & Demsetz, H. (1972). Production, information costs, and economic organization. *American Economic Review*, *62*, 777–795.

Allen, T. D., McManus, S. E., & Russell, J. E. A. (1999). Newcomer socialization and stress: Formal peer relationships as a source of support. *Journal of Vocational Behavior*, *54*, 453–470.

Alliance for Board Diversity. (2010). *Missing pieces: Women and minorities on Fortune 500 boards: 2010 Alliance for board diversity census*. Alliance for Board Diversity. Retrieved from http://www.abd.org

Anderson, C. A., & Bushman, B. J. (2002). Media violence and the American public revisited. *American Psychologist*, *57*(6–7), 448–450. doi:10.1037/0003-066X.57.6-7.448

Andersson, L. M., & Pearson, C. M. (1999). Tit for tat? The spiraling effect of incivility in the workplace. *Academy of Management Review*, *24*, 452–471.

Aquino, K., & Thau, S. (2009). Workplace victimization: Aggression from the target's perspective. *Annual Review of Psychology*, *60*, 717–741. doi:10.1146/annurev.psych.60.110707.163703

Ashford, S., Rothbard, N., Piderit, S., & Dutton, J. (1998). Out on a limb: The role of context and impression management in selling gender-equity issues. *Administrative Science Quarterly*, *43*, 23–57.

Bauer, T. N., Morrison, E. W., & Callister, R. R. (1998). Organizational socialization: A review and directions for future research. In G. R. Ferris (Ed.), *Research in personnel and human resources management* (Vol. 16, pp. 149–214). Stamford, CT: JAI Press.

Baumeister, R. F., Twenge, J. M., & Nuss, C. K. (2002). Effects of social exclusion on cognitive processes: Anticipated aloneness reduces intelligent thought. *Journal of Personality and Social Psychology*, *83*(4), 817–827. doi:10.1037/0022-3514.83.4.817

Bell, E. L. (1990). The bicultural life experience of career-oriented black women. *Journal of Organizational Behavior*, *11*, 461–464.

Bell, E. L. J., & Nkomo, S. M. (2001). *Our separate ways: Black and white women and the struggle for professional identity*. Boston, MA: Harvard Business School Press.

Berry, J. W. (1990). Psychology of acculturation. In R. W. Brislin (Ed.), *Applied cross-cultural psychology* (Vol. 14, pp. 233–253). Newbury Park, CA: Sage Publications.

Bilimoria, D., & Piderit, S. K. (1994). Board committee membership: Effects of sex-based bias. *Academy of Management Journal*, *37*, 1453–1477.

Blake-Beard, S., Murrell, A. J., & Thomas, D. A. (2007). Unfinished business: The impact of race on understanding mentoring relationships. In B. Rose-Ragins & K. Kram (Eds.), *Handbook on mentoring* (pp. 223–247). Thousand Oaks, CA: Sage Publications.

Blass, F. R., Brouer, R. L., Perrewé, P. L., & Ferris, G. R. (2007). Politics understanding and networking ability as a function of mentoring: The role of gender and race. *Journal of Leadership & Organizational Studies*, *14*, 93–105.

Brass, D. J. (1995). A social network perspective on human resources management. In G. R. Ferris (Ed.), *Research in personnel and human resources management* (Vol. 13, pp. 39–79). Greenwich, CT: JAI Press.

Brief, A. P., Aldag, R. J., Van Sell, M., & Melone, N. (1979). Anticipatory socialization and role stress among registered nurses. *Journal of Health and Social Behavior*, *20*, 161–166.

Brief, A. P., & Hayes, E. L. (1997). The continuing "American dilemma": Studying racism in organizations. In C. L. Cooper & D. M. Rousseau (Eds.), *Trends in organizational behavior* (pp. 89–106). Chichester, UK: Wiley.

Burt, R. S. (1997). The contingent value of social capital. *Administrative Science Quarterly*, *42*, 339–365.

Chao, G. T., O'Leary-Kelly, A. M., Wolf, S., Klein, H. J., & Gardner, P. D. (1994). Organizational socialization: Its content and consequences. *Journal of Applied Psychology*, *79*, 730–743.

Charles, A. C., & Nkomo, S. M. (2012). The intersection of race and politics: A framework for racialized organizational politics perceptions. In G. R. Ferris & D. C. Treadway (Eds.), *Politics in organizations: Theory and research considerations* (pp. 451–486). New York, NY: Routledge/Taylor and Francis.

Colella, A. J., McKay, P. F., Daniels, S. R., & Signal, S. M. (2012). *Employment discrimination*. New York, NY: Oxford University Press. Retrieved from http://search.proquest.com/docview/1285631396?accountid=4840

Cortina, L. M. (2008). Unseen injustice: Incivility as modern discrimination in organizations. *Academy of Management Review*, *33*(1), 55–75.

Cox, T. (2004). Problems with research by organizational scholars on issues of race and ethnicity. *Journal of Applied Behavioral Science*, *40*(2), 124–145.

Cox, T., & Nkomo, S. M. (1990). Invisible men and women: A status report on race as a variable in organization behavior research. *Journal of Organizational Behavior*, *11*(6), 419.

Cox, T. H., & Nkomo, S. M. (1986). Differential performance appraisal criteria: A field study of black and white managers. *Group & Organization Studies*, *11*, 101–119.

Daily, C. M., Certo, S. T., & Dalton, D. R. (1999). A decade of corporate women: Some progress in the boardroom, none in the executive suite. *Strategic Management Journal*, *20*, 93–99.

Davis, G., & Watson, G. (1982). *Black life in corporate America*. Garden City, NY: Anchor Books.

Dickens, F., Jr., & Dickens, J. B. (1982). *The black managers: Making it in the corporate world*. New York, NY: AMACOM.

Dipboye, R. L., & Halverson, S. K. (2004). Subtle (and not so subtle) discrimination in organizations. In R. W. Griffin & A. M. O'Leary (Eds.), *The dark side of organizational behavior* (pp. 131–158). San Francisco, CA: Jossey-Bass.

Domhoff, G. W. (2002). *Who rules America? Power and politics*. New York, NY: Harper and Row.

Dovidio, J. F., & Gaertner, S. L. (2000). Aversive racism in selection decisions: 1989 and 1999. *Psychological Science*, *11*, 315–319.

Erkut, S., Kramer, V. W., & Konrad, A. M. (2008). Critical Mass: Does the number of women on a corporate board make a difference? In S. Vinnicombe, R. J. Burke, D. Bilimoria & M. Huse (Eds.), *Women on corporate boards of directors: International research and practice* (pp. 350–366). Cheltenham, MA: Edward Edgar.

Fairhurst, G. T., & Snavely, B. K. (1983). A test of the social isolation of male tokens. *The Academy of Management Journal*, *26*(2), 353–361.

Ferdman, B. M., & Cortes, A. C. (1992). Culture and identity among Hispanic managers in an Anglo business. In S. B. Kanouse, P. Rosenfeld, & A. L. Culbertson (Eds.), *Hispanics and work* (pp. 247–277). Newbury Park, CA: Sage Publications.

Fernandez, J. P. (1981). *Racism and sexism in corporate life*. Lexington, MA: Lexington Books.

Ferris, D. L., Brown, D. J., Berry, J. W., & Lian, H. (2008). The development and validation of the workplace ostracism scale. *Journal of Applied Psychology*, *93*, 1348–1366. doi:10.1037/a0012743

Ferris, G. R., Bhawuk, D. P. S., Frink, D. D., Keiser, J. D., Gilmore, D. C., & Canton, R. C. (1996). The paradox of diversity in organizations. In A. Gutschelhofer & J. Scheff (Eds.), *Paradoxical management: Contradictions in management – A management of contradictions* (pp. 203–229). Vienna, Austria: Linde Verlag.

Ferris, G. R., Davidson, S. L., & Perrewé, P. L. (2005). *Political skill at work: Impact on work effectiveness*. Mountain View, CA: Davies-Black Publishing.

Ferris, G. R., Frink, D. D., Bhawuk, D. P. S., Zhou, J., & Gilmore, D. C. (1996). Reactions of diverse groups to politics in the workplace. *Journal of Management*, *22*, 23–44.

Ferris, G. R., Frink, D. D., & Galang, M. C. (1993). Diversity in the workplace: The human resources management challenges. *Human Resource Planning*, *16*, 41–51.

Ferris, G. R., Frink, D. D., Galang, M. C., Zhou, J., Kacmar, K. M., & Howard, J. L. (1996). Perceptions of organizational politics: Predictors, stress-related implications, and outcomes. *Human Relations*, *49*, 233–266.

Ferris, G. R., & Hochwarter, W. A. (2011). Organizational politics. In S. Zedeck (Ed.), *APA handbook of industrial and organizational psychology* (Vol. 3, pp. 435–459). Washington, DC: American Psychological Association.

Ferris, G. R., & Judge, T. A. (1991). Personnel/human resources management: A political influence perspective. *Journal of Management*, *17*, 447–488.

Ferris, G. R., Kane, R. E., Summers, J. K., & Munyon, T. P. (2011). Physiological and psychological health and well-being implications of political skill: Toward a multi-mediation organizing framework. In P. L. Perrewé & D. C. Ganster (Eds.), *The role of individual differences in occupational stress and well being* (Vol. 9, pp. 63–107). Research in Occupational Stress and Well Being. Bingley, UK: Emerald Group Publishing Limited.

Ferris, G. R., & King, T. R. (1992). The politics of age discrimination in organizations. *Journal of Business Ethics*, *11*, 341–350.

Ferris, G. R., King, T. R., Judge, T. A., & Kacmar, K. M. (1991). The management of shared meaning: Opportunism in the reflection of attitudes, beliefs, and values. In R. A. Giacalone & P. Rosenfeld (Eds.), *Applied impression management: How image making affects managerial decisions* (pp. 41–64). Newbury Park, CA: Sage Publications.

Ferris, G. R., Russ, G. S., & Fandt, P. M. (1989). Politics in organizations. In R. A. Giacalone & P. Rosenfeld (Eds.), *Impression management in the organization* (pp. 143–170). Hillsdale, NJ: Lawrence Erlbaum.

Ferris, G. R., Treadway, D. C., Kolodinsky, R. W., Hochwarter, W. A., Kacmar, C. J., Douglas, C., & Frink, D. D. (2005). Development and validation of the political skill inventory. *Journal of Management*, *31*, 126–152.

Ferris, G. R., Treadway, D. C., Perrewé, P. L., Brouer, R. L., Douglas, C., & Lux, S. (2007). Political skill in organizations. *Journal of Management*, *33*, 290–320.

Fisher, C. D. (1986). Organizational socialization: An integrative review. In K. M. Rowland & G. R. Ferris (Eds.), *Research in personnel and human resources management* (Vol. 4, pp. 101–145). Greenwich, CT: JAI Press.

Fried, Y., Rowland, K. M., & Ferris, G. R. (1984). The physiological measurement of work stress: A critique. *Personnel Psychology*, *37*, 583–615.

Friedman, R. A. (1996). Defining the scope and logic of minority and female network groups: Can separation enhance integration? In G. R. Ferris (Ed.), *Research in personnel and human resources management* (Vol. 14, pp. 307–349). Greenwich, CT: JAI Press.

Friedman, R. A., Kane, M., & Cornfield, D. R. (1998). Social support and career optimism: Examining the effectiveness of network groups among black managers. *Human Relations*, *51*, 1155–1177.

Gee, G. C. (2002). A multilevel analysis of the relationship between institutional and individual racial discrimination and health status. *American Journal of Public Health*, *92*, 615–623.

Geletkanycz, M. A., & Hambrick, D. C. (1997). The external ties of top executives: Implications for strategic choice and performance. *Administrative Science Quarterly*, *42*, 654–681.

Gerber, J., & Wheeler, L. (2009). On being rejected: A meta-analysis of experimental research on rejection. *Perspectives on Psychological Science*, *4*(5), 468–488.

Gottlieb, B. H. (1997). Conceptual and measurement issues in the study of coping with chronic stress. In B. H. Gottlieb (Ed.), *Coping with chronic stress* (pp. 3–40). New York, NY: Plenum Press.

Graves, J. L. (2003). *The emperor's new clothes: Biological theories of race at the millennium.* Piscataway, NJ: Rutgers University Press.

Hambrick, D. C., Finkelstein, S., & Mooney, A. C. (2005). Executive job demands: New insights for explaining strategic decisions and leader behaviors. *Academy of Management Review*, *30*, 472–491.

Hambrick, D. C., & Fukutomi, G. D. S. (1991). The seasons of a CEO's tenure. *Academy of Management Review*, *16*, 719–742.

Hayes, E. L. (1995). It's not what you know, it's who you know: The effects of human and social capital on race differences in promotion and support. *Dissertation Abstracts International*, *56*, 2383.

Hershcovis, M. S., Reich, T. C., Parker, S. K., & Bozeman, J. (2012). The relationship between workplace aggression and target deviant behaviour: The moderating roles of power and task interdependence. *Work & Stress*, *26*(1), 1–20. doi:10.1080/02678373.2012.660770

Hewlin, P. F. (2003). And the award for best actor goes to …: Facades of conformity in organizational settings. *The Academy of Management Review*, *28*(4), 633–642. doi:10.2307/30040752

Hewlin, P. F. (2009). Wearing the cloak: Antecedents and consequences of creating facades of conformity. *Journal of Applied Psychology*, *94*(3), 727–741. doi:10.1037/a0015228

Higgins, E. T. (1989). Self-discrepancy theory: What patterns of self-beliefs cause people to suffer? In L. Berkowitz (Ed.), *Advances in experimental social psychology* (Vol. 22, pp. 93–136). San Diego, CA: Academic Press.

Hillman, A. J., Cannella, A. A., & Harris, I. C. (2002). Women and racial minorities in the boardroom: How do directors differ? *Journal of Management*, *28*, 747–763.

Hillman, A. J., Shropshire, C., & Cannella, A. A. (2007). Organizational predictors of women on corporate boards. *Academy of Management Journal*, *50*, 941–952.

Hirschman, A. (1970). *Exit, voice, and loyalty: Responses to decline in firms, organizations, and states*. Cambridge, MA: Harvard University Press.

Hitlan, R. T., Cliffton, R. J., & DeSoto, M. C. (2006). Perceived exclusion in the workplace: The moderating effects of gender on work-related attitudes and psychological health. *North American Journal of Psychology*, *8*(2), 217–236. Retrieved from http://search.proquest.com/docview/621357191?accountid=4840

Hochwarter, W. A., Ferris, G. R., Zinko, R., Arnell, B., & James, M. (2007). Reputation as a moderator of political behavior–work outcomes relationships: A two-study investigation with convergent results. *Journal of Applied Psychology*, *92*, 567–576.

Huang, L., Frideger, M., & Pearce, J. L. (2013). Political skill: Explaining the effects of nonnative accent on managerial hiring and entrepreneurial investment decisions. *Journal of Applied Psychology*, *98*(6), 1005–1017.

Ibarra, H. (1993). Personal networks of women and minorities in management: A conceptual framework. *Academy of Management Review*, *18*, 56–87.

Ilgen, D. R., & Youtz, M. A. (1986). Factors affecting the evaluation and development of minorities in organizations. In K. M. Rowland & G. R. Ferris (Eds.), *Research in personnel and human resources management* (Vol. 4, pp. 307–337). Greenwich, CT: JAI Press.

Jackall, R. (1988). *Moral mazes: The world of corporate managers*. New York, NY: Oxford University Press.

James, E. H. (2000). Race-related differences in promotions and support: Underlying effects of human and social capital. *Organization Science*, *11*, 493–508.

James, K., Lovato, C., & Khoo, G. (1994). Social identity correlates of minority workers' health. *Academy of Management Journal*, *37*, 383–396.

Jex, S. M., & Beehr, T. A. (1991). Emerging theoretical and methodological issues in the study of work-related stress. In G. R. Ferris & K. M. Rowland (Eds.), *Research in personnel and human resources management* (Vol. 9, pp. 311–365). Greenwich, CT: JAI Press.

Johnson, P. R., & Indvik, J. (2001). Rudeness at work: Impulse over restraint. *Public Personnel Management*, *30*(4), 457–465.

Kanter, R. M. (1977). *Men and women of the corporation*. New York, NY: Basic Books.

Karasek, R. A. (1979). Job demands, job decision latitude, and mental strain: Implications for job redesign. *Administrative Science Quarterly*, *24*, 285–308.

Karasek, R. A. (1998). Demand/control model: A social, emotional, and physiological approach to stress risk and active behavior development. In J. M. Stellman (Ed.), *Encyclopedia of occupational health and safety* (pp. 34.06–34.14). Geneva, Switzerland: ILO.

Kelly, R., & Kaplan, J. (1993). How Bell labs creates star performers. *Harvard Business Review*, *71*, 128–132.

Kesner, I. F. (1988). Directors' characteristics and committee membership: An investigation of type, occupation, tenure, and gender. *Academy of Management Journal*, *31*, 66–84.

Lankau, M. J., & Scandura, T. A. (2002). An investigation of personal learning in mentoring relationships: Content, antecedents, and consequences. *Academy of Management Journal*, *45*, 779–790.

Lee, P. M., & James, E. H. (2007). She'-E-OS: Gender effects and investor reactions to the announcements of top executive appointments. *Strategic Management Journal*, *28*, 227–241.

LePine, J. A., & Wilcox-King, A. (Eds.). (2010). Editor's comments: Developing novel theoretical insight from reviews of existing theory and research, *Academy of Management Review*, 35, 506–509.

Marger, M. N. (2005). *Race and ethnic relations: American and global perspectives*. Belmont, CA: Cengage Learning, Inc.

McDonald, M. L., & Westphal, J. D. (2013). Access denied: Low mentoring of women and minority first-time directors and its negative effects on appointments to additional boards. *Academy of Management Journal*, *56*(4), 1169–1198.

Miller, T., & del Carmen Triana, M. (2009). Demographic diversity in the boardroom: Mediators of the board diversity–firm performance relationship. *Journal of Management Studies*, *46*, 755–786.

Miller, V. D., & Jablin, F. M. (1991). Information seeking during organizational entry: Influences, tactics, and a model of the process. *Academy of Management Review*, *16*, 92–120.

Mintzberg, H. (1983). *Power in and around organizations*. Englewood Cliffs, NJ: Prentice-Hall.

Morris, J. A., & Feldman, D. C. (1996). The dimensions, antecedents, and consequences of emotional labor. *Academy of Management Review*, *21*(4), 986–1010.

Morrison, E. W. (1993). Newcomer information seeking: Exploring types, modes, sources, and outcomes. *Academy of Management Journal*, *36*, 557–589.

Munyon, T. P., Summers, J. K., Buckley, M. R., Ranft, A. L., & Ferris, G. R. (2010). Executive work design. New perspectives and future directions. *Journal of Organizational Behavior*, *31*, 432–447.

Munyon, T. P., Summers, J. K., Thompson, K. W., & Ferris, G. R. (in press). Political skill and work outcomes: A theoretical extension, meta-analytic investigation, and agenda for the future. *Personnel Psychology*.

Nelson, D. L. (1987). Organizational socialization: A stress perspective. *Journal of Occupational Behavior*, *8*, 311–324.

Nkomo, S. M. (1992). The emperor has no clothes: Rewriting "race in organizations". *Academy of Management Review*, *17*(3), 487–513.

Nkomo, S. M. (2009). The sociology of race: The contributions of W.E.B. DuBois. In P. Adler (Ed.), *Handbook of sociology and organization studies: Classical foundations* (pp. 375–398). London: Oxford Press.

Nkomo, S. M., & Stewart, M. (2006). Diverse identities in organizations. In S. Clegg, C. Hardy, T. Lawrence, & W. Nord (Eds.), *The Sage handbook of organizational studies* (pp. 520–540). London: Sage Publications.

Noe, R. A., Greenberger, D. B., & Wang, S. (2002). Mentoring: What we know and where we might go. In G. R. Ferris & J. J. Martocchio (Eds.), *Research in personnel and human resources management* (Vol. 21, pp. 129–173). Bingley, UK: Emerald Group Publishing Limited.

Ostroff, C., & Kozlowski, S. W. J. (1992). Organizational socialization as a learning process: The role of information acquisition. *Personnel Psychology*, *45*, 849–874.

Ostroff, C., & Kozlowski, S. W. J. (1993). The role of mentoring in the information gathering process of newcomers during early organizational socialization. *Journal of Vocational Behavior*, *42*, 170–183.

Pearson, C. M., Andersson, L. M., & Wegner, J. W. (2001). When workers flout convention: A study of workplace incivility. *Human Relations*, *54*(11), 1387–1419. doi:10.1177/00187267015411001

Perrewé, P. L., & Nelson, D. L. (2004). Gender and career success: The facilitative role of political skill. *Organizational Dynamics*, *33*, 366–378.

Perrewé, P. L., Young, A. M., & Blass, F. R. (2002). Mentoring within the political arena. In G. R. Ferris, M. R. Buckley, & D. B. Fedor (Eds.), *Human resources management: Perspectives, context functions, and outcomes* (4th ed., pp. 343–355). Upper Saddle River, NJ: Prentice-Hall.

Perrewé, P. L., & Zellars, K. L. (1999). An examination of attributions and emotions in the transactional approach to the organizational stress process. *Journal of Organizational Behavior*, *20*, 739–752.

Perrewé, P. L., Zellars, K. L., Ferris, G. R., Rossi, A. M., Kacmar, C. J., & Ralston, D. A. (2004). Neutralizing job stressors: Political skill as an antidote to the dysfunctional consequences of role conflict stressors. *Academy of Management Journal*, *47*, 141–152.

Peterson, C. A., & Philpot, J. (2006). Women's roles on US Fortune 500 boards: Director expertise and committee memberships. *Journal of Business Ethics*, *72*, 177–196.

Pettigrew, T. F., & Martin, J. (1987). Shaping the organizational context for black American inclusion. *Journal of Social Issues*, *43*(1), 41–78.

Pfeffer, J. (1981). *Power in organizations*. Boston, MA: Pitman.

Proudford, K., & Nkomo, S. M. (2006). Race in organizations. In A. M. Konrad, P. Prasad, & J. K. Pringle (Eds.), *Handbook of workplace diversity* (pp. 323–345). London: Sage Publications.

Richman, L. S., & Leary, M. R. (2009). Reactions to discrimination, stigmatization, ostracism, and other forms of interpersonal rejection: A multi-motive model. *Psychological Review*, *116*(2), 365–383.

Roberson, L., & Block, C. J. (2001). Racioethnicity and job performance: A review and critique of theoretical perspectives on the causes of group differences. In B. M. Staw & R. I. Sutton (Eds.) *Research in organizational behavior* (Vol. 23, pp. 247–325). Oxford, UK: JAI Press/Elsevier Science.

Roberts, R. K., Swanson, N. G., & Murphy, L. R. (2004). Discrimination and occupational mental health. *Journal of Mental Health*, *13*(2), 129–142. doi:10.1080/09638230410001669264

Rosen, B. (1982). Career progress of women: Getting in and staying in. In J. Sgro & H. J. Bernardin (Eds.), *Women in the workplace* (pp. 210–227). New York, NY: Praeger.

Rosen, B., & Lovelace, K. (1991). Piecing together the diversity puzzle. *HR Magazine*, *36*, 78–84.

Rothenberg, P. S. (2005). *White privilege: Essential readings on the other side of racism*. New York, NY: Worth Publishers.

Ryan, R. M., & Deci, E. L. (2000). Self-determination theory and the facilitation of intrinsic motivation, social development, and well-being. *American Psychologist*, *55*(1), 68–78.

Segrest Purkiss, S. L., Perrewé, P. L., Gillespie, T. L., Mayes, B. T., & Ferris, G. R. (2006). Implicit sources of bias in employment interview judgments and decisions. *Organizational Behavior and Human Decision Processes*, *101*, 152–167.

Siebert, S. E., Kraimer, M. L., & Liden, R. C. (2001). A social capital theory of career success. *Academy of Management Journal*, *44*(2), 219–237.

Terjesen, S., Sealy, R., & Singh, V. (2009). Women directors on corporate boards: A review and research agenda. *Corporate Governance: An International Review*, *17*, 320–337.

Thau, S., Aquino, K., & Poortvliet, P. M. (2007). Self-defeating behaviors in organizations: The relationship between thwarted belonging and interpersonal work behaviors. *Journal of Applied Psychology*, *92*(3), 840–847. doi:10.1037/0021-9010.92.3.840

Thomas, D. A. (1989). Mentoring and irrationality: The role of racial taboos. *Human Resource Management*, *28*(2), 279–290.

Treadway, D. C., Breland, J. W., Williams, L. M., Cho, J., Yang, J., & Ferris, G. R. (2013). Social influence and interpersonal power in organizations: Roles of performance and political skill in two studies. *Journal of Management*, *39*(6), 529–1553.

U.S. Census Bureau. (2004). *Evidence from Census 2000 about earnings by detailed occupation for men and women*. Special Report. U.S. Department of Commerce, Washington, DC.

Van Maanen, J. (1978). Police organization: A longitudinal examination of job attitudes in an urban police department. *Administrative Science Quarterly*, *20*, 207–228.

Van Maanen, J., & Schein, E. H. (1979). Toward a theory of organizational socialization. In B. M. Staw (Ed.), *Research in Organizational Behavior* (Vol. 1, pp. 209–264). Greenwich, CT: JAI Press.

Wanberg, C. R., Welsh, E. T., & Hezlett, S. A. (2003). Mentoring research: A review and dynamic process model. In J. J. Martocchio & G. R. Ferris (Eds.), *Research in personnel and human resources management* (Vol. 22, pp. 39–124). Bingley, UK: Emerald Group Publishing Limited.

Westphal, J. D., & Stern, I. (2006). The other pathway to the boardroom: Interpersonal influence behavior as a substitute for elite credentials and majority status in obtaining board appointments. *Administrative Science Quarterly*, *51*, 169–204.

Williams, D. R., Yu, Y., Jackson, J. S., & Anderson, N. B. (1997). Racial differences in physical and mental health: Socio-economic status, stress, and discrimination. *Journal of Health Psychology*, *2*, 335–351.

Williams, K. D. (2007). Ostracism: The kiss of social death. *Social and Personality Psychology Compass*, *1*, 236–2247.

A REVIEW OF MINORITY STRESS RELATED TO EMPLOYEES' DEMOGRAPHICS AND THE DEVELOPMENT OF AN INTERSECTIONAL FRAMEWORK FOR THEIR COPING STRATEGIES IN THE WORKPLACE

Thomas Köllen

ABSTRACT

Every employee embodies manifestations of every demographic that attach to him or her different minority and majority statuses at the same time. As these statuses are often related to organizational hierarchies, employees frequently hold positions of dominance and subordination at the same time. Thus, a given individual's coping strategies (or coping behavior) in terms of minority stress due to organizational processes of hierarchization, marginalization, and discrimination, are very often a simultaneous coping in terms of more than one demographic. Research

The Role of Demographics in Occupational Stress and Well Being
Research in Occupational Stress and Well Being, Volume 12, 41–82

ISSN: 1479-3555/doi:10.1108/S1479-355520140000012000

on minority stress mostly focuses on single demographics representing only single facets of workforce diversity. By integrating the demographics of age, disability status, nationality, ethnicity, race, sexual orientation, and religion into one framework, the intersectional model proposed in this chapter broadens the perspective on minorities and related minority stress in the workplace. It is shown that coping with minority stress because of one demographic must always be interpreted in relation to the other demographics. The manifestation of one demographic can limit or broaden one's coping resources for coping with minority stress because of another dimension. Thus, the manifestation of one demographic can determine the coping opportunities and coping behavior one applies to situations because of the minority status of another demographic. This coping behavior can include disclosure decisions about invisible demographics. Therefore, organizational interventions aiming to create a supportive workplace environment and equal opportunities for every employee (e.g., diversity management approaches) should include more demographics instead of focusing only on few.

Keywords: Minority stress; coping resources; intersectionality; stigma; workforce diversity; diversity management

INTRODUCTION

In society, as well as in the workplace, specific manifestations for each demographic can be identified that tend to confront employees with different layers and intensities of "minority stress." This "minority stress" is due to the stigmatizing effect of these manifestations, such as being homosexual in terms of "sexual orientation" or being, for example, Black or African-American in terms of race. In the workplace, this stress is primarily based on the experience of prejudice events and related mechanisms of discrimination, the expectations of rejection, internalized marginalization, and the related ameliorative processes of coping with the situation. Most of the research on "minority stress" attempts, somewhat one-dimensionally, to understand the structure and the impact of this minority stress alongside one specific manifestation of "being a minority," for example, of being homosexual (DiPlacido, 1998; Waldo, 1999), or, more specifically, of being gay (Kimmel & Mahalik, 2005; Meyer 1995) or lesbian (Brooks, 1981). These examples already evince that gender is an important demographic that, in isolation, can have an impact on an employee's workplace situation (Basford, Offermann, & Behrend, in press; Miner-Rubino & Cortina, 2004). Nevertheless, whilst in the context of a wider society, men or women as gendered groups cannot perforce be seen as a "minority" per se, in certain workplace settings they can, for example, men working as pre-school teachers (Cameron, 2001; Nordberg, 2002) or women working in engineering or technological professions (Hanappi-Egger, 2013; Wallace & Sheldon, 2014). Against this background, research focusing on multiple historically oppressed groups often utilized the term "women and minorities" (Krook & O'Brien, 2010; McDonald & Westphal, 2013). Thus, when developing an interconnected framework for coping with minority stress related to employees' demographics, this dimension has to be considered as well, although the focus will be on age, mental and physical capabilities, sexual orientation, ethnicity/race, nationality, and religion. As an adequate approach to conjointly considering these demographics, this chapter builds on an intersectional perspective. An intersectional framework, in this context, allows a consideration of the issues of race/ethnicity, age, sexual orientation, disability, nationality, and religion "as they are simultaneously expressed" (Talwar, 2010, p. 15). Social hierarchies amongst the manifestations of each demographic are interconnected and also ingrained in the organizations that employees are working for. Within these organizations employees hold positions of subordination or dominance, and, very often, both simultaneously (Talwar, 2010; Weber, 2001). Thus, coping with these hierarchies is frequently a simultaneous coping, in terms of more than one demographic, as different demographics assume different degrees of relevance in different situations and settings. In order to develop a conceptual framework for these interdependencies and their impact for different coping strategies, this chapter will be structured as detailed here: in the following, a more nuanced outline of the concept of intersectionality will be given. This is then followed by a short introduction to Goffman's (1963) concept of "stigma" and to the related "identity threat model of stigma" from Major and O'Brien (2005). These concepts will theoretically frame the coping strategies for handling minority stress available to an employee that can be related to his or her demographics. Subsequently, a structured review of minority stress issues and related coping strategies alongside the aforementioned demographics will provide the empirical insights to develop the intersectional framework that is proposed in this chapter. This chapter ends by discussing future applications of this model, as well as its limitations and connecting points for its further development.

INTERSECTIONALITY, STIGMA, AND MINORITY STRESS

Intersectionality

Intersectionality, as a concept or a research paradigm, has emerged from critical gender studies and feminist studies, taking into account that it is no longer possible to assume that every woman is confronted with the same kinds of societal or organizational oppression or marginalization. Historically, the first step toward an intersectional approach to studying different demographics and their interplay arose from the political interventions of "black feminism" (Taylor, 1998), which analyzed the intersection of gender and race (or skin color) (Crenshaw, 1991; Jordan-Zachery, 2007). These studies were often referred to as "post-colonial studies" or "post-colonial feminist analyses" (Mohanty, 1988), as most of these studies were on black US American women (Brah & Phoenix, 2004). Furthermore, literature increasingly criticized feminist studies as being too centered on the middle classes (Collins, 1993). These studies started adding the category of "social class" (Mahony & Zmroczek, 1997), noting that women do not only experience oppression and marginalization because of their gender, and race, but also because of their social class (e.g., Acker, 2006; Holvino, 2010; Knapp, 2005). Later studies also started taking into account the social categories of sexual orientation (e.g., Bowleg, Huang, Brooks, Black, & Burkholder, 2003) and age (e.g., Kertzner, Meyer, Frost, & Stirratt, 2009) too. Thus, at least from an historical perspective, intersectionality emerged as a specification, fragmentation and further development of gender and women studies. Nevertheless, an intersectional framework should not maintain this predominance of gender as a demographic criterion or social category, since, determined by situation and setting, every social category can potentially be a key category for processes of inclusion and exclusion. Thus, as every employee represents at least one manifestation of every social category, there is no reason for prioritizing gender as a category.

Yuval-Davis (2006) identifies influential processes of naturalization working on both the societal and the organizational level that discursively constitute these social categories:

> They tend to homogenize social categories and to treat all who belong to a particular social category as sharing equally the particular natural attributes (positive or negative) specific to it. Categorical attributes are often used for the construction of inclusionary/exclusionary boundaries that differentiate between self and other, determining what is

> "normal" and what is not, who is entitled to certain resources and who is not. In this way the interlinking grids of differential positionings in terms of class, race and ethnicity, gender and sexuality, ability, stage in the life cycle and other social divisions, tend to create, in specific historical situations, hierarchies of differential access to a variety of resources – economic, political and cultural. (Yuval-Davis, 2006, p. 199)

Each demographic consists of different manifestations or social categories that constitute hierarchies that legitimize certain allocations of resources and other kinds of privileges and general positioning and social standing (Ferrall, 1997; Tsui, Egan, & Iii, 1992). As an example, the related mechanisms of inclusion and exclusion for the demographic of sexual orientation work alongside its manifestations hetero-, homo-, or bisexual; those for the demographic nationality alongside domestic and non-domestic, and there may be further hierarchies among the non-domestic nationalities in addition to this.

For individuals that do not represent the dominant manifestation of one demographic (whatever that may be in a certain setting), this means coping with possible mechanisms of exclusion or marginalization. Often a certain demographic has more relevance than another in a given situation or in a certain context, especially when minority and majority statuses are in flux because of shifting constellations within teams (Coston & Kimmel, 2012; Mumby & Stohl, 1991). A lesbian Indian bookkeeper in one project team, consisting otherwise only of male colleagues, could be more subject to those stereotypes based on her gender. In contrast in, say, a predominantly Italian project team, stereotypes about being Indian could be more relevant. The same could hold true in terms of her sexual orientation, age, skin color, accent, disability status, and any other demographic in any other given situation or environment. Nevertheless, although certain demographics are more relevant than others in certain settings, each individual always represents manifestations of every demographic, and the attributed stereotypes can strengthen, weaken, or contradict each other. Stereotypes attached to demographics are, by and large, neither wholly negative nor wholly positive. Stereotypic images of, for example, nationalities usually have both negative and positive facets (Glick & Fiske, 2001). Furthermore, not every minority manifestation has to be perceived as necessarily predominantly negative. Nevertheless, negative attributions are more often related to minority than to majority manifestations of demographics. Thus, employees representing one or more of these minority manifestations (e.g., being non-domestic and gay) often especially struggle with coping with the related mechanisms of exclusion and marginalization (Bowleg et al., 2003). These negative attributions to primarily minority manifestations of demographics can be conceptualized as having a "stigmatizing" effect.

Stigma, Minority Stress and Coping Resources

Although Goffman (1963) conceptualizes stigma as a societal phenomenon with a certain shared consensus across the members of a certain society, any manifestation of any demographic, in a certain setting or situation, can act as a stigma with negative consequences for those who represent this stigmatizing category. Goffman (1963) explains the way stigma works as follows: "We believe the person with a stigma is not quite human. On this assumption we exercise varieties of discrimination, through which we effectively, if often un-thinkingly, reduce his [or her] life chances. We construct a stigma theory, an ideology to explain his [or her] inferiority […] We tend to impute a wide range of imperfections" (Goffman, 1963, p. 14).

The public perception of the "stigma" radiates all the other possible characteristics that could describe a person. Goffman (1963) distinguishes between discredited and discreditable stigmas. Discredited stigmas are already known or visible, such as gender, race, and a physical disability, whereas discreditable stigmas are not directly visible, such as HIV status, mental illness, or homosexuality. He conceptualizes five basic strategies for dealing with a stigma:

1. The "direct attempt to correct what he [or she] sees as the objective basis of his [or her] failing" (*ibid.*, p. 18). As an example of such an attempt, in terms of "sexual orientation," and without evaluating its prospects of success, Goffman gives the example of homosexual psychotherapy (*ibid.*, p. 18).
2. The attempt to correct the stigma indirectly "by devoting much private effort to the mastery of areas of activity ordinarily felt to be closed on incidental and physical grounds to one with his [or her] shortcoming" (*ibid.*, p. 19).
3. Breaking "with what is called reality, and obstinately attempt[ing] to employ an unconventional interpretation of the character of [her or] his social identity" (*ibid.*, p. 20).
4. Using the "stigma for 'secondary gains', as an excuse for ill success that has come his way for other reasons" (*ibid.*, p. 20).
5. The avoidance of any contact with "non-stigmatized" persons to avoid the anticipated disrespect (Goffman, 1963).

The stigma-based processes of marginalization, exclusion and disrespect occurring in the workplace can lead to a massive destabilizing and threatening of the individual's personal and social identity. Although stigmatized employees often utilize variations of the aforementioned self-protective coping strategies, stigmatization generally has the potential to undermine stigmatized individuals' self-esteem (Crocker & Major, 1989). Besides the negative effects on one's self worth, stress in general, and, by extension, stigma-related minority stress, undermines the individual's feelings of control or mastery (Caplan, 1981). The perception of having a certain kind of control, or being able to predict events in which one is involved enhances an individual's coping resources. The same goes for the individual's self-esteem, whereas, conversely, shrinking coping resources can also negatively affect one's self-esteem (Thoits, 2013). The "identity threat model of stigma" from Major and O'Brien (2005) states that "identity threat results when stigma-relevant stressors are appraised as potentially harmful to one's social identity and as exceeding one's coping resources. Identity threat [...] motivates attempts at threat reduction through coping strategies" (Major & O'Brien, 2005, p. 393). Thus the coping strategy applied by stigmatized employees (that is, mostly by minority employees), is determined by the intensity of the perceived "identity threat." The individual estimation of this threat as potentially destabilizing for one's identity is, in turn, dependent on two factors. The first is the personal estimation of the harmfulness of the experienced stressors; the second is the individual coping resources. Both factors are interrelated and they might intensify when it comes to multiple stigmatization, for example because of multiple minority statuses. In order to develop a framework that conceptualizes these multiple coping strategies intersectionally, minority stress for the demographics of age, mental, and physical capabilities, sexual orientation, ethnicity/race, nationality, and religion will be considered more closely in the following paragraphs.

DEMOGRAPHICS

As previously mentioned, dependent on the setting or the situation, every demographic can become crucial for the allocation of resources amongst employees. These resources can be any kind of resources, ranging from information (Bygren, 2013), opportunities (Schmidt & Müller, 2013), and voice and agency (Kamenou & Fearfull, 2006; Meares, Oetzel, Torres,

Derkacs, & Ginossar, 2004), to job promotions and money. Stereotype-based organizational mechanisms of exclusion that frequently keep minority employees away from these resources force those representing one or more, often stigmatized, minority statuses, to cope with these marginalizing mechanisms. In order to gain a deeper understanding of the situation of multiple stigmatization, six demographics are looked at more closely below.

Religion

Having a religious belief can be a source of strength (Bozard & Sanders, 2011) that positively influences the individual's subjective well-being, as religious persons seem to be happier on average, and more satisfied with life, than individuals who are non-religious (Chamberlain & Zika, 1988; Lewis & Cruise, 2006), at least in religious environments (Eichhorn, 2012; Stavrova, Fetchenhauer, & Schlosser, 2013). Nevertheless, most nations have one predominant religion that leaves other religions with a minority status. Non-laicistic societies, where certain religions are very strong, often tend to categorize other religions in an antagonistic way. For example, societies that define themselves as strongly Christian often tend to develop an antagonistic attitude toward Islam (Schiffauer, 2004). States where is the use of religious value systems is legitimate or sanctioned in politics tend to have a higher level of discrimination against religious minorities, as these discriminations then also have political legitimacy (Fox, 2000). Besides these antagonistic tendencies, smaller religious communities, often referred to as in diaspora (Baumann, 2000), are often an especial focus of certain types of marginalization and discrimination by the majority religion. The main reason for this is that the majority religion often feels threatened by the mere existence of the minority religions. "Religious beliefs, among other things, give people the ability to find meaning and understanding about the world and their place in it. Such beliefs constitute psychological walls that individuals and groups use to defend their individual and collective psyche. Accordingly, such walls of belief are political and will be defended" (Fox, 2000, p. 427). Thus, the mere existence of a minority religion has the potential to challenge the worldview of the majority. Religious discrimination, often founded in these processes of demarcation, or sometimes merely founded in ignorance, also occurs in the workplace. Employees who do not want to hide their minority religion, and who also want to practice their religion in the workplace, often feel a strong pressure to justify their religion in front of non-religious colleagues, or colleagues who belong to the majority religion (Ghumman, Ryan, Barclay, & Markel, 2013; Huang & Kleiner, 2001).

Coping with Religion-Related Minority Stress

As coping strategies, all five of those proposed by Goffman (1963) can be applied. Correcting the stigma could seemingly be done easily by converting to the majority faith (Lofland & Skonovd, 1981). In reality, religious people would rarely do this, because having a personal spiritual worldview seems, to the majority of people, not to be a matter of choice. Furthermore, minority religions in particular tend to have very tight social ties between members (Ferriss, 2002), a factor that augments the cost of converting and, potentially, might cause sanctions from the individual's own family and community. Another issue related to religious conversion that might deter people from converting, is that converts are sometimes not accepted as equals by those "born into" the religion. This kind of "second class" treatment of converts is especially noticeable in religions that have a non-missionary self-understanding (Sharma, 2012). At the time of writing, no study has been published about the interrelation of perceived stigmatization and converting. An indirect correction of a potential stigmatizing impact of one's religion through participating in activities performed by members of the majority religion is possible, if there is no formal exclusion attached to the activities. As religion itself means the construction of a certain reality, the coping strategy of creating a "reality" of one's own is the essence of religion anyhow. Religions can be described as systems of meaning "that influence all aspects of life and constitute central resources for the construction of identity, on the individual as well as on the collective level. Because of their global scope, they are especially helpful when people have to cope with distress, fears and identity destabilization" (Brandt, 2013, pp. 301–302). Thus religions can also help in coping with identity destabilization and minority stress that might be due to the stigmatizing impact of other demographics. "Secondary gains" of one's religion are mainly due to the strong networks attached to religions that also help members with non-spiritual issues (Traunmüller, 2009). The avoidance of any contact with "non-stigmatized" persons to prevent the anticipated disrespect is a side-effect of strong religious community building (Lim & Putnam, 2010). This coping mechanism is primarily applied by ultra-religious people to whom their minority religion is a central element of their identity. In doing so, these individuals can maintain the positive image they hold of their religion, and avoid the emergence of minority effectively.

Intersections with Other Demographics

In terms of intersections with other demographics, negative interrelations can be identified with gender and sexual orientation, as many religions do not attach the same societal status to women or homosexual persons as they do to men and heterosexual persons (Kubicek et al., 2009). Thus participating in non-affirming religious settings can be associated with higher levels of internalized homophobia (Barnes & Meyer, 2012; Rowen & Malcolm, 2003; Shilo & Savaya, 2012). Religious lesbians and gay men, therefore, often experience identity conflicts in integrating their sexual and religious identities. As a coping strategy to handle the related minority stress, gays and lesbian frequently choose not to disclose their homosexuality to other members of their religious community (Anderton, Pender, & Asner-Self, 2011; Ginicola & Smith, 2011; Tozer & Hayes, 2004). The negative side effects of this can be their general psychological destabilizing and a massive shrinking of their coping resources (Schuck & Liddle, 2001). Another coping mechanism, that is only rarely applied nowadays, is accepting spiritual "help" from one's religious community to "convert" one's homosexuality into heterosexuality. The effectiveness of this is highly questionable, but in the past it was partially practiced by several Christian churches, that offered help for this conversion through prayer or even through exorcism (Ross & Stålström, 1979; Silverstein, 2003; Spitzer, 2003). Religious women that do not conform to "traditional" gender roles, sometimes also struggle to reconcile their gender identity and religious identity (Dhruvarajan, 1988), an issue that can lead to a shrinking of one's coping resources for handling minority stress that might be due to other demographics (Garber, 2013). In terms of age, most religions explicitly value older people and circumscribe rules for taking care of them and keeping them integrated in society (Koenig, Kvale, & Ferrel, 1988). The same is true for disabled people (Selway & Ashman, 1998). Thus, for older and disabled people religiosity can broaden their coping resources and reduce their potential minority stress. Nationality only has a direct relation to religion when the state defines itself as a religious state, or when a certain religion is predominantly present in a certain state, such as Judaism in Israel (Juergensmeyer, 1994). Ethnicity and religion are often intertwined, especially when religion becomes a descriptive characteristic of an ethnicity (Smith, 1978). In these cases minority stress because of one's religion coincides with potential minority stress that is perceived with one's ethnicity or nationality.

Ethnicity, Race, and Nationality

There are several reasons for and against a joint consideration of the demographics race, ethnicity and nationality. A distinct discussion of ethnicity and race is often legitimized by these arguments:

> Race is said to be involuntary, ethnicity voluntary; race to be a matter of external categorization, ethnicity of internal self-identification; race to be based on differences of phenotype or nature, ethnicity on differences of culture; race to be rigid, ethnicity flexible; race to involve super – and subordinate, ethnicity coordinate groups; race to arise from processes of exclusion, ethnicity from processes of inclusion; race to have grown out of the European colonial encounter with the non-European world, ethnicity out of the history of nation-state formation. (Brubaker, 2009, pp. 25–26)

Brubaker's literature review shows that all of these criteria do not allow ethnicity and race to be sharply distinguished:

> People may voluntarily identify with ostensibly racial categories and resist attempts to downplay them; conversely, external categorization is central to what is ordinarily considered ethnicity in many settings. "Racial" differences are in some instances based on ancestry, way of life, or even class rather than on phenotype; conversely, phenotypical differences are often implicated in "ethnic" categorization. "Racial" categories are sometimes flexible, and "ethnic" categories sometimes rigid. "Racial" categories may be coordinate, "ethnic" categories super – and subordinate. "Racial" categories may be invoked in struggles for inclusion, "ethnic" categories in processes of exclusion. Some "racial" categories have histories largely independent of European colonial expansion. (Brubaker, 2009, p. 26)

The category of ethnicity has an especially strong relation to nationality. Nations are a relatively new territorial concept, and the issue of developing a national identity emerged over the last few centuries. National borders, as they exist today, are mainly the result of wars, political negotiations, or of colonial occupations by European states. The border-shaping wars and negotiations, for example, those within Europe, often ran alongside or between ethnic groups. Thus, nations are often the national territory for an ethnic group, or they are a territory where a certain ethnic group comprises the majority of the inhabitants (Connor, 1990; Hutchinson, 2000). There are, however, many examples of ethnicities that do not have a national territory, such as Kurds (Bruinessen, 1998), or of nations that consist of different ethnicities, this often being the mainspring for social conflicts (Sheth, 1989). However, if people of these ethnicities migrate between the countries, they are often categorized by their assumed nationality, such as Turks or Iraqis.

The potentially stigmatizing attributions to race, ethnicity, and nationality that minority employees are confronted with in terms of these categories are therefore both interrelated and interdependent. In their everyday work, minority employees are confronted with different intensities of racist, nationalist and ethnicity-based discriminatory behavior (Dunn, Loosemore, Phua, & Ozguc, 2011; Köllen, 2012). This can cause severe stress for these employees, especially when their nation, race, or ethnicity works as an anchor for their identity (Schuh, Dick, Wegge, & Haslam, 2013).

Coping with Nationality-, Ethnicity-, and Race-Related Minority Stress
Coping strategies, related to the health-damaging minority stress (Vega & Rumbaut, 1991) that is inherent in these race-, ethnicity-, and nationality-induced experiences of exclusion and marginalization are discussed alongside Goffman's (1963) five coping strategies. A direct attempt to correct a stigmatizing demographic in terms of race is hardly possible, as one cannot change one's skin color. Changing one's ethnicity is not possible, as it is related to the unchangeable elements of personal appearance. As an attempt to correct a stigma indirectly, cultural elements estimated to be crucial for the ethnic (or also racial) majority can be adopted. To a certain extent one can adapt clothing, hair style, personal taste, habitus, languages, and argot in order to not be perceived, or at any rate less perceived, as a member of a stigmatized minority ethnic group (DeVos, 1980; Nagel, 1994). These processes are often similar to acculturation processes, which can also be utilized to adapt the cultural elements of a certain nationality (Ward, Fox, Wilson, Stuart, & Kus, 2010). These processes can, conversely, enhance minority stress or a particular "acculturative stress" (Berry, 1970). This stress is mainly due to the struggles one may experience in integrating one cultural identity into another, or by on the wholesale replacement of one cultural identity with another, while simultaneously seeking to maintain one's self integrity (Berry, 2006; Cuéllar, 2000). Thus, acculturation processes can work in both directions: they may both reduce and enhance one's minority stress. One's nationality can be formally changed according to the relevant national laws. That said, if one does indeed choose, and is legally allowed to change his or her national minority status into a majority status, it does not necessarily follow that the potentially stigmatizing effect of the former nationality totally disappears. Identifiers like accent, appearance, or also canonic knowledge might hint at the former nationality and provoke stigma-related minority stress (Spinner, 1994). The coping strategy of creating a new positively connoted social identity that contrasts the negative attributions by majority race, ethnicity, or nationality can be done

by accentuating more prominently the traditional myths and history of one's ethnicity, race or nationality. Ethnicities and nationalities tend especially to have strong myths and histories presenting them in a positive light (Smith, 1987). As, for the individual, these accentuations need a certain confirmation from others, and this coping strategy is closely related to the strategy of avoiding any contact with non-stigmatized persons, to avoid the anticipated disrespect. Thus stigmatized minority ethnicities or minority nationalities often tend to build strong communities in hostile places. One function of these communities is, by mutual confirmation, to stabilize a positive self-image that is potentially threatened by everyday experiences with the majority nationality or ethnicity. Thus, in contrast to the regions or nations where they are the majority ethnicity or nationality, the myths, history, and related rites are even more important to the members of a certain ethnicity or nationality where they are the minority, than they are in their "home" regions. This is mainly because members of these groups need them to an even greater degree in order to stabilize a positive self-image in environments that are perceived as tending to destabilize this image and causing minority stress (Wimmer, 2008). Secondary gains of these strong communities are due to the social capital that is inherent in these networks, which provide their members with a strong basis of mutual help and support. Secondary gains one can earn from the stereotypes attached to one's ethnicity, nationality, or race are, similar to the other demographics, derived from the fact that, usually, there are also stereotypes that can be utilized in a positive way for one's career development. If, for example, a certain nationality is perceived as especially disciplined, or artistic, a national can utilize this presupposition about his or her abilities when this capability is requested in a certain job context. By overemphasizing one's nationality (through applying a related accent, for example), one can also suggest the possession of the requested stereotypic national characteristics for a given job or promotion. On the other hand, positive stereotypes, such as performance-related stereotypes, can work as stressors for minorities, as they can create a permanent pressure to conform to these stereotypes and to prove the truth of them. In terms of performance-related stereotypes, this stress is especially high for employees who are less capable of representing these stereotypes (Cheryan & Bodenhausen, 2000; Cocchiara & Quick, 2004).

Intersections with Other Demographics

In terms of intersections with other demographics, strong relations can occur between religion and ethnicity or nationality, especially when a certain religious aspect is part of one's ethnic or national identity (Marty & Appleby, 1997). In these cases stigma-related minority stress has to be considered conjointly, as a destabilization of one category also destabilizes the other. In terms of gender, some ethnicities or nations might pass on constitutive myths that do not conform with gender equality, and therefore might cause an identity struggle for some men and women of these ethnicities or nationalities (Allen, 1998). Older or disabled people, similar to religious communities, can often rely on the support of their ethnic or national community that broadens their coping resources and helps to reduce minority stress. Sexual orientations other than heterosexuality are often not accepted in these communities, especially when they have a strong religious component (Nagel, 2000), because most religions still do not provide affirming environments toward homosexuality (Barnes & Meyer, 2012). Thus gay and lesbians might sometimes struggle to reconcile both their ethnic and/or religious identity, and their sexual identity. This struggle might aggravate their minority stress due to both categories and reduce their coping resources (Yinger, 1994).

Age

Grossmann et al. (2010) find that older people seem to have a higher capability for coping with conflict situations. As one reason for this, they suggest that older people are more capable of keeping their distance from conflicts, and succeed in not getting emotionally involved in them (Grossmann et al., 2010). In general, it seems that, compared to younger adults, older adults "solve emotionally salient and interpersonal problems in more effective ways" (Blanchard-Fields, 2007, p. 26). Furthermore, older people tend to have a more stable personality (Worthy, Gorlick, Pacheco, Schnyer, & Maddox, 2011). Therefore it can be assumed that since older people have more coping resources at their disposal, potential stigma-relevant stressors might be estimated as less harmful to them.

Age itself can have a stigmatizing effect in different situations. Stereotype-based marginalization and exclusion because of one's age, especially against older people, is often referred to as ageism (Nelson, 2002). In the context of the United States, Nelson (2005) states that older adults "tend to be marginalized, institutionalized, and stripped of responsibility, power, and, ultimately, their dignity" (Nelson, 2005, p. 208). Ageism manifests itself primarily in patronizing language toward older people.

The language younger people use when speaking with older people often becomes overly polite, louder, slower, and the sentences used become more simplistic (Fox & Giles, 1993). Nelson (2005) names this phenomenon over-accommodation. Another ageist issue is infantilization and the related insulting usage of baby talk, connoting a relationship of dependency (Nelson, 2005). An ageist issue related to this infantilization is the downplay of serious thoughts, feelings and concerns that older people express (Biggs & Haapala, 2013). These types of language-based ageism also occur in the workplace and, as a massive mechanism of marginalization, can have negative consequences for older employees' working conditions and climate (Iweins, Desmette, Yzerbyt, & Stinglhamber, 2013; Nussbaum, Pitts, Huber, Krieger, & Ohs, 2005).

Ageist behavior is mostly based on the stereotypical assumption that older people are physically and mentally less capable than younger people. Furthermore, age is often associated with less willingness to embrace new developments and trends. Another motive for ageism is the fact that elderly people can remind other people of their mortality, thus ageist behavior can also be a defensive reaction to being confronted with one's own future death (Martens, Greenberg, Schimel, & Landau, 2004). Older employees have to face the related mechanisms of exclusion and marginalization at their workplaces (Branine & Glover, 1997; Rupp, Vodanovich, & Credé, 2006). As a severe type of ageism, age discrimination occurs in contact with colleagues as well as with supervisors, and can manifest itself in decisions about employment, retirement, job termination, training, benefits, and promotion opportunities (Dennis & Thomas, 2007). Age is, however, not easily categorized. What is considered old or young may differ between industries and occupations, and also between societies (Amrhein, 2013; Vincent, 2006). For example, in developed societies, people are living longer; therefore what is considered to be "middle age" in these societies may be considered old in developing countries. What is considered old in high-tech industries may not considered old in politics (Brooke & Taylor, 2005). Thus, age has subjective components in addition to its objective components (Fried, Grant, Levi, Hadani, & Slowik, 2007; Posthuma & Guerrero, 2013). Nevertheless, every occupational setting has scales that categorize employees as old or young (Schabracq, 2003). Older employees, as well as other "stigmatized groups, are harmed by their devalued social identity and that they try to cope with their predicament" (Desmette & Gaillard, 2008, p. 169). Alongside Goffman's coping strategies the elderly have different possibilities to cope with the potentially stigmatizing impact of their age.

Coping with Age-Related Minority Stress

It is not possible to correct one's stigmatizing age directly. But the trigger for age-related mechanisms of marginalization or exclusion is mostly the perception of one's age by others. Most of the time people do not assume someone's age because they know, for example, because they read it in one's passport or in other official documents.

Usually people treat other people "age-specifically" because they draw their conclusions because from appearance. This includes, amongst others, clothing, bodily and mental posture, or other bodily symptoms of age. As one indirect attempt to try to avoid ageism, at least to a certain degree, one can counteract these symptoms, for example, with younger clothing or "younger" opinions. A strategy that corresponds to the strategy of avoiding contact to non-stigmatized persons (i.e., younger colleagues), aiming to reduce the perceived minority stress at the workplace, is an early retirement. The development of this intention can in itself help reduce stigma-related stress. For the actual time of retirement, this means a definite ending of this stress. For the time that remains until retirement, after having made this decision, the related disengagement means "devaluing the domain where they are stigmatized" (Desmette & Gaillard, 2008, p. 171), and thus it can reduce the perceived stigma-related stress. On the other hand, the retiree might perceive his or her decision to retire as an involuntary exit that is mainly due to the organizational stigmatizing pressure that has forced him or her into this decision. The perception of treading a path of an involuntary transition into retirement because of external pressure can cause a reduction in life satisfaction (Hershey & Henkens, 2014) and may actually increase stigma-related stress (Negrini, Panari, Simbula, & Alcover, 2013). Thus, the decision to retire earlier can impact minority stress in both directions for the time remaining in the job. However, as an earlier retirement is usually related to a partial loss of income, and as, additionally, not every employer offers this option in the same way, not every older employee can afford to apply this coping behavior. Lower paid workers, especially, can only rarely choose this option. Highlighting some age-related positive attributions can be part of a coping strategy of creating a new positively connoted age identity that contrasts the negative attributions through younger colleagues. Such attributes can be "being more experienced," or "having had success in the past." To stabilize this self-image it can be useful to establish an inner circle of other colleagues of the same age, to mutually confirm this self-image. Adequate settings for this can be round-tables, conjoint tennis – and golf-club memberships, or joint bowling evenings or trips. Secondary gains of this coping behavior, similar to other constitutions of networks around a certain demographic manifestation, are the mutual dependencies that are created with these networks, and that are the basis for mutual help and support.

Intersections with Other Demographics

As an intersection with other demographics, older people tend to become more religious. One reason for this is the more intense involvement with one's own mortality, due to the experience of the weakening of one's physical state and an increased confrontation with death in one's closer environment. Religions help to attach sense to these cases and also to one's own anticipated death and weakening body (Hunsberger, 1985; Koenig et al., 1988). As outlined earlier on religion, being religious can strengthen an individual's coping resources for stigma-related stress in general. This is because religions can help to attach meaning to stigma-related negative experiences, rendering them less grave. On the other hand, belonging to a minority religion can also create additional minority stress because of the religion itself. Thus religious older people may feel less stress because of stigmatization by others, but they may have an additional stress-trigger that can be inherent in their religion itself. As the deterioration of one's health that is a concomitant of aging often means the need for assistance in certain situations, there is also a strong intersection with the demographic disability. However, as older people are more likely to be expected to need assistance, this might not trigger additional stigma-related minority stress. The intersection of age and sexual orientation resides in the myth that sexuality and having a sexual life is a privilege for younger people (Hodson & Skeen, 1994). Added to this is the persistent societal perception of gays and lesbians as (over)sexualized persons, in comparison to heterosexuals (Buba & Vaskovics, 2001). Thus, openly gay or lesbian elderly might additionally be confronted with prejudices because of their assumed non-age-appropriate sexual activity, no matter whether they are sexually active or not. This might increase their age-related stress.

Disability

Disabled people, in the workplace as well as in everyday life, are often confronted with stereotype-based discriminatory behavior. This behavior is often referred to as disablism.

"Disablism is a set of assumptions and practices promoting the differential or unequal treatment of people because of actual or presumed disabilities" (Campbell, 2008, p. 152). In this context disablism can be defined as "discriminatory, oppressive or abusive behavior arising from the belief that disabled people are inferior to others" (Miller, Parker, & Gillinson, 2004, p. 9). From a social constructionist viewpoint, disablism can be described as the everyday production of disability. In contrast, as another term for discriminatory behavior toward disabled persons, "ableism can be associated with the production of ableness, the perfectible body and, by default, the creation of a neologism that suggests a falling away from ableness that is disability" (Campbell, 2008, pp. 152–153). However, both concepts stigmatize disabled people as deficient and very often transfer a certain physical or mental impairment to many more facets of personal deficiency.

Employers and colleagues alike often attach very concrete stereotypic attributes to disabled people, such as the expectation of low productivity, the perception that employing disabled people is a risk in terms of absence rates and availability, and the perception that the presence of disabled people in the workplace might provoke existential anxiety in colleagues and customers (Kregel & Unger, 1993; Roulstone & Williams, 2013). Thus, employers often estimate disabled people as being less employable (Bricout & Bentley, 2000; Waltz, Santuzzi, & Finkelstein, 2013) and they are less likely to be hired than non-disabled applicants (Bordieri & Drehmer, 1986), especially when applying for jobs involving a higher level of interpersonal contact (Louvet, 2007) Disabled persons are less likely to be chosen as business partners (Colella, DeNisi, & Varma, 1998), and in professional contexts disabled employees tend to be estimated as "warmer" but less competent than non-disabled colleagues (Louvet, Rohmer, & Dubois, 2009). As with other minorities or women, for disabled people the phenomenon of a "glass ceiling" is observable, keeping them away from leadership or management positions (Braddock & Bachelder, 1994).

In the workplace there is a hierarchy observable between the different types of disability. Employers continue to view employees or candidates with physical disabilities more positively than those with psychiatric or intellectual disabilities (Hernandez, 2000). This is even more unfortunate, as employment, especially when it is competitive, can improve one's self-esteem and thereby can contribute to recovery from mental illnesses, such as depression, whereas unemployment or poor quality jobs may actually worsen such illnesses (Bezborodovs & Thornicroft, 2013). Thus, admitting to having mental health problems in the workplace carries a certain danger of losing one's job and activating a negative spiral of internalizing stigmatizing attributions, as well as aggravating one's mental health problems (Drapalski et al., 2013; Krupa, Kirsh, Cockburn, & Gewurtz, 2009).

Many Western countries have certain legislation, like disabilities acts, that force employers to employ a certain quota of disabled people. Furthermore, many countries promote the employment of disabled persons with different kinds of financial support (Hotchkiss, 2004; Maschke, 2008). These supportive legal settings are still contrasted by "principal barriers to employing workers with disabilities [that] are a lack of awareness of disability and accommodation issues, concern over costs, and fear of legal liability" (Kaye, Jans, & Jones, 2011, p. 526). However, refusing to employ a disabled person, as a blatant form of direct discrimination, is becoming increasingly uncommon in Western societies. Nevertheless, subtle forms of prejudices against disabled persons still persist, and they are still the basis for more subtle forms of disablism in the workplace; in this context Deal (2006) introduced the term "aversive disablism."

Coping with Disability-Related Minority Stress

Following Goffman's classification, disabilities may be either discreditable or discrediting stigmata, depending upon the severity and nature of the disability and on the individual's response to it. This is true for both physical and mental disabilities. Directly correcting a disability might be possible only if it is curable or temporary, but mostly this is not possible. Indirectly, the stigma of disability can be corrected by devoting much effort to proving that the stereotypic ascriptions to disabled persons are false. The assumption of being less productive, for example, can be falsified by working even harder. That said, if one permanently has to work harder merely in order to prove a certain persistent stereotype to be wrong, and without receiving other kinds of additional resources that exceed the compensation any less hard working non-disabled colleagues receive, this might actually cause a strong feeling of unfair treatment. According to equity theory (Adams, 1965), this might increase one's minority stress and lead to ceasing working hard, or to other behavioral changes, in response to this perceived unfairness. Using a disability for "secondary gains" by using it as an excuse for a lack of success can be applied as well, but this, potentially, would contribute to stabilizing the stereotypic assumption, that the personal impairment exceeds the mere disability. As many disabilities are not visible to everyone, people can often choose whether to disclose their disability or not. Based on Goffman (1963), Holmes and River (1998) summarize the possibilities available to persons with mental illnesses for handling their discreditable stigma with "social withdrawal, secrecy, selective disclosure, indiscriminate disclosure, education, and social action (Goffman, 1963). Briefly, social withdrawal is a retreat from social interaction. Persons choose to avoid most people rather than risk being found out. Secrecy means individuals hide their mental illness from others. Indiscriminate disclosure implies 'coming out' about one's condition to most contacts. Selective disclosure involves coming out judiciously to specific individuals. Social action means lobbying for change in the treatment of persons with mental illness at the level of the individual, the community, or the government." These strategies can be applied at the workplace as well and they are transferable to physical disabilities that are not directly visible as well, such as for a positive HIV status, for cardiac conditions, or for diabetes (Fesko, 2001; Petrides et al., 1995). It can be assumed that the availability of more coping resources (because one is representing majority manifestations of other demographics), is related to more open coping mechanisms in terms of one's disability. It is very difficult to say what he best way of dealing with one's concealable disability in order to reduce one's stigma-related stress level to a minimum may be. It may be that the concealment of a disability from one's colleagues merely replaces one from of stress with another; the stress of having to maintain a false self-image merely supplants the stress that is due to the situation where colleagues cannot handle this new knowledge (von Schrader, Malzer, & Bruyère, 2013). This is especially often the case with mental disabilities (MacDonald-Wilson et al., 2011; Russinova, Griffin, Bloch, Wewiorski, & Rosoklija, 2011). The insecurity and discomfort felt by colleagues when approaching disabled persons might also negatively affect the disabled persons themselves, and increase their minority stress.

Intersections with Other Demographics

In terms of intersections with other demographics, disability status and frailty are often closely related to age, as, with aging, the level of disability rises in most cases (Gilleard & Higgs, 2011). As this interrelation potentially describes the future development of every individual, disabilities might be more acceptable at an older age than at a younger age. Nevertheless, even for older people their disability status can generate additional minority stress, as society favors an aging that masks all facets of weakness and dependency as long as possible (Overall, 2006). As with the intersection of the demographics of age and religion, so the intersection of disability and religion works in the same way. In a threefold way, religion can act as a stress deterrent or stress buffer for disabled people

(Siegel, Anderman, & Schrimshaw, 2001). Firstly, as a response to the destabilizing question "why me?" religions can offer explanation patterns for individual's disabilities that allow people to find some kind of sense or meaning in their disabilities. Such explanations can be a confiding "God has a reason" (Bulman & Wortman, 1977), or "God wants me to prove myself, and test my faith." Furthermore, disabilities can be interpreted as a divine punishment of personal misbehavior (Reinders, 2011), or as a "help" to focus one's attention on other, maybe more essential, things. These patterns help reduce the stigma-related stress that is potentially inherent in disabilities (Park, 2010). Secondly, a religious belief can enhance an individual's coping resources for handling their disability-related stress, as they allow the individual to keep "feelings of mastery or control and of self-worth" (Siegel et al., 2001, p. 641). Thirdly, religions can promote social integration and facilitate access to social support. Most religious communities offer a certain kind of social infrastructure, such as weekly groups or the organization of special events (Idler, 1987). Religious groups are often based on mutual responsibility and solidarity, and thus often have a broad supportive infrastructure (George, Ellison, & Larson, 2002). Support provided by the religious community broadens one's general coping resources and can range from support for grocery shopping to religious community hospitals.

Sexual Orientation

The sexual orientation of an individual is not a directly visible demographic. Thus, according to Goffman (1963), one's sexual orientation is a potentially discreditable stigma. In most societies homosexuality and bisexuality can still have an stigmatizing impact (Breen & Karpinski, 2013; Frost, 2011). Heterosexuality is usually normatively anticipated for every individual, and homosexuality, as a break with these expectations, is often deemed an "unnatural" deficiency (Herek, 2010). As in society as a whole, in the workplace co-workers and colleagues are also initially assumed to be heterosexual. Employees who do not meet that expectation are often confronted with different stigma-related stereotypes that can be the basis for certain barriers in the workplace (Croteau, 1996; Waldo, 1999). The intensity and shape of these stereotypes can differ across cultures, and, at least for Western societies, the stigmatizing effect of bisexuality and homosexuality is demonstrably shrinking in recent times (Keleher & Smith, 2012; McCormack, 2012). Nevertheless, these stereotypes do persist, even in Western countries. Furthermore, there are still many, many countries left where these stereotypes are the basis for politically and societally excluding practices for gays and lesbians, such as some Eastern European or African countries (Binnie & Klesse, 2013; Tamale, 2013).

One important field of stereotypes that works within organizations is related to the stereotypic shift of femininity and masculinity that is attached to homosexuality (Kite & Deaux, 1987). In this context, the tendency is often to attribute masculine characteristics to lesbians and feminine ones to gay men (Allen & Smith, 2011). As a result, organizational mechanisms of inclusion and exclusion that operate alongside the category of gender work also on the level of sexuality or sexual orientation (Bobbitt-Zeher, 2011; Reskin, 1993). Based on these stereotypes, creative competencies, or competencies that are presupposed to require a high degree of social skills are very often attributed to gay men. They are given less credit for having competencies in calculative and leading areas (cf. Madon, 1997; Sanchez & Vilain, 2012). The same mechanism leads to the attribution of certain stereotypic characteristics to lesbians that seemingly qualify them for work areas that would not be intended for heterosexual women (Peplau & Fingerhut, 2004). Another field of stereotypes is a latent over-sexualization of lesbians and gay men. In occupational life this reduction of homosexual employees to their sexuality often turns upon the fiction of asexuality as a crucial characteristic of a productive workplace (cf. Burrell, 1984; Rastetter, 1999). The high level of tabooing sexuality in the workplace and in economical practice (Riach & Wilson, 2007), combined with their over-sexualization, can lead to a latent resistance to assign those tasks to lesbians and gays that seemingly require a high degree of economic rationality (Giuffre, Dellinger, & Williams, 2008; Haddock, Zanna, & Esses, 1993). Besides these concrete attributions, more workplace-related barriers derive from the societal phenomenon of heterosexism that also operates on the organizational level. Heterosexism describes the societal tendency to generally attach a higher value to heterosexuality than, for example, to homosexuality. This devaluation of homosexuality (and furthermore of individuals that are perceived to be homosexual), often leads to specific discriminations that can be interpreted as expressions of this supposed inferiority (Swim, Pearson, & Johnston, 2007; Walls, 2008). For example, in application processes this can manifest itself in a lower probability for obviously homosexual applicants to be invited to an application talk compared to equally qualified, obviously heterosexual applicants (Adams, Cahill, & Ackerlind, 2005; Drydakis, 2011; Pichler, Varma, & Bruce, 2010; Tilcsik, 2011; Weichselbaumer, 2003). In the long run this can lead to lower occupational status attainments for lesbians and gay men (Ueno, Peña-Talamantes, & Roach, 2013). In the workplace discrimination can, for example, occur as an exclusion from the flow of information, as social isolation, or the permanent denial of promotions. Aggravated types of discrimination can extend to the threat or use of violence (Bilgehan Ozturk, 2011; Willis, 2012). Bisexual employees are additionally confronted with different layers of biphobia, a hostile attitude toward bisexual persons that occurs among heterosexual as well as homosexual people (Köllen, 2013).

Coping with "Sexual Orientation"-Related Minority Stress

As being homosexual or being bisexual are not a matter of choice or will (Horowitz & Newcomb, 2002; Reiter, 1989), one cannot directly change this potential stigma. Indirectly this stigma can be corrected by devoting much effort to counter-stereotypic behavior. Gay employees, for example, can try to show how tough they are, in order to prove the stereotype that gays are weak and less masculine wrong (Blashill & Powlishta, 2009). Using the stigma of homosexuality for secondary gains can be done by overemphasizing sexual orientation-related stereotypes that, in a positive way, can help the individual's career. Such examples can be the stereotype of gays as being creative (Madon, 1997) or lesbians as being tough and strong-willed (Eliason, Donelan, & Randall, 1992). Generally the invisibility of one's sexual orientation leaves open several options for dealing with one's homosexuality or bisexuality at work, such as the degree and type of openness one encounters in one's colleagues in everyday work life. On the other hand, the way of dealing with one's homosexuality is determined by the way stereotypic presuppositions are internalized (Chow & Cheng, 2010; Lingiardi, Baiocco, & Nardelli, 2012; Szymanski, Kashubeck, & Meyer, 2008) and integrated into one's self-image, and how they provide directions of action. The avoidance of any contact with "non-stigmatized" heterosexual persons to potentially avoid anticipated disrespect is a coping strategy that can be undertaken by a general social withdrawal in the workplace, or by choosing a workplace because it has a majority of gay or lesbian colleagues (Frohn, 2013). Equivalent to what is valid for concealable disabilities, it can be assumed that the availability of more coping resources (because one is representing majority manifestations of other demographics), is related to more open coping mechanisms in terms of one's homosexuality. It is difficult to estimate the effectiveness of a certain coping behavior, but several studies show that a more covert coping behavior carries the inherent danger of destabilizing the lesbian and gay individual (DeJordy, 2008) and harming his or her achievement potential

(Barreto, Ellemers, & Banal, 2006). Thus, it can be assumed that more open gays and lesbians have a higher amount of coping resources, stabilized through that openness itself.

Intersections with Other Demographics

One important intersection of the demographic of sexual orientation is this with religion: "Institutional religions derive much of their power from controlling and ordering human behavior. Sexual behaviors, in particular, are often the focus of intense attention because of their potential both to stabilize and to destabilize societies. Decisions about whom to have sex with, about the status of one's relationship to that person, and about specific sex acts are consequential ones" (Kalbian, 2013, p. 1). Against this background most religions and related ethnic communities do not accept homosexuality and bisexuality, especially male homo and bisexuality, or they make it at least a divisive issue (Hurteau, 2013). This might cause struggles in integrating sexual and ethnic or religious identities (Levy & Reeves, 2011) and it might negatively affect the individual's coping resources in terms of handling stigma-related minority stress deriving from one's homosexuality or bisexuality (Ganzevoort, van der Laan, & Olsman, 2010). In terms of gender, several studies show that boys and men have stronger homophobic attitudes than girls and women (Hooghe, Claes, Harell, Quintelier, & Dejaeghere, 2010). This is in line with findings that lesbian and gay employees experience more frequent and more intense discriminatory behavior from male than from female colleagues (Ragins & Cornwell, 2001). Thus, it might be assumed that working together with predominantly female colleagues constitutes a less stressful working atmosphere for gays and lesbians than working together with predominantly male colleagues. Furthermore, as homosexuality seems to challenge one's masculine identity more than it does one's feminine or female identity (Reese, Steffens, & Jonas, 2013), gay men who perceive their masculinity as an important element of their identity construction might struggle in reconciling their homosexuality and masculinity.

DEVELOPMENT OF AN INTERSECTIONAL FRAMEWORK

In summary it can be stated that for each demographic there is one manifestation that works as a dominant norm, and to other manifestations, that diverge from this norm, are attached – at least by trend – the image of deficiency. This is a societal phenomenon as well as a phenomenon that takes effect in the workplace. Gender aside, these ascribed values or hierarchical positionings of each manifestation, run parallel with their numerical appearance in societies, and subsequently at the workplace. Usually, the majority manifestations of demographics set the standard, bringing minority manifestations in marginalized positions. For Western societies, Table 1 gives an overview of the demographics considered in this chapter.

In Western societies, being white is still the racial manifestation that provokes the least pressure to have to justify itself in the workplace. At the same time, it is also the manifestation that occurs most often in these societies. When working in higher positions especially, this can pressurize non-white employees. As one's race can usually be identified by one's skin color, the direct visibility of one's race is very high. For those aging Western societies that, for the purpose of stabilizing their pension systems, are motivating people to retire later, one can hardly define "older" people as a minority in the workplace. Additionally, the seniority principle that requires a certain age for reaching higher positions is an important argument against this categorization of "older" employees as marginalized group. Furthermore, as noted above, the meaning and threshold of "being old" can differ between industries and societies. Nevertheless, the older one gets, the higher the pressure to show that one is still capable of those tasks related to the job, and the more intensely one is confronted with ageist behavior, especially when over pensionable age. Although there are certain medical or cosmetic possibilities available for retarding the visibility of one's age, all in all, age is a very visible demographic. As most Western societies are very achievement-oriented societies, to a certain extent they are also ableist. This places disabled persons in a deficient minority

Table 1. Dominant Manifestations and Minority Statuses of Demographics in Western Workplaces.

Demographic	Dominant Manifestation	Minority Status	Visibility
Gender	Male	–	
Race	White	Non-white	
Age	Young/middle aged	Older aged	
Disability status	Without disability	Mentally/physical disabled	
Nationality/ethnicity	Domestic	Non-domestic	
Religion	Majority religion	Minority religion	
Sexual orientation	Heterosexual	Homo-/bisexual	

position, in which there are huge differences between the different kinds of mental and physical disabilities. Some disabilities are directly visible, but there are many non-visible disabilities, that leave it open to the disabled person whether, and to whom, to disclose them. Nationality and ethnicity are much less visible on first appearance, but, as they are often related to different mother tongues, they are often assumed because of someone's accent or language. Most societies, and also their subsystems such as organizations, attach the highest value to their majority nationality or ethnicity. Very often, the "foreign" nationalities or ethnicities are valued considerably lower than the majority. Sometimes there are attributed hierarchies attached to an order of "foreign" nationalities or ethnicities that are due to perceived cultural distances or historical events and legends. Such constructions of specific pasts are important for the maintenance of a certain national or ethnical identity, and they often contain denigrations of other specific ethnicities or nationalities. Related processes of demarcation can also occur in workplaces and seriously narrow down career prospects for non-domestic employees. Although many Western societies are becoming more and more laicist and secular, Christian religions are frequently estimated as being more acceptable than other religions. Though one's religious belief is not per se a visible demographic, certain religious practices can make it visible in the workplace. These practices can range from wearing religious symbols, or rituals that have to be accomplished while at work, to certain kinds of dress. In the workplace, this can generate a certain pressure to justify themselves for employees of these religions. While in strongly laicist societies any kind of religious belief can provoke this pressure, in most Western societies this pressure only targets non-Christian minority religions. In terms of sexual orientation, a societal shift is observable toward a higher level of acceptance of homosexuality and bisexuality in most Western countries. Nevertheless, heterosexuality is still seen as the predominant standard which every individual is usually assumed to meet. Deviations from this are in a minority position that is still estimated to be deficient. As one's sexual orientation is an invisible demographic, gay, lesbian, and bisexual employees can chose, up to a point, to whom they disclose their sexuality, but the pressure remains to keep a consistent image of oneself in the workplace. This pressure can be an enormous source of minority stress.

Due to the fact that each demographic has a different degree of direct visibility, the possibilities of coping in the workplace with the stress deriving from minority manifestations of each demographic differ. All these coping strategies have in common that they need coping resources, as coping always means intentionally setting certain actions. Employees do not have to concern themselves about how to handle their majority manifestations in everyday work, as these manifestations bring them into an advantageous position anyhow. This allows them a certain kind of "thoughtlessness" about these issues, although this "thoughtlessness" can include the marginalization of minorities. In contrast, employees do have to actively concern themselves about their minority manifestations, as they bear the inherent danger – beside concrete discriminatory issues related to individuals' careers – of destabilizing and harming their psychological condition, and thus minority-related marginalization experiences can have a negative impact that goes beyond the workplace. Fig. 1 shows the interrelation of demographic minority statuses, coping resources and coping strategies. As some demographics leave open the possibility of gradual disclosure, disclosure status is a mediating parameter between coping resources and coping strategy or coping behavior.

The bottom of Fig. 1 visualizes the different demographics considered for this model. Each of them can be equally relevant to an individual's experiences and behavior in the workplace, because each of them provides manifestations that attach minority statuses to the employees representing one of these manifestations. As every employee represents manifestations

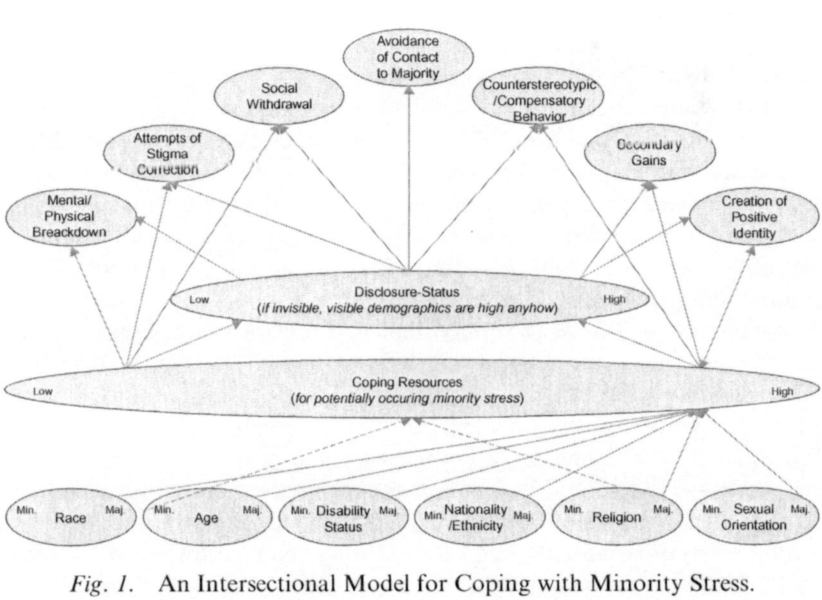

Fig. 1. An Intersectional Model for Coping with Minority Stress.

of every demographic, employees can accumulate minority statuses. As already discussed above, in the workplace one's minority status is often connected with different types and intensities of marginalization. For proactively handling this marginalization, individuals need coping resources. Having a majority status can help to augment these resources, as majority manifestations are not usually under pressure to have to justify themselves, and therefore they support an individual's self-esteem and perception of having control of their workplace situation. Thus majority statuses in one or more demographic can provide coping resources for handling minority statuses in one or more other demographics. The age of older employees can affect their coping resources in two directions. On the one hand, several studies show that being old can often be associated with becoming more stable and having greater equanimity (e.g., Brose, Scheibe, & Schmiedek, 2013), and thus this can affect one's coping resources in a positive way. On the other hand being older also involves the danger of being confronted with ageist behavior in the workplace, and thus potentially having a weakening impact. Religion is the second demographic that can impact one's coping resources in a twofold way: having a religious faith usually provides individuals with a strong worldview and a strong pattern of interpreting everyday issues that affect one's life (Moreira-Almeida, Lotufo Neto, & Koenig, 2006). For employees this can be a very stabilizing factor that enhances their coping resources for handling minority stress situations. But, since religions can also have the status of a minority or a majority religion in one's workplace settings, religion can also be a demographic that generates minority stress or majority support.

Table 1 illustrates that different demographics themselves have different degrees of direct visibility. Thus, the disclosure status in terms of one's minority status is an important parameter for some demographics. This disclosure status is never a fixed event, as it can vary amongst colleagues and also vary over time. Telling some colleagues about one's depression, for example, does not mean that everybody is aware of it, nor does it necessarily mean that in future the individual will tell more, or new, colleagues. Nevertheless, having disclosed a minority status – as well as having a visible minority status – one has exposed oneself to a potentially marginalizing treatment from those colleagues that are aware, or able to perceive it. However, it also opens up an opportunity to experience support or at least reactions considerably less negative than were anticipated. Whatever the case, disclosing one's invisible, potentially stigmatizing minority status to others requires, at the time of disclosing, coping resources, if only to handle anticipated negative reactions as they might be foreseen in a possible worst-case scenario. Thus, a high level of coping resources and a high degree of disclosure can be positively interrelated, as well as a low level of coping resources and a low level of disclosure. In terms of coping strategies – or stigma management strategies (Goffman, 1963) – the causalities between the different strategies and visible minority statuses is akin to those between the different strategies and disclosed minority statuses. The creation or maintenance of a positive minority identity requires a high level of coping resources, and it can also enhance one's coping resources. Furthermore, it can support a positive self-image, if invisible demographics are disclosed. Earning secondary gains from a minority status, for example, by building on useful stereotypes, or by emphasizing one's minority status to excuse other things, is only possible if the status is disclosed or visible. The same is true for the strategy of applying counter-stereotypic or compensatory behavior. This strategy also requires a high level of coping resources. If employees applying this strategy have more than one minority status they might struggle in reconciling different counter-stereotypes and maintaining a consistent image. If one has only a low level of coping resources, a possible strategy is to try to avoid contacts with non-stigmatized majority group members. In doing so, one can try to avoid anticipated marginalization because of one's minority status. This strategy becomes harder the more minority statuses someone combines, as the amount of possible colleagues that fit into one's demographic pattern will shrink. This can be "solved" by a general social withdrawal. By trying to minimize contact to others, one can also minimize potential marginalization experiences in everyday workplace encounters. A strategy that is not limited to the workplace is to try to change or to "correct" one's stigmatizing minority status. Formally this is possible for only a few demographics (religion and nationality), but in practice, even for these demographics it is hard to "convince" one's environment that one has really renounced the former minority status. A consequence rather than a strategy can be the result of low coping resources and a related low level of disclosure about one's invisible minority statuses: a mental and physical breakdown. This can be due to the stress related to the maintenance of a disclosure status as well as to the permanent experience of stigma-based discriminatory events.

CONCLUSION, DISCUSSION, AND OUTLOOK

The major contribution of the intersectional model proposed in this chapter is to broaden the perspective on minorities and related minority stress in the workplace. By bringing together the demographics age, nationality, ethnicity, race, sexual orientation, disability status, and religion, it is apparent that coping with minority stress because of one demographic has to be seen and interpreted in relation to the other demographics as well. By considering one's coping resources for minority stress as pooled resources that can provide the energy for coping with minority stress in terms of any demographic, it becomes obvious that coping with single minority statuses cannot be understood in isolation. Every employee simultaneously embodies manifestations of any demographic that attach to him or her different minority and majority statuses. As these statuses are often related to organizational hierarchies, employees very often simultaneously hold positions of dominance and subordination (Talwar, 2010; Weber, 2001). Thus, an individual's coping strategies or coping behavior within organizational processes of hierarchization, marginalization, and discrimination are very often simultaneous coping in terms of more than one demographic. Furthermore, since minority and majority constellations can change between different workplace settings, different demographics can gain different degrees of relevance in different settings and situations. Nevertheless, every demographic always has the potential to become the crucial demographic for allocating relevant minority and majority statuses. Depending on the manifestations of other demographics one has, this can mean different levels of coping resources available for coping with potential minority stress. This can limit or broaden one's coping opportunities and thus the manifestation of one demographic can determine the coping behavior one applies, because of the minority status of another demographic. Depending on the type of demographic, this coping behavior can include disclosure decisions about invisible demographics.

Future research could empirically test parts of the model in different contexts or conceptually extend it. It would be interesting to add a cultural component to this model that might reflect the ways in which different demographics gain different degrees of importance in different cultural contexts. As gender is not considered in this model it would also be interesting to find a way of integrating it; for example, by not building on minority stress, but on something adequate that makes its inclusion possible. Furthermore, although the six demographics considered in this model are the most popular demographics in organizational research, many more relevant demographics could be envisaged for an extension of this model, such as family background, education or physical attractiveness. As this chapter focuses on minority stress, future research could also try to gain a deeper understanding of potential elements of "majority stress" and its interrelation with "minority stress." It might be that insecurity about how to treat or to approach minorities can provoke stress for the majorities. If an individual is confronted with a transsexual person, a person with depression or any other minority for the first time, that individual might be unsure about how to act without seeming impolite, curious, or stigmatizing. This insecurity might create an uncomfortable atmosphere between minorities and majorities, and the majority stress might react upon the minorities and may increase their stress level. Future research on this potential reciprocal stress alongside the different demographics might allow an extension of the proposed model.

Another connecting point for future research is deepening the insight into the potential certain demographics might have to enhance one's coping resources of their own accord. In the model or the framework proposed, religion and age are pointed out as just such demographics, as having a religion as well as being older can provide higher coping resources. In the case of religion, these coping resources derive from the strength an individual can gain from the fact that religions usually seek to provide explanations, and make minority stress situations explainable and sometimes even meaningful to the religious individual. Furthermore, the strong communities that are often based on a common religious belief can provide coping resources by providing social support and a stable platform where one is definitively not in a minority position because of one's religion. However, both factors can vary between individuals. The degree one believes in the whole religious explanatory model in terms of the world and life in general, as well as the degree to which one is attached and committed to the religious community might differ between individuals. Thus, the coping resources one receives from one's religious belief might also differ. Future research can try to understand these interrelations more deeply in order to extend the proposed model in an important way. The same applies to age. The line of argumentation as to why older people might have a higher level of coping resources reasons that, due to their life experience, they are able to confront stressful situations more calmly. As individual biographies differ, so the experiences of minority stress and the experiences of having handled and "survived" these situations will differ. Thus, on the individual level, there might be big differences as to what extent these life experiences really work in stabilizing when being confronted with such situations again. Future research could target these issues and try to understand the influence of individual and biographical components for the level of individual's coping resources.

Future research could also focus on the contribution employers and organizations themselves could make to enhance employees' coping resources. Under the aegis of diversity management strategies, especially, it might be asked to what extent a one-dimensional approach that only focuses on single dimensions of employee diversity, mostly gender and race, should be replaced by more comprehensive approaches. As the model suggests, employees' coping behavior with, for example, racial minority stress is also influenced by their other demographics. Thus targeting the dimensions of, for example, religion and sexual orientation might also strengthen employees for coping with minority statuses beyond religion and sexual orientation.

REFERENCES

Acker, J. (2006). Inequality regimes: Gender, class, and race in organizations. *Gender & Society*, *20*(4), 441–464.

Adams, E. M., Cahill, B. J., & Ackerlind, S. J. (2005). A qualitative study of Latino lesbian and gay youths' experiences with discrimination and the career development process. *Journal of Vocational Behavior*, *66*(2), 199–218.

Adams, J. S. (1965). Inequity in social exchange. In L. Berkowitz (Ed.), *Advances in experimental social psychology* (Vol. 2, pp. 267–299). New York, NY: Academic Press.

Allen, J., & Smith, J. L. (2011). The influence of sexuality stereotypes on men's experience of gender-role incongruence. *Psychology of Men & Masculinity*, *12*(1), 77–96.

Allen, S. (1998). Identity: Feminist perspectives on "race," ethnicity and nationality. In N. Charles & H. Hintjens (Eds.), *Gender, ethnicity and political ideologies* (pp. 46–67). New York, NY: Routledge.

Amrhein, L. (2013). Die soziale Konstruktion von "Hochaltrigkeit" in einer jungen Altersgesellschaft. *Zeitschrift fur Gerontologie und Geriatrie*, *46*(1), 10–15.

Anderton, C. L., Pender, D. A., & Asner-Self, K. K. (2011). A review of the religious identity/sexual orientation identity conflict literature: Revisiting Festinger's cognitive dissonance theory. *Journal of LGBT Issues in Counseling*, *5*(3–4), 259–281.

Barnes, D. M., & Meyer, I. H. (2012). Religious affiliation, internalized homophobia, and mental health in lesbians, gay men, and bisexuals. *American Journal of Orthopsychiatry*, *82*(4), 505–515.

Barreto, M., Ellemers, N., & Banal, S. (2006). Working under cover: Performance-related self-confidence among members of contextually devalued groups who try to pass. *European Journal of Social Psychology*, *36*(3), 337–352.

Basford, T. E., Offermann, L. R., & Behrend, T. S. (in press). Do you see what I see? Perceptions of gender microaggressions in the workplace. *Psychology of Women Quarterly*.

Baumann, M. (2000). Diaspora: Genealogies of semantics and transcultural comparison. *Numen*, *47*(3), 313–337.

Berry, J. W. (1970). Marginality, stress and ethnic identification in an acculturated aboriginal community. *Journal of Cross-Cultural Psychology*, *1*, 239–252.

Berry, J. W. (2006). Acculturative stress. In P. T. P. Wong & L. C. J. Wong (Eds.), *Handbook of multicultural perspectives on stress and coping* (pp. 287–298). New York, NY: Springer.

Bezborodovs, N., & Thornicroft, G. (2013). Stigmatisation of mental illness in the workplace: Evidence and consequences. *Die Psychiatrie*, *10*, 102–107.

Biggs, S., & Haapala, I. (2013). Elder mistreatment, ageism, and human rights. *International Psychogeriatrics*, *25*(8), 1299–1306.

Bilgehan Ozturk, M. (2011). Sexual orientation discrimination: Exploring the experiences of lesbian, gay and bisexual employees in Turkey. *Human Relations*, *64*(8), 1099–1118.

Binnie, J., & Klesse, C. (2013). Like a bomb in the gasoline station: East–West migration and transnational activism around lesbian, gay, bisexual, transgender and queer politics in Poland. *Journal of Ethnic and Migration Studies*, *39*(7), 1107–1124.

Blanchard-Fields, F. (2007). Everyday problem solving and emotion: An adult developmental perspective. *Current Directions in Psychological Science*, *16*(1), 26–31.

Blashill, A., & Powlishta, K. (2009). Gay stereotypes: The use of sexual orientation as a cue for gender-related attributes. *Sex Roles*, *61*(11–12), 783–793.

Bobbitt-Zeher, D. (2011). Gender discrimination at work: Connecting gender stereotypes, institutional policies, and gender composition of workplace. *Gender & Society*, *25*(6), 764–786.

Bordieri, J. E., & Drehmer, D. E. (1986). Hiring decisions for disabled workers: Looking at the cause. *Journal of Applied Social Psychology*, *16*(3), 197–208.

Bowleg, L., Huang, J., Brooks, K., Black, A., & Burkholder, G. (2003). Triple Jeopardy and beyond: Multiple minority stress and resilience among black lesbians. *Journal of Lesbian Studies*, *7*(4), 87–108.

Bozard, R. L., & Sanders, C. J. (2011). Helping Christian lesbian, gay, and bisexual clients recover religion as a source of strength: Developing a model for assessment and integration of religious identity in counseling. *Journal of LGBT Issues in Counseling*, *5*(1), 47–74.

Braddock, D., & Bachelder, L. (1994). *The glass ceiling and persons with disabilities*. Washington, DC: Glass Ceiling Commission, U.S. Department of Labor.

Brah, A., & Phoenix, A. (2004). Ain't I a woman? Revisiting intersectionality. *Journal of International Women's Studies*, *5*(3), 75–86.

Brandt, P.-Y. (2013). Psychological aspects of the role of religion in identity construction. *Integrative Psychological and Behavioral Science*, *47*(2), 299–303.

Branine, M., & Glover, I. (1997). Ageism in work and employment: Thinking about connections. *Personnel Review*, *26*(4), 233–244.

Breen, A. B., & Karpinski, A. (2013). Implicit and explicit attitudes toward gay males and lesbians among heterosexual males and females. *The Journal of Social Psychology*, *153*(3), 351–374.

Bricout, J. C., & Bentley, K. J. (2000). Disability status and perceptions of employability by employers. *Social Work Research*, *24*(2), 87–95.

Brooke, L., & Taylor, P. (2005). Older workers and employment: Managing age relations. *Ageing & Society*, *25*(03), 415–429.

Brooks, V. R. (1981). *Minority stress and lesbian women*. Lanham, MD: Lexington Books.

Brose, A., Scheibe, S., & Schmiedek, F. (2013). Life contexts make a difference: Emotional stability in younger and older adults. *Psychology and Aging*, *28*(1), 148–159.

Brubaker, R. (2009). Ethnicity, race, and nationalism. *Annual Review of Sociology*, *35*(1), 21–42.

Bruinessen, M. V. (1998). Shifting national and ethnic identities: The Kurds in Turkey and the European diaspora. *Journal of Muslim Minority Affairs*, *18*(1), 39–52.

Buba, H. P., & Vaskovics, L. A. (2001). *Benachteiligung gleichgeschlechtlich orientierter Personen und Paare*. Köln, Germany: Bundesanzeiger Verlags.m.b.H.

Bulman, R. J., & Wortman, C. B. (1977). Attributions of blame and coping in the "real world": Severe accident victims react to their lot. *Journal of Personality and Social Psychology*, *35*(5), 351–363.

Burrell, G. (1984). Sex and organizational analysis. *Organization Studies*, *5*(2), 97.

Bygren, M. (2013). Unpacking the causes of segregation across workplaces. *Acta Sociologica*, *56*(1), 3–19.

Cameron, C. (2001). Promise or problem? A review of the literature on men working in early childhood services. *Gender, Work & Organization*, *8*(4), 430–453.

Campbell, F. A. K. (2008). Exploring internalized ableism using critical race theory. *Disability & Society*, *23*(2), 151–162.

Caplan, G. (1981). Mastery of stress: Psychosocial aspects. *The American Journal of Psychiatry*, *138*(4), 413–420.

Chamberlain, K., & Zika, S. (1988). Religiosity, life meaning and wellbeing: Some relationships in a sample of women. *Journal for the Scientific Study of Religion*, *27*(3), 411–420.

Cheryan, S., & Bodenhausen, G. V. (2000). When positive stereotypes threaten intellectual performance: The psychological hazards of "model minority" status. *Psychological Science*, *11*(5), 399–402.

Chow, P. K. Y., & Cheng, S. T. (2010). Shame, internalized heterosexism, lesbian identity, and coming out to others: A comparative study of lesbians in Mainland China and Hong Kong. *Journal of Counseling Psychology*, *57*(1), 92–104.

Cocchiara, F. K., & Quick, J. C. (2004). The negative effects of positive stereotypes: Ethnicity-related stressors and implications on organizational health. *Journal of Organizational Behavior*, *25*(6), 781–785.

Colella, A., DeNisi, A. S., & Varma, A. (1998). The impact of ratee's disability on performance judgments and choice as partner: The role of disability–job fit stereotypes and interdependence of rewards. *Journal of Applied Psychology*, *83*(1), 102–111.

Collins, P. H. (1993). Toward a new vision: Race, class, and gender as categories of analysis and connection. *Race, Sex & Class*, *1*(1), 25–45.

Connor, W. (1990). When is a nation? *Ethnic and Racial Studies*, *13*(1), 92–103.

Coston, B. M., & Kimmel, M. (2012). Seeing privilege where it isn't: Marginalized masculinities and the intersectionality of privilege. *Journal of Social Issues*, *68*(1), 97–111.

Crenshaw, K. (1991). Mapping the margins: Intersectionality, identity politics, and violence against women of color. *Stanford Law Review*, *43*(6), 1241–1299.

Crocker, J., & Major, B. (1989). Social stigma and self-esteem: The self-protective properties of stigma. *Psychological Review*, *96*(4), 608–630.

Croteau, J. M. (1996). Research on the work experiences of lesbian, gay, and bisexual people: An integrative review of methodology and findings. *Journal of Vocational Behavior*, *48*(2), 195–209.

Cuéllar, I. (2000). Acculturation and mental health: Ecological transactional relations of adjustment. In I. Cuéllar & F. A. Paniagua (Eds.), *Handbook of multicultural mental health: Assessment and treatment of diverse populations* (pp. 45–62). San Diego, CA: Academic Press.

Deal, M. (2006). Aversive disablism: Subtle prejudice toward disabled people. *Disability & Society*, *22*(1), 93–107.

DeJordy, R. (2008). Just passing through: Stigma, passing, and identity decoupling in the work place. *Group & Organization Management*, *33*(5), 504–531.
Dennis, H., & Thomas, K. (2007). Ageism in the workplace. *Generations*, *31*(1), 84–89.
Desmette, D., & Gaillard, M. (2008). When a "worker" becomes an "older worker": The effects of age-related social identity on attitudes towards retirement and work. *The Career Development International*, *13*(2), 168–185.
DeVos, G. A. (1980). Ethnic adaptation and minority status. *Journal of Cross-Cultural Psychology*, *11*(1), 101–124.
Dhruvarajan, V. (1988). Religious ideology and interpersonal relationships within the family. *Journal of Comparative Family Studies*, *19*, 273–285.
DiPlacido, J. (1998). Minority stress among lesbians, gay men, and bisexuals: A consequence of heterosexism, homophobia, and stigmatization. In G. M. Herek (Ed.), *Stigma and sexual orientation: Understanding prejudice against lesbians, gay men, and bisexuals* (pp. 138–159). Thousand Oaks, CA: Sage Publications.
Drapalski, A. L., Lucksted, A., Perrin, P. B., Aakre, J. M., Brown, C. H., DeForge, B. R., & Boyd, J. E. (2013). A model of internalized stigma and its effects on people with mental illness. *Psychiatric Services*, *64*(3), 264–269.
Drydakis, N. (2011). Women's sexual orientation and labor market outcomes in Greece. *Feminist Economics*, *17*(1), 89–117.
Dunn, K., Loosemore, M., Phua, F., & Ozguc, U. (2011). Everyday ethnic diversity and racism on Australian construction sites. *International Journal of Diversity in Organisations, Communities & Nations*, *10*(6), 129–147.
Eichhorn, J. (2012). Happiness for believers? Contextualizing the effects of religiosity on life-satisfaction. *European Sociological Review*, *28*(5), 583–593.
Eliason, M., Donelan, C., & Randall, C. (1992). Lesbian stereotypes. *Health Care for Women International*, *13*(2), 131–144.
Ferrall, C. (1997). Empirical analysis of occupational hierarchies. *The Journal of Human Resources*, *32*(1), 1–34.
Ferriss, A. L. (2002). Religion and the quality of life. *Journal of Happiness Studies*, *3*(3), 199–215.
Fesko, S. L. (2001). Disclosure of HIV status in the workplace: Considerations and strategies. *Health & Social Work*, *26*(4), 235–244.
Fox, J. (2000). Religious causes of discrimination against ethno-religious minorities. *International Studies Quarterly*, *44*(3), 423–450.
Fox, S., & Giles, H. (1993). Accommodating intergenerational contact: A critique and theoretical model. *Journal of Aging Studies*, *7*(4), 423–451.
Fried, Y., Grant, A. M., Levi, A. S., Hadani, M., & Slowik, L. H. (2007). Job design in temporal context: A career dynamics perspective. *Journal of Organizational Behavior*, *28*(7), 911–927.
Frohn, D. J. T. (2013). Subjective theories of lesbian, gay, bisexual, and transsexual employees concerning how they deal with their sexual or gender identity in the workplace – An exploratory qualitative study. *Forum: Qualitative Social Research*, *14*(3), 1–82.
Frost, D. M. (2011). Social stigma and its consequences for the socially stigmatized. *Social and Personality Psychology Compass*, *5*(11), 824–839.
Ganzevoort, R. R., van der Laan, M., & Olsman, E. (2010). Growing up gay and religious. Conflict, dialogue, and religious identity strategies. *Mental Health, Religion & Culture*, *14*(3), 209–222.

Garber, M. B. (2013). The intersection of spiritual, sexual, and national identity: A qualitative study of mature Dutch women. *Journal of Religion, Spirituality & Aging*, *25*(2), 177–204.

George, L. K., Ellison, C. G., & Larson, D. B. (2002). Explaining the relationships between religious involvement and health. *Psychological Inquiry*, *13*(3), 190–200.

Ghumman, S., Ryan, A., Barclay, L., & Markel, K. (2013). Religious discrimination in the workplace: A review and examination of current and future trends. *Journal of Business and Psychology*, *28*(4), 439–454.

Gilleard, C., & Higgs, P. (2011). Frailty, disability and old age: A re-appraisal. *Health: An Interdisciplinary Journal for the Social Study of Health, Illness and Medicine*, *15*(5), 475–490.

Ginicola, M. M., & Smith, C. (2011). The church, the closet, and the couch: The counselor's role in assisting clients to integrate their sexual orientation and religious identity. *Journal of LGBT Issues in Counseling*, *5*(3–4), 304–326.

Giuffre, P., Dellinger, K., & Williams, C. L. (2008). No retribution for being gay?: Inequality in gay-friendly workplaces. *Sociological Spectrum*, *28*(3), 254–277.

Glick, P., & Fiske, S. T. (2001). Ambivalent stereotypes as legitimizing ideologies: Differentiating paternalistic and envious prejudice. In J. T. Jost & B. Major (Eds.), *The psychology of legitimacy: Emerging perspectives on ideology, justice, and intergroup relations* (pp. 278–306). New York, NY: Cambridge University Press.

Goffman, E. (1963). *Stigma: Notes on the management of spoiled identity*. Englewood Cliffs, NJ: Prentice-Hall.

Grossmann, I., Na, J., Varnum, M. E. W., Park, D. C., Kitayama, S., & Nisbett, R. E. (2010). Reasoning about social conflicts improves into old age. *Proceedings of the National Academy of Sciences*, *107*(16), 1–5.

Haddock, G., Zanna, M. P., & Esses, V. M. (1993). Assessing the structure of prejudicial attitudes – The case of attitudes toward homosexuals. *Journal of Personality and Social Psychology*, *65*(6), 1105–1118.

Hanappi-Egger, E. (2013). Backstage: The organizational gendered agenda in science, engineering and technology professions. *European Journal of Women's Studies*, *20*(3), 279–294.

Herek, G. M. (2010). Sexual orientation differences as deficits: Science and stigma in the history of American psychology. *Perspectives on Psychological Science*, *5*(6), 693–699.

Hernandez, B. (2000). Employer attitudes toward workers with disabilities and their ADA employment rights: A literature review. *Journal of Rehabilitation*, *66*(4), 4–16.

Hershey, D. A., & Henkens, K. (2014). Impact of different types of retirement transitions on perceived satisfaction with life. *The Gerontologist*, *54*(2), 232–244.

Hodson, D. S., & Skeen, P. (1994). Sexuality and aging: The hammerlock of myths. *Journal of Applied Gerontology*, *13*(3), 219–235.

Holmes, E. P., & River, L. P. (1998). Individual strategies for coping with the stigma of severe mental illness. *Cognitive and Behavioral Practice*, *5*(2), 231–239.

Holvino, E. (2010). Intersections: The simultaneity of race, gender and class in organization studies. *Gender, Work & Organization*, *17*(3), 248–277.

Hooghe, M., Claes, E., Harell, A., Quintelier, E., & Dejaeghere, Y. (2010). Anti-gay sentiment among adolescents in Belgium and Canada: A comparative investigation into the role of gender and religion. *Journal of Homosexuality*, *57*(3), 384–400.

Horowitz, J. L., & Newcomb, M. D. (2002). A multidimensional approach to homosexual identity. *Journal of Homosexuality*, *42*(2), 1–19.

Hotchkiss, J. L. (2004). A closer look at the employment impact of the Americans with disabilities act. *Journal of Human Resources*, *39*(4), 887–911.

Huang, C.-C., & Kleiner, B. H. (2001). New developments concerning religious discrimination in the workplace. *International Journal of Sociology and Social Policy*, *21*(8/9/10), 128–136.

Hunsberger, B. (1985). Religion, age, life satisfaction, and perceived sources of religiousness: A study of older persons. *Journal of Gerontology*, *40*(5), 615–620.

Hurteau, P. (2013). *Male homosexualities and world religions*. Basingstoke, UK: Palgrave Macmillan.

Hutchinson, J. (2000). Ethnicity and modern nations. *Ethnic and Racial Studies*, *23*(4), 651–669.

Idler, E. L. (1987). Religious involvement and the health of the elderly: Some hypotheses and an initial test. *Social Forces*, *66*(1), 226–238.

Iweins, C., Desmette, D., Yzerbyt, V., & Stinglhamber, F. (2013). Ageism at work: The impact of intergenerational contact and organizational multi-age perspective. *European Journal of Work and Organizational Psychology*, *22*(3), 331–346.

Jordan-Zachery, J. S. (2007). Am I a black woman or a woman who is black? A few thoughts on the meaning of intersectionality. *Politics & Gender*, *3*(02), 254–263.

Juergensmeyer, M. (1994). *The new cold war? Religious nationalism confronts the secular state*. Berkeley, CA: University of California Press.

Kalbian, A. H. (2013). Sexuality in religions. *International Encyclopedia of Ethics*. Oxford: Blackwell Publishing Ltd.

Kamenou, N., & Fearfull, A. (2006). Ethnic minority women: A lost voice in HRM. *Human Resource Management Journal*, *16*(2), 154–172.

Kaye, H. S., Jans, L., & Jones, E. (2011). Why don't employers hire and retain workers with disabilities? *Journal of Occupational Rehabilitation*, *21*(4), 526–536.

Keleher, A., & Smith, E. R. A. N. (2012). Growing support for gay and lesbian equality since 1990. *Journal of Homosexuality*, *59*(9), 1307–1326.

Kertzner, R. M., Meyer, I. H., Frost, D. M., & Stirratt, M. J. (2009). Social and psychological well-being in lesbians, gay men, and bisexuals: The effects of race, gender, age, and sexual identity. *American Journal of Orthopsychiatry*, *79*(4), 500–510.

Kimmel, S. B., & Mahalik, J. R. (2005). Body image concerns of gay men: The roles of minority stress and conformity to masculine norms. *Journal of Consulting and Clinical Psychology*, *73*(6), 1185–1190.

Kite, M. E., & Deaux, K. (1987). Gender belief systems: Homosexuality and the implicit inversion theory. *Psychology of Women Quarterly*, *11*(1), 83–96.

Knapp, G.-A. (2005). Race, class, gender: Reclaiming baggage in fast travelling theories. *European Journal of Women's Studies*, *12*(3), 249–265.

Koenig, H. G., Kvale, J. N., & Ferrel, C. (1988). Religion and well-being in later life. *The Gerontologist*, *28*(1), 18–28.

Köllen, T. (2012). European disintegration: Tendencies of renationalization within the European union and its impact on the common labor market and EU consumer markets. *The International Journal of Diversity in Organizations, Communities, and Nations*, *11*(5), 117–138.

Köllen, T. (2013). Bisexuality and diversity management – Addressing the B in LGBT as a relevant "sexual orientation" in the workplace. *Journal of Bisexuality*, *13*(1), 122–137.

Kregel, J., & Unger, D. (1993). Employer perceptions of the work potential of individuals with disabilities: An illustration from supported employment. *Journal of Vocational Rehabilitation*, *3*(4), 17–25.

Krook, M. L., & O'Brien, D. Z. (2010). The politics of group representation: Quotas for women and minorities worldwide. *Comparative Politics*, *42*(3), 253–272.

Krupa, T., Kirsh, B., Cockburn, L., & Gewurtz, R. (2009). Understanding the stigma of mental illness in employment. *Work*, *33*(4), 413–425.

Kubicek, K., McDavitt, B., Carpineto, J., Weiss, G., Iverson, E. F., & Kipke, M. D. (2009). God made me gay for a reason: Young men who have sex with men's resiliency in resolving internalized homophobia from religious sources. *Journal of Adolescent Research*, 24(5), 601–633.

Levy, D. L., & Reeves, P. (2011). Resolving identity conflict: Gay, lesbian, and queer individuals with a Christian upbringing. *Journal of Gay & Lesbian Social Services*, *23*(1), 53–68.

Lewis, C. A., & Cruise, S. M. (2006). Religion and happiness: Consensus, contradictions, comments and concerns. *Mental Health, Religion & Culture*, *9*(3), 213–225.

Lim, C., & Putnam, R. D. (2010). Religion, social networks, and life satisfaction. *American Sociological Review*, *75*(6), 914–933.

Lingiardi, V., Baiocco, R., & Nardelli, N. (2012). Measure of internalized sexual stigma for lesbians and gay men: A new scale. *Journal of Homosexuality*, *59*(8), 1191–1210.

Lofland, J., & Skonovd, N. (1981). Conversion motifs. *Journal for the Scientific Study of Religion*, *20*(4), 373–385.

Louvet, E. (2007). Social judgment toward job applicants with disabilities: Perception of personal qualities and competences. *Rehabilitation Psychology*, *52*(3), 297–303.

Louvet, E., Rohmer, O., & Dubois, N. (2009). Social judgment of people with a disability in the workplace: *How to make a good impression on employers*, *68*, 153–159.

MacDonald-Wilson, K. L., Russinova, Z., Rogers, E. S., Lin, C. H., Ferguson, T., Dong, S., & MacDonald, M. K. (2011). Disclosure of mental health disabilities in the workplace. In I. Z. Schultz & E. S. Rogers (Eds.), *Work accommodation and retention in mental health* (pp. 191–217). New York, NY: Springer.

Madon, S. (1997). What do people believe about gay males? A study of stereotype content and strength. *Sex Roles*, *37*(9–10), 663–685.

Mahony, P., & Zmroczek, C. (1997). *Class matters: "Working Class" women's perspectives on social class*. Oxford: Taylor & Francis.

Major, B., & O'Brien, L. T. (2005). *The social psychology of stigma annual review of psychology* (Vol. 56, pp. 393–421). Palo Alto, CA: Annual Reviews.

Martens, A., Greenberg, J., Schimel, J., & Landau, M. J. (2004). Ageism and death: Effects of mortality salience and perceived similarity to elders on reactions to elderly people. *Personality and Social Psychology Bulletin*, *30*(12), 1524–1536.

Marty, M. E., & Appleby, R. S. (1997). *Religion, ethnicity, and self-identity: Nations in turmoil*. Lebanon, NH: University Press of New England.

Maschke, M. (2008). *Behindertenpolitik In der Europäischen Union: Lebenssituation behinderter Menschen und nationale Behindertenpolitik in 15 Mitgliedstaaten*. Wiesbaden, Germany: VS Verlag.

McCormack, M. (2012). *The declining significance of homophobia: How teenage boys are redefining masculinity and heterosexuality*. New York, NY: Oxford University Press.

McDonald, M. L., & Westphal, J. D. (2013). Access denied: Low mentoring of women and minority first-time directors and its negative effects on appointments to additional boards. *Academy of Management Journal*, *56*(4), 1169–1198.

Meares, M. M., Oetzel, J. G., Torres, A., Derkacs, D., & Ginossar, T. (2004). Employee mistreatment and muted voices in the culturally diverse workplace. *Journal of Applied Communication Research*, *32*(1), 4–27.

Meyer, I. H. (1995). Minority stress and mental health in gay men. *Journal of Health and Social Behavior*, *36*(1), 38–56.

Miller, P., Parker, S., & Gillinson, S. (2004). *Disablism: How to tackle the last prejudice*. London, UK: Demos.

Miner-Rubino, K., & Cortina, L. M. (2004). Working in a context of hostility toward women: Implications for employees' well-being. *Journal of Occupational Health Psychology*, *9*(2), 107–122.

Mohanty, C. T. (1988). Under western eyes: Feminist scholarship and colonial discourses. *Feminist Review*, *30*(3), 61–88.

Moreira-Almeida, A., Lotufo Neto, F., & Koenig, H. G. (2006). Religiousness and mental health: A review. *Revista Brasileira de Psiquiatria*, *28*, 242–250.

Mumby, D. K., & Stohl, C. (1991). Power and discourse in organization studies: Absence and the dialectic of control. *Discourse & Society*, *2*(3), 313–332.

Nagel, J. (1994). Constructing ethnicity: Creating and recreating ethnic identity and culture. *Social Problems*, *41*(1), 152–176.

Nagel, J. (2000). Ethnicity and sexuality. *Annual Review of Sociology*, *26*(1), 107–133.

Negrini, A., Panari, C., Simbula, S., & Alcover, C. M. (2013). The push and pull factors related to early retirees' mental health status: A comparative study between Italy and Spain. *Revista de Psicologia del Trabajo y de Las Organizaciones*, *29*(2), 51–58.

Nelson, T. D. (2002). *Ageism: Stereotyping and prejudice against older persons*. Cambridge, MA: MIT Press.

Nelson, T. D. (2005). Ageism: Prejudice against our feared future self. *Journal of Social Issues*, *61*(2), 207–221.

Nordberg, M. (2002). Constructing masculinity in women's worlds: Men working as preschool teachers and hairdressers. *NORA: Nordic Journal of Women's Studies*, 10(1), 26–37.

Nussbaum, J. F., Pitts, M. J., Huber, F. N., Krieger, J. L. R., & Ohs, J. E. (2005). Ageism and ageist language across the life span: Intimate relationships and non-intimate interactions. *Journal of Social Issues*, *61*(2), 287–305.

Overall, C. (2006). Old age and ageism, impairment and ableism: Exploring the conceptual and material connections. *NWSA Journal*, *18*(1), 126–137.

Park, C. L. (2010). Making sense of the meaning literature: An integrative review of meaning making and its effects on adjustment to stressful life events. *Psychological Bulletin*, *136*(2), 257–301.

Peplau, L. A., & Fingerhut, A. (2004). The paradox of the lesbian worker. *Journal of Social Issues*, *60*(4), 719–735.

Petrides, P., Petermann, F., Henrichs, H. R., Petzoldt, R., Rölver, K. M., Schidlmeter, A., Weber, B., & Wendt, A. (1995). Coping with employment discrimination against diabetics: Trends in social medicine and social psychology. *Patient Education and Counseling*, *26*(1–3), 203–208.

Pichler, S., Varma, A., & Bruce, T. (2010). Heterosexism in employment decisions: The role of job misfit. *Journal of Applied Social Psychology*, *40*(10), 2527–2555.

Posthuma, R. A., & Guerrero, L. (2013). Age stereotypes in the workplace: Multidimensionality, cross-cultural applications, and directions for future research. *The Sage Handbook of Aging, Work and Society* (pp. 250–265). Thousand Oaks, CA: Sage Publications.

Ragins, B. R., & Cornwell, J. M. (2001). Pink triangles: Antecedents and consequences of perceived workplace discrimination against gay and lesbian employees. *Journal of Applied Psychology*, *86*(6), 1244–1261.

Rastetter, D. (1999). Die entsexualisierung der organisation. *Soziale Welt*, *50*(2), 169–185.

Reese, G., Steffens, M. C., & Jonas, K. J. (2013). Religious affiliation and attitudes towards gay men: On the mediating role of masculinity threat. *Journal of Community & Applied Social Psychology*, *24*(4), 340–355.

Reinders, H. (2011). Is there meaning in disability? Or is it the wrong question? *Journal of Religion, Disability & Health*, *15*(1), 57–71.

Reiter, L. (1989). Sexual orientation, sexual identity, and the question of choice. *Clinical Social Work Journal*, *17*(2), 138–150.

Reskin, B. (1993). Sex segregation in the workplace. *Annual Review of Sociology*, *19*, 241–270.

Riach, K., & Wilson, F. (2007). Don't screw the crew: Exploring the rules of engagement in organizational romance. *British Journal of Management*, *18*(1), 79.

Ross, M., & Stålström, O. (1979). Exorcism as psychiatric treatment: A homosexual case study. *Archives of Sexual Behavior*, *8*(4), 379–383.

Roulstone, A., & Williams, J. (2013). Being disabled, being a manager: "Glass partitions" and conditional identities in the contemporary workplace. *Disability & Society*, *29*(1), 16–29.

Rowen, C. J., & Malcolm, J. P. (2003). Correlates of internalized homophobia and homosexual identity formation in a sample of gay men. *Journal of Homosexuality*, *43*(2), 77–92.

Rupp, D. E., Vodanovich, S. J., & Credé, M. (2006). Age bias in the workplace: The impact of ageism and causal attributions. *Journal of Applied Social Psychology*, *36*(6), 1337–1364.

Russinova, Z., Griffin, S., Bloch, P., Wewiorski, N. J., & Rosoklija, I. (2011). Workplace prejudice and discrimination toward individuals with mental illnesses. *Journal of Vocational Rehabilitation*, *35*(3), 227–241.

Sanchez, F. J., & Vilain, E. (2012). Straight-acting gays: The relationship between masculine consciousness, anti-effeminacy, and negative gay identity. *Archives of Sexual Behavior*, *41*(1), 111–119.

Schabracq, M. J. (2003). Issues of the second career half. In M. J. Schabracq, J. A. M. Winnubst, & C. L. Cooper (Eds.), *The handbook of work and health psychology* (2nd ed., pp. 333–348). Chichester, UK: Wiley.

Schiffauer, W. (2004). Vom Exil- zum Diaspora-Islam. Muslimische Identitäten in Europa. *Soziale Welt*, *55*(4), 347–368.

Schmidt, W., & Müller, A. (2013). Social integration and workplace industrial relations: Migrant and native employees in German industry. *Industrial Relations*, *68*(3), 361–386.

Schuck, K. D., & Liddle, B. J. (2001). Religious conflicts experienced by lesbian, gay, and bisexual individuals. *Journal of Gay & Lesbian Psychotherapy*, *5*(2), 63–82.

Schuh, S. C., Dick, R., Wegge, J., & Haslam, S. A. (2013). Soziale Identität und Stresserleben. In P. Genkova, T. Ringeisen, & F. T. L. Leong (Eds.), *Handbuch Stress und Kultur* (pp. 113–125). Wiesbaden, Germany: Springer Fachmedien Wiesbaden.

Selway, D., & Ashman, A. F. (1998). Disability, religion and health: A literature review in search of the spiritual dimensions of disability. *Disability & Society*, *13*(3), 429–439.

Sharma, A. (2012). Religions: Missionary and non-missionary. In A. Sharma (Ed.), *Problematizing religious freedom* (Vol. 9, pp. 175–195). Dordrecht, The Netherlands: Springer.

Sheth, D. L. (1989). Nation-building in multi-ethnic societies: The experience of South Asia. *Alternatives, 14*(4), 379–388.

Shilo, G., & Savaya, R. (2012). Mental health of lesbian, gay, and bisexual youth and young adults: Differential effects of age, gender, religiosity, and sexual orientation. *Journal of Research on Adolescence, 22*(2), 310–325.

Siegel, K., Anderman, S. J., & Schrimshaw, E. W. (2001). Religion and coping with health-related stress. *Psychology & Health, 16*(6), 631–653.

Silverstein, C. (2003). The religious conversion of homosexuals: Subject selection is the voir dire of psychological research. *Journal of Gay & Lesbian Psychotherapy, 7*(3), 31–53.

Smith, A. D. (1987). *The ethnic origins of nations*. Oxford: Blackwell.

Smith, T. L. (1978). Religion and ethnicity in America. *The American Historical Review, 83*(5), 1155–1185.

Spinner, J. (1994). *The boundaries of citizenship: Race, ethnicity, and nationality in the liberal state*. Baltimore, MD: Johns Hopkins University Press.

Spitzer, R. (2003). Can some gay men and lesbians change their sexual orientation? 200 participants reporting a change from homosexual to heterosexual orientation. *Archives of Sexual Behavior, 32*(5), 403–417.

Stavrova, O., Fetchenhauer, D., & Schlosser, T. (2013). Why are religious people happy? The effect of the social norm of religiosity across countries. *Social Science Research, 42*(1), 90–105.

Swim, J. K., Pearson, N. B., & Johnston, K. E. (2007). Daily encounters with heterosexism: A week in the life of lesbian, gay, and bisexual individuals. *Journal of Homosexuality, 53*(4), 31–48.

Szymanski, D. M., Kashubeck, S., & Meyer, J. (2008). Internalized heterosexism: Measurement, psychosocial correlates, and research directions. *Counseling Psychologist, 36*(4), 525–574.

Talwar, S. (2010). An intersectional framework for race, class, gender, and sexuality in art therapy. *Art Therapy, 27*(1), 11–17.

Tamale, S. (2013). Confronting the politics of nonconforming sexualities in Africa. *African Studies Review, 56*(02), 31–45.

Taylor, U. Y. (1998). Making waves: The theory and practice of black feminism. *Black Scholar, 28*(2), 18.

Thoits, P. (2013). Self, identity, stress, and mental health. In C. Aneshensel, J. Phelan, & A. Bierman (Eds.), *Handbook of the sociology of mental health* (pp. 357–377). Dordrecht, The Netherlands: Springer.

Tilcsik, A. (2011). Pride and prejudice: Employment discrimination against openly gay men in the United States. *American Journal of Sociology, 117*(2), 586–626.

Tozer, E. E., & Hayes, J. A. (2004). Why do individuals seek conversion therapy?: The role of religiosity, internalized homonegativity, and identity development. *The Counseling Psychologist, 32*(5), 716–740.

Traunmüller, R. (2009). Religion und Sozialintegration. *Berliner Journal für Soziologie, 19*(3), 435–468.

Tsui, A. S., Egan, T. D., & Iii, C. A. O. R. (1992). Being different: Relational demography and organizational attachment. *Administrative Science Quarterly, 37*(4), 549–579.

Ueno, K., Peña-Talamantes, A. E., & Roach, T. A. (2013). Sexual orientation and occupational attainment. *Work and Occupations*, *40*(1), 3–36.

Vega, W. A., & Rumbaut, R. G. (1991). Ethnic minorities and mental health. *Annual Review of Sociology*, *17*(1), 351–383.

Vincent, J. A. (2006). Ageing contested: Anti-ageing science and the cultural construction of old age. *Sociology*, *40*(4), 681–698.

von Schrader, S., Malzer, V., & Bruyère, S. (2013). Perspectives on disability disclosure: The importance of employer practices and workplace climate. *Employee Responsibilities and Rights Journal*, *25*(1), 1–19.

Waldo, C. R. (1999). Working in a majority context: A structural model of heterosexism as minority stress in the workplace. *Journal of Counseling Psychology*, *46*(2), 218–232.

Wallace, M., & Sheldon, N. (2014). Women and engineering: A workforce development issue. In R. Harris & T. Short (Eds.), *Workforce development* (pp. 113–129). Singapore: Springer.

Walls, N. E. (2008). Toward a multidimensional understanding of heterosexism: The changing nature of prejudice. *Journal of Homosexuality*, *55*(1), 20–70.

Waltz, P. R., Santuzzi, A. M., & Finkelstein, L. M. (2013). Focusing on employability through the lens of stigma. *Industrial and Organizational Psychology*, *6*(1), 28–31.

Ward, C., Fox, S., Wilson, J., Stuart, J., & Kus, L. (2010). Contextual influences on acculturation processes: The roles of family, community and society. *Psychological Studies*, *55*(1), 26–34.

Weber, L. (2001). *Understanding race, class, gender, and sexuality: A conceptual framework*. New York, NY: McGraw-Hill.

Weichselbaumer, D. (2003). Sexual orientation discrimination in hiring. *Labour Economics*, *10*(6), 629–642.

Willis, P. (2012). Witnesses on the periphery: Young lesbian, gay, bisexual and queer employees witnessing homophobic exchanges in Australian workplaces. *Human Relations*, *65*(12), 1589–1610.

Wimmer, A. (2008). The making and unmaking of ethnic boundaries: A multilevel process theory. *American Journal of Sociology*, *113*(4), 970–1022.

Worthy, D. A., Gorlick, M. A., Pacheco, J. L., Schnyer, D. M., & Maddox, W. T. (2011). With age comes wisdom: Decision making in younger and older adults. *Psychological Science*, *22*(11), 1375–1380.

Yinger, J. M. (1994). *Ethnicity: Source of strength? Source of conflict?* Albany, NY: State University of New York Press.

Yuval-Davis, N. (2006). Intersectionality and feminist politics. *European Journal of Women's Studies*, *13*(3), 193–209.

AGE, OCCUPATIONAL STRAIN, AND WELL-BEING: A PERSON-ENVIRONMENT FIT PERSPECTIVE

Hannes Zacher, Daniel C. Feldman and Heiko Schulz

ABSTRACT

We develop a conceptual model, based on person-environment fit theory, which explains how employee age affects occupational strain and well-being. We begin by explaining how age directly affects different dimensions of objective and subjective P-E fit. Next, we illustrate how age can moderate the relationship between objective P-E fit and subjective P-E fit. Third, we discuss how age can moderate the relationships between P-E fit, on one hand, and occupational strain and well-being on the other. Fourth, we explain how age can impact occupational strain and well-being directly independent of P-E fit. The chapter concludes with implications for future research and practice.

Keywords: Age; aging; lifespan; person-environment fit; strain; well-being

The Role of Demographics in Occupational Stress and Well Being
Research in Occupational Stress and Well Being, Volume 12, 83–111

ISSN: 1479-3555/doi:10.1108/S1479-355520140000012002

INTRODUCTION

As the proportion of the workforce comprised of older employees continues to grow, researchers in the behavioral sciences have paid increasing attention to relationships between employee age and important work outcomes, including occupational strain and well-being (Kooij, De Lange, Jansen, & Dikkers, 2013; Scheibe & Zacher, 2013). Most previous research in this area has attempted to explain associations of age with occupational strain and well-being through two theoretical lenses. One stream of research has focused on how within-person changes associated with aging affect occupational strain and well-being. For instance, Scheibe and Zacher (2013) describe how employees' capacity and motivation to display and regulate emotions change across the lifespan and, in turn, influence their occupational strain and well-being. The second stream of research has focused on how changes in the workplace itself affect the levels of occupational strain and well-being experienced by older employees. This research stream, for example, suggests that increased age discrimination along with changing job demands (e.g., greater pressure to maintain IT proficiency) lead to heightened occupational strain and poorer well-being for older employees (von Hippel, Kalokerinos, & Henry, 2012; White & Spector, 1987).

In this chapter, we integrate these two research streams by utilizing person-environment fit (P-E fit) to explore the relationships among age, occupational strain, and well-being. The P-E fit perspective is particularly germane to understanding how age affects occupational strain and well-being because it integrates the two separate approaches into a person-by-situation framework (Edwards & Shipp, 2007; Schmitt, Zacher, & Frese, 2012).

The concept of P-E fit has a long history in the fields of psychology and management. Broadly, P-E fit is defined as the degree of compatibility or match between the characteristics of an employee and the characteristics of his or her work environment (French, Caplan, & Van Harrison, 1982; Kristof, 1996). When P-E fit is high, employees typically exhibit more positive job attitudes (Edwards, 1991) and higher job performance (Kristof-Brown & Billsberry, 2013; Kristof-Brown, Zimmerman, & Johnson, 2005). Conversely, when employees' characteristics do not mesh with work demands, low levels of P-E fit are associated with greater occupational strain and poorer well-being (Edwards & Cooper, 1990; Edwards & Rothbard, 1999; French et al., 1982; Harrison, 1978; von Hippel et al., 2012).

There has been virtually no research integrating theories and findings on aging, P-E fit, and occupational strain and well-being. Indeed, only two book chapters have discussed the relationship between age and P-E fit

(Feldman & Vogel, 2009; Perry, Dokko, & Golom, 2012), and these two chapters do not discuss occupational strain and well-being as outcome variables. Consistent with the holistic approach used in both the scientific and applied occupational health literature (Keyes, 2007; World Health Organization, 2004), we conceptualize occupational strain and well-being in terms of individuals' physical health (e.g., psychosomatic complaints and physical energy), attitudes and perceptions (e.g., emotional exhaustion, job satisfaction, and perceived meaningfulness of work), and social relationships (e.g., discrimination and marginalization). In the long run, occupational strain and well-being may lead to more severe and chronic physical health problems (e.g., coronary heart disease), emotional problems (e.g., clinical depression), performance problems (e.g., counterproductive behavior), and interpersonal problems (e.g., social isolation).

We begin this chapter by exploring age-related changes that occur both within individuals and across work environments over time. Next, we consider the environmental demands placed on employees as well as the environmental supplies which help employees achieve their goals. We then address P-E fit theory, highlighting the different types and levels of fit this theory addresses.

Using P-E fit theory, in the following section we posit five inter-related propositions about the relationships among age, occupational strain, and

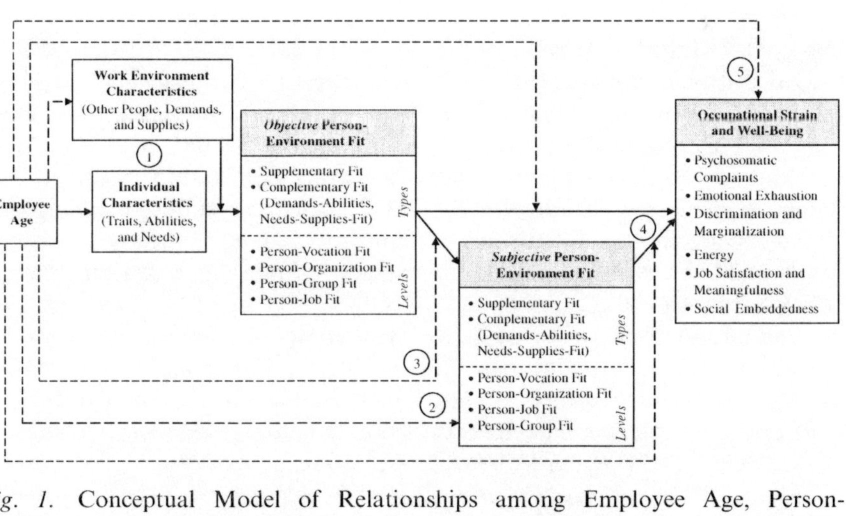

Fig. 1. Conceptual Model of Relationships among Employee Age, Person-Environment Fit, and Occupational Strain and Well-Being. *Note*: Numbers in circles refer to the research propositions.

well-being. We start by explaining how aging directly affects objective P-E fit (Proposition 1) and subjective P-E fit (Proposition 2). Next, we illustrate how age can moderate the relationship between objective and subjective P-E fit (Proposition 3). Then, we discuss how age can moderate the relationships of P-E fit with occupational strain and well-being (Proposition 4). Finally, we describe how age influences occupational strain and well-being directly, that is, independently of P-E fit processes (Proposition 5). Fig. 1 provides an overview of our conceptual model and research propositions.

AGE-RELATED CHANGES WITHIN INDIVIDUALS AND ACROSS WORK ENVIRONMENTS

Within-Person Changes

Several recent review articles have summarized how age-related, intraindividual changes influence employees' work motivation, performance, occupational strain, and well-being (Farr & Ringseis, 2002; Hedge & Borman, 2012; Kanfer, Beier, & Ackerman, 2013; Ng & Feldman, 2013b; Scheibe & Zacher, 2013; Warr, 2001). Aging can lead to declines, increases, or sustained levels in these outcome variables. Moreover, the process of aging forces many individuals to reorganize or reorder their career and personal life goals (Kanfer & Ackerman, 2004).

Ng and Feldman (2013b) identify five specific areas in which age-related changes in individuals occur. First, there is a broad consensus in the literature that employees' *cognitive abilities* change with age, such that "fluid intelligence" (e.g., short-term information processing and memory retrieval) tends to decline with age. On the other hand, "crystallized intelligence" (e.g., experience-based knowledge, skill, and judgment) tends to be relatively stable or even increase with age (Baltes, Staudinger, & Lindenberger, 1999; Salthouse, 2012).

Second, there is some evidence that some *personality characteristics* change across the adult lifespan. In particular, conscientiousness, emotional stability, and agreeableness typically increase with age, while extraversion and openness to experience tend to decrease with age (Roberts, Walton, & Viechtbauer, 2006; Warr, Miles, & Platts, 2001).

Third, employees' *goal orientations* tend to change across the lifespan. The research in this area suggests that, over the course of a career, individuals shift from a desire to maximize gains in young adulthood (e.g., through acquiring more human and social capital) to a desire to maintain resources and prevent resource losses in middle and late adulthood (Baltes & Baltes, 1990; Ebner, Freund, & Baltes, 2006; Lang & Carstensen, 2002).

Fourth, *socio-emotional experiences* change with age. Older employees appear to value emotionally positive events and meaningful relationships more highly than their younger colleagues (Charles & Carstensen, 2010; Kooij, De Lange, Jansen, Kanfer, & Dikkers, 2011) and tend to remember emotionally positive events more clearly than emotionally negative events.

Fifth, numerous studies have examined the association between employees' age and their *physical and mental health* (Maertens, Putter, Chen, Diehl, & Huang, 2012). A recent meta-analysis shows that older employees do not differ from younger employees with regard to mental health and self-reported physical health, but have somewhat lower scores on clinical measures of physical health (Ng & Feldman, 2013a). Other meta-analytic results suggest that older employees report lower levels of unfavorable job attitudes like emotional exhaustion and job dissatisfaction (Ng & Feldman, 2010), although a meta-analysis conducted by Rauschenbach, Krumm, Thielgen, and Hertel (2013) did not find a significant relationship between age and irritation.

Further, it should be noted that these age-related changes in employee characteristics may affect P-E fit both individually and in combination with each other (Feldman & Vogel, 2009). For instance, increases in crystallized intelligence can help compensate for declines in cognitive functioning related to short-term recall. Similarly, older employees' attention to positive emotional experiences may help buffer them from some of the detrimental effects of declines in physical health.

Environmental Changes

As individuals move through the various stages of their careers, numerous elements of their work environments change. Employees' P-E fit may increase or decrease over time for reasons besides age; changes in the work environment also impact P-E fit.

Employees' jobs and vocations may become more demanding due to increases in the number of tasks and the level of responsibility given to them over time (Hurrell & Lindström, 1992). This may lead to declines in P-E fit unless older employees compensate by utilizing greater experience-based judgment and knowledge. In addition, the social context at work may change as individuals age; they may face different social expectations and stereotypes that could either increase or decrease P-E fit. While extrinsic rewards such as pay and benefits typically increase as employees accrue more years of seniority, this is not necessarily the case for intrinsic rewards such as recognition from coworkers and supervisors (Noonan, 2005). Moreover, changes in human resource policies and practices (e.g., training opportunities and performance evaluation standards) and in organizational cultures and climates (e.g., organizational norms and senior management's values) might decrease the likelihood that older employees will achieve P-E fit, too (Farr & Ringseis, 2002; Feldman & Vogel, 2009).

By and large, there has been less research conducted on age-related environmental changes than on age-related within-person changes. Prior research in this area, however, does reveal several interesting patterns. For example, research on career stages has shown that job demands are higher in mid-career compared to early and late career (Hurrell & Lindström, 1992; Lindström, 1988) because employees at this career stage assume more responsible supervisory positions yet still do not have full job autonomy (Ng & Feldman, 2010). Another set of studies suggests that as employees get closer to retirement they face decreasing work demands either because they receive less challenging job assignments or voluntarily withdraw into part-time positions (Feldman & Ng, 2007). Research in the area of work-family balance suggests that while older employees enjoy the increased flexibility of having "empty nests," others are equally, if not more, constricted by responsibilities for aging parents (Allen & Shockley, 2012; Baltes & Young, 2007; Zacher, Jimmieson, & Winter, 2012).

There has also been considerable research on age stereotypes. The findings in this research stream highlight that older employees face more negative perceptions from their supervisors about their abilities to perform and more negative attitudes from their colleagues about their contributions to the firm, although there is some evidence that the level of negative age stereotyping has stabilized or diminished somewhat in recent years (Hassell & Perrewe, 1995; Posthuma & Campion, 2009). Several negative age stereotypes, however, appear to be rather widely held (Ng & Feldman, 2012). For example, one negative stereotype impacting older employees is the assumption they will have trouble working for younger supervisors (Tsui, Porter, & Egan, 2002). In a similar vein, research on relational demography and organizational age norms shows that colleagues' and supervisors' expectations of an individual's performance decrease as an individual ages (Lawrence, 1988; Tsui & O'Reilly, 1989). In particular, older employees are often seen as less capable of learning new technology and adjusting to organizational change.

Equally important, employees' perceptions of their own social environments also change as they age. For instance, because older employees particularly value emotionally positive and meaningful experiences, they may interpret interactions with their coworkers, supervisors, and customers differently from their younger counterparts. While older employees might be less attuned to negative cues being sent from coworkers, they might also be more likely to withdraw from social interactions when they do receive such negative cues.

Environmental Demands and Supplies

Last here, we draw an important distinction on the "environment" side of the equation. In particular, we distinguish environmental demands from environmental supplies.

Environmental demands refer to the requirements and expectations that vocations, organizations, work groups, and jobs place on employees. *Environmental supplies*, in contrast, refer to intrinsic and extrinsic resources provided to individuals by their vocations, organizations, work groups, and jobs. These supplies help satisfy employees' desires and needs, for example, by providing them with pay, recognition, social support, and job autonomy.

The aging process can affect both the environmental demands and environmental supplies of older employees. Changing environmental demands may challenge older employees to reorder their priorities or reorient how they perform their jobs (Kanfer & Ackerman, 2004). In some cases, environmental demands increase as employees hold more responsible jobs; in other cases, environmental demands decrease as older employees are marginalized into less challenging assignments. By the same token, employees may receive more environmental supplies as they age (e.g., more flexible schedules or more staff as individuals gain seniority) or fewer environmental supplies (as changes in job responsibilities lead to lower job status).

P-E FIT THEORY

Researchers have identified various forms of P-E fit which are relevant to understanding the relationships among age, P-E fit, and occupational strain and well-being. The theoretical framework presented by Edwards and

Shipp (2007) is particularly helpful in this regard. They highlight three different forms of fit – objective versus subjective, supplementary versus complementary, and static versus dynamic – as well as four different levels of fit: vocation, organization, group, and job.

Objective versus Subjective Fit

Researchers in this area make an important distinction between objective P-E fit and subjective P-E fit (Edwards, Cable, Williamson, Lambert, & Shipp, 2006). *Objective P-E fit* refers to an explicit comparison between the characteristics of an employee and the characteristics of his or her environment. To assess objective P-E fit, employee and environmental characteristics are assessed separately (Kristof, 1996). *Subjective P-E fit*, in contrast, refers to employees' self-perceptions and assessments of their fit with the work environment (Kristof, 1996). In making these subjective assessments, individuals rely on their own feelings and perceptions about their past experiences, present situations, and future expectations (Shipp & Jansen, 2011).

While objective and subjective P-E fit tend to be correlated, their links to outcome variables (such as job attitudes and job performance) may vary in strength. In particular, Edwards and Shipp (2007) note that employees' "contact with reality" and "accuracy of self-assessment" influence whether objective P-E fit and subjective P-E fit tend to converge.

Supplementary versus Complementary Fit

Edwards and Shipp (2007) also make a distinction between supplementary and complementary fit. *Supplementary fit* occurs when an employee has similar characteristics to other employees in the work environment (e.g., same kind of education, experience, and worldview). *Complementary fit*, by contrast, occurs when the exchange between the person and the environment is asymmetrical.

There are two subtypes of complementary P-E fit. *Demands-abilities fit* occurs when work demands can be met with the employee's abilities, knowledge, and experience. In contrast, *needs-supplies fit* occurs when employees' desires and needs are fulfilled by environmental supplies (Caplan, Cobb, French, Van Harrison, & Pinneau, 1975; Kristof-Brown et al., 2005; Muchinsky & Monahan, 1987).

The distinctions described here are important to consider because older employees are less likely to be similar to the majority of other employees in their units (i.e., supplementary fit) and, as such, might be more likely to experience occupational strain and well-being (Avery, McKay, & Wilson, 2007; von Hippel et al., 2012). In addition, age-related changes in employees' traits, abilities, and needs may lead to increased strain and poorer well-being if changes in individual characteristics do not mesh with, or are accompanied by, appropriate changes in characteristics of the work environment.

Static versus Dynamic Fit

P-E fit researchers have also made a distinction between static P-E fit and dynamic P-E fit (Feldman & Vogel, 2009; Ostroff, Shin, & Feinberg, 2002). *Static P-E fit* is concerned with those aspects of the person and the environment that are relatively stable over time. Most prior research on P-E fit has measured person and environment factors simultaneously at one point in time, implicitly treating P-E fit as a largely static construct.

In contrast, conceptualizing *dynamic P-E fit* entails examining how aspects of individuals and environments change over time; studying dynamic P-E fit requires researchers to study person and environmental factors across multiple time periods. In the context of aging, examining dynamic P-E fit is particularly relevant because within-person changes and changes in the social environment create opportunities and challenges for individuals striving to achieve fit as they age (Feldman & Vogel, 2009). For instance, as individuals age, they may perceive bridge employment as better fits for their needs (Adams & Rau, 2004), but jobs entailing up-to-date technology as poorer fits for their abilities. In the present chapter, our focus is on dynamic fit since we are concerned with age-related changes within individuals and across environments over time. For that reason, our conceptual model in Fig. 1 does not explicitly distinguish between static and dynamic fit.

Levels of Fit

Last here, Edwards and Shipp (2007) identify different *levels* of the work environment with which P-E fit can be achieved. These levels include the vocation (or profession) as a whole, the organization, the work group, and the job (Feldman & Vogel, 2009; Kristof, 1996). In Fig. 1, the four different levels of P-E fit appear below the dotted lines.

It should be noted that there can be different forms of fit at different levels of fit (Edwards & Shipp, 2007). For instance, person-organization fit can be supplementary in nature; in this case, employees' traits and values are similar to the characteristics of other people in the firm. Alternatively, person-organization fit can be complementary in nature; in this case, individuals bring new and different kinds of skills and experience to their employers.

Further, there can be spillover effects from one level of fit to another. For example, if there is poor fit at the occupational level, it is much more difficult for individuals to achieve fit at the organizational level. Cascading levels of poor fit can be particularly stressful for older employees because their employment alternatives in the external labor market are fewer and their ability to recoup job retraining and job relocation costs in a two-to-five-year period is lower as well (Feldman & Vogel, 2009).

Occupational Strain and Well-Being as Outcomes of P-E Fit

There has been considerable research using P-E fit theory to explain occupational strain and well-being. In particular, this literature has examined how individual differences and situational characteristics *interact* to influence these stress-related variables. Further, researchers in this area have examined the reciprocal and dynamic relationships of occupational strain and well-being with P-E fit (Caplan et al., 1975; Edwards, Caplan, & Harrison, 1998; Edwards & Cooper, 1990; French et al., 1982; Harrison, 1978). That is, just as individual differences and situational characteristics affect occupational strain and well-being over time, employees' experiences of occupational strain and well-being lead them to reassess their P-E fit.

Edwards and Shipp (2007) summarize some of the most salient findings in this literature. First, objective P-E fit can affect occupational strain and well-being either directly or indirectly (by changing individuals' perceptions of subjective fit). Second, needs-supplies fit is typically the most proximal determinant of occupational strain and well-being; employees are most likely to experience greater occupational strain and poorer well-being when supplies in their work environments do not meet their needs (Edwards & Shipp, 2007). In contrast, demands-abilities fit is a more distal or indirect determinant of occupational strain and well-being. Further, environmental supplies are highly determined by demands-ability fit; employees who have high demands-abilities fit are most likely to demonstrate stronger performance, receive greater extrinsic rewards in return, and enjoy a greater sense of accomplishment about their work (Shipp & Jansen, 2011).

Third, supplementary fit is more likely to have indirect effects on occupational strain and well-being. Here the argument is that similarity to others in the work environment fulfills individuals' needs for affiliation and social support, which in turn lead to greater role clarity and greater trust and communication with group members. In effect, the fulfillment of affiliation needs not only facilitates employees performing their role requirements more effectively, but also buffers employees against the potentially deleterious effects of stressful work demands (Edwards & Shipp, 2007; Feldman & Vogel, 2009).

Another set of findings suggests that the effects of P-E fit on occupational strain and well-being will be strongest when employee characteristics, work environment factors, and job outcomes all share the same domain content. Domain-specific fit assesses P-E fit in terms of broad categories of variables (e.g., personality traits). For instance, employees' emotional strain is greatest when the emotion regulation demands of their jobs exceed their emotion regulation abilities. This alignment of domains of employee characteristics, work environment factors, and job outcomes has been called the "triple-match principle" (de Jonge & Dormann, 2006).

Along the same lines, it should be noted that the strength of findings in this area is somewhat dependent upon the level of specificity or generality in which P-E fit is defined (Edwards & Shipp, 2007). At a theoretical level, several of the distinctions among different types of fit described above are assumed to be orthogonal to each other. However, in practice, various researchers in the field have used different combinations of types and levels of fit in their empirical studies, making inferences across studies more difficult. As a consequence, global fit – defined as overall P-E fit across numerous levels, types, and dimensions of the construct – is most frequently used as a predictor of occupational health and well-being (Edwards & Shipp, 2007).

Last here, it is important to recognize that the relationships of P-E fit with occupational strain and well-being are not linear (Edwards & Shipp, 2007). Occupational strain decreases when environmental supplies increase to meet employees' needs. However, excess supplies that go beyond "equilibrium fit" might not lead to any greater sense of well-being. Along the same lines, occupational strain is likely to increase when the demands of the work environment exceed employees' abilities to satisfy those demands. However, when employees' abilities exceed those needed to perform their work effectively, increasing employees' skills is unlikely to lead to further decreases in occupational strain (Edwards et al., 2006).

THEORETICAL MODEL

The conceptual model in Fig. 1 presents five propositions derived from P-E fit theory. We discuss each of these five propositions in greater detail below.

Age and Objective P-E Fit

In their review of the literature, Feldman and Vogel (2009) concluded that age-related changes can have significant consequences for employees' objective P-E fit. They argue that age is generally negatively related to person-vocation, person-organization, and person-job fit because changes in individual and environmental characteristics over time lead to greater discrepancies between individuals' needs and organizations' resources. In other words, as employees age there is an increased likelihood that their abilities and needs will fall out of sync with the demands and supplies of their work environments.

Moreover, individuals may be less able and less motivated to re-establish high levels of person-vocation, person-organization, and person-job fit as they age. First, older employees often find the job search process aversive, in large part because they are aware of age discrimination in the workplace. Second, older employees may view their remaining time in the workforce as rather limited and therefore decide to remain in vocations or jobs with poor fit until retirement. Third, older employees are often embedded in their communities and may be willing to sacrifice some level of P-E fit at work to maintain high levels of person-community fit (Feldman, Ng, & Vogel, 2012).

In contrast, Feldman and Vogel (2009) proposed that age is positively related to person-group fit because older employees have higher needs for socio-emotional gratification than younger employees. As such, older employees are willing to invest more energy into building and maintaining strong interpersonal relationships with others in their work group. However, Feldman and Vogel (2009) also suggest that as increasing numbers of older colleagues retire from the workforce, older employees' supplementary person-group fit might start to decline nonetheless.

Below, we extend these ideas by taking a more detailed look at how different forms of age-related changes impact different types and levels of objective P-E fit. In doing so, we assume that P-E fit is dynamic and that age-related changes in employees interact with changes in workplace environment to determine objective P-E fit.

In Propositions 1a and 1b, we posit that age-related changes in cognitive and physical abilities have a particularly strong impact on employees' demands-abilities fit. In jobs and vocations which require high levels of fluid intelligence (e.g., air traffic controllers) or physical abilities (e.g., construction workers), person-job and person-vocation demands-abilities fit are likely to decline with age. In contrast, in jobs and vocations which require high levels of crystallized intelligence (e.g., counselors or academics), person-job and person-vocation demands-abilities fit are likely to increase with age.

As noted by Kanfer and Ackerman (2004), most jobs in today's economy require a combination of both fluid and crystallized intelligence. Consequently, the declines in person-vocation and person-job fit due to decreases in fluid intelligence may be compensated for by increases in crystallized intelligence (Bäckman & Dixon, 1992). Further, as economies move from primarily manufacturing to service industries, there may be fewer older employees who experience declining person-vocation and person-job demands-abilities fit due to losses in physical strength and endurance.

Proposition 1a. In jobs and vocations where employees' fluid intelligence and physical abilities are critical work demands, person-job and person-vocation demands-abilities fit will decrease with age.

Proposition 1b. In jobs and vocations where employees' crystallized intelligence is a critical work demand, person-job and person-vocation demands-abilities fit will increase with age.

Further, age-related changes in employees' personality may also influence demands-abilities fit across the lifespan (Propositions 1c and 1d). In jobs and vocations which require high levels of conscientiousness, agreeableness, and emotional stability (e.g., negotiators and mediators), employees' person-job and person-vocation demands-abilities fit are likely to increase with age. In contrast, in jobs and vocations which require high levels of extraversion and openness to experience (e.g., consultants), person-job and person-vocation demands-abilities fit are generally likely to decrease with age. Because we expect that age-related declines in extraversion are likely to be largely offset by increases in agreeableness, we do not predict significant effects of age on person-group or person-organization fit.

Proposition 1c. In jobs and vocations where employees' conscientiousness, agreeableness, and emotional stability are critical work demands, person-job and person-vocation demands-abilities fit will increase with age.

Proposition 1d. In jobs and vocations where employees' extraversion and openness to experience are critical work demands, person-job and person-vocation demands-abilities fit will decrease with age.

Generally, researchers have assumed that needs-supplies fit will be higher for older employees because they are more interested in achieving and maintaining positive interpersonal relations and social affirmation (Feldman & Vogel, 2009). Thus, in Propositions 1e and 1f, we posit that age-related changes in employees' goal orientations and socio-emotional preferences will be related to person-vocation, person-organization, person-group, and person-job needs-supplies fit. In early adulthood, individuals are focused on acquiring new skills and on achieving future-oriented goals. However, as employees enter middle and late adulthood, they are more likely to focus on maintaining or preventing the loss of resources they already possess (Carstensen, Isaacowitz, & Charles, 1999; Ebner et al., 2006). As a result, in organizations and groups that emphasize the acquisition of new knowledge and the achievement of future-oriented goals, needs-supplies fit is likely to decline with age.

On the other hand, because people place a higher emphasis on having positive social relationships and emotional experiences as they age (Ebner et al., 2006; Lang & Carstensen, 2002), individuals who work in vocations, organizations, groups, and jobs that emphasize positive and meaningful social interactions (e.g., kindergarten teachers) are more likely to have high levels of needs-supplies fit. In large part, this relationship is driven by the fact that such individuals' needs are amply matched by the supplies of these work environments.

Proposition 1e. In work environments that emphasize the acquisition of new knowledge and achievement of future-oriented goals, needs-supplies fit will decline with age.

Proposition 1f. In work environments that emphasize the development and maintenance of positive social relationships, needs-supplies fit will increase with age.

Our last tenet of Proposition 1 considers the moderating effect of work and career centrality in the relationship between employee age and needs-supplies fit (Proposition 1g). It is possible, for instance, that older employees might increase their focus on interpersonal relationships by having more intense relationships with spouses, children, extended family members, and friends outside work rather than with people inside the workplace (Feldman et al., 2012; Lang & Carstensen, 2002). Thus, the effects of age on objective P-E fit may be moderated by employees' levels of work and career centrality (i.e., the importance employees attach to their work and careers; Paullay, Alliger, & Stone-Romero, 1994). When work and career centrality are high, needs-supplies P-E fit is likely to increase with age; in contrast, when work and career centrality are low, employees' needs-supplies P-E fit is likely to decrease with age.

> **Proposition 1g.** The relationship between employee age and needs-supplies fit is moderated by work and career centrality. The relationship is positive among individuals with high work and career centrality and negative among individuals with low work and career centrality.

Age and Subjective P-E Fit

While objective P-E fit and subjective P-E fit are likely to be correlated, there are several reasons why age might influence subjective P-E fit differently than it influences objective P-E fit. The underlying argument here is that aging might not only change the criteria that individuals use to assess P-E fit but also how they receive and interpret feedback from the environment.

First, older employees are less likely to focus on the acquisition of new knowledge and social ties for future use than younger employees (Jansen & Shipp, 2013; Shipp & Jansen, 2011). Instead, older employees are more likely to concentrate on having meaningful work and positive social relationships in the present (Charles & Carstensen, 2010; Scheibe & Carstensen, 2010). Whatever disappointments older employees might have about past career failures are more likely to dissipate in emotional intensity over time. Moreover, any anxiety individuals might have about future P-E fit is likely to decline as older employees close in on retirement. Thus, in Proposition 2a, we posit that younger employees' subjective assessments are more likely to be based on their evaluations of future or potential fit, while older employees' subjective assessments are more likely to be based on current fit (Jansen & Shipp, 2013; Shipp & Jansen, 2011).

Consistent with Carstensen et al.'s (1999) socioemotional selectivity theory, we further posit in Propositions 2b and 2c that these age-related shifts in the evaluative basis of subjective P-E fit are adaptive in terms of occupational well-being and strain. Older employees who focus on the present in assessing P-E fit will have higher levels of occupational well-being and lower levels of strain than older employees who focus predominantly on their past or future P-E fit, as a focus on the present is more consistent with older employees' age-related abilities and needs. In contrast, younger employees who focus on future subjective P-E fit should have higher levels of occupational well-being and lower levels of strain than younger employees who focus predominantly on their past or present P-E fit; for younger employees, a future focus is more consistent with their developmental abilities and needs (Carstensen et al., 1999; Lang & Carstensen, 2002).

Proposition 2a. Older employees' subjective P-E fit is more heavily based on evaluations of present fit, whereas younger employees' subjective P-E fit is more heavily based on expectations of future P-E fit.

Proposition 2b. Older employees who base their subjective P-E fit on evaluations of present fit will have higher levels of occupational well-being and lower levels of strain than older employees who base their subjective P-E fit on evaluations of past or future fit.

Proposition 2c. Younger employees who base their subjective P-E fit on evaluations of future fit will have higher levels of occupational well-being and lower levels of strain than younger employees who base their subjective P-E fit on evaluations of past and present fit.

In Proposition 2d, we posit that older employees will exhibit more positive bias in making subjective assessments of P-E fit. In general, we would expect some positive bias on both the part of younger and older employees in assessing subjective P-E fit because people are generally inclined to have self-enhancing perceptions of themselves and their abilities. However, this positive bias is likely to increase as people age. Older employees are more likely to shift their subjective assessments of P-E fit to those criteria on which they see themselves as scoring high. For example, older employees are less likely to judge P-E fit on the basis of their technical skills because doing so would be more threatening to their self-esteem and identity. Rather, older employees are more likely to assess subjective fit in terms of judgment, savvy, and contributions to their colleagues and their firms more broadly. Older employees are also less likely to focus on negative events in their environments and to concentrate on current successes and contributions. Socioemotional selectivity theory (Carstensen et al., 1999) and the literature on emotional aging (Scheibe & Carstensen, 2010) suggest that this positive bias will be especially strong for person-group needs-supplies fit because it is central in fulfilling individuals' affiliation and relatedness needs.

Proposition 2d. Older employees' evaluations of subjective P-E fit are more positive than younger employees' evaluations, particularly for person-group needs-supplies fit.

The Moderating Effect of Age on the Relationship between Objective and Subjective P-E Fit

Based on both theory and empirical findings in the lifespan development literature, we also predict that age will moderate the relationship between objective and subjective P-E fit. As noted earlier, there are often discrepancies between these two constructs due to what Edwards and Shipp (2007) label employees' "contact with reality" and "accuracy of self-assessment." In effect, the less accurate employees' perceptions of their environments and themselves, the more likely there is to be a discrepancy between objective and subjective P-E fit.

In Proposition 3a, we suggest that individuals' capabilities and motivations to process information accurately vary across the lifespan. For younger adults, the need to process information accurately is critical to career survival and career growth; however unpleasant the feedback from the environment might be, the costs of ignoring such feedback have long-term impact. In short, young adults are more motivated to obtain accurate feedback about vocational P-E fit because it helps them evaluate whether they made good initial employment choices. In contrast, older employees have less incentive to seek out disconfirming negative feedback about vocational P-E fit and are less likely to incorporate that feedback into their self-images. Consequently, compared to younger employees, older employees' subjective assessments of P-E fit are more likely to diverge from objective P-E fit.

Proposition 3a. The positive relationship between objective and subjective person-vocation fit is moderated by age, such that this relationship is stronger for younger employees than for older employees.

In a similar vein, we argue that the relationship between objective person-job demands-abilities fit and subjective person-job demands-abilities fit will be moderated by age, such that the relationship will be stronger for younger employees than for older employees (Proposition 3b). Younger employees have to be especially attuned to feedback on their demands-abilities fit because it is the dimension along which they are most likely to be evaluated on in terms of important extrinsic rewards (e.g., salary increases and promotions). Furthermore, older employees are less able and willing than younger employees to retrieve negative feedback from memory (Scheibe & Carstensen, 2010) – and it is in the area of person-job demands-abilities fit in which older employees are most likely to receive negative feedback (Posthuma & Campion, 2009).

Proposition 3b. The positive relationship between objective person-job demands-abilities fit and subjective person-job demands-abilities fit is moderated by age such that this relationship is stronger for younger employees than for older employees.

In addition, we expect that the relationship between objective person-group fit and subjective group fit will be stronger for older employees than for younger employees (Proposition 3c). Because older employees are particularly attuned to having positive socio-emotional relationships with their colleagues, they will exert more energy to achieve both supplementary and complementary fit on the person-group dimension. Further, older employees will be more sensitive to cues from their work environment about their current person-group fit as well as potential changes in person-group fit (Lang & Carstensen, 2002).

In contrast, younger employees are more closely attuned to feedback on their skills and abilities and are more likely to change vocations, organizations, and jobs on that basis. For that reason, younger employees have less incentive to ensure person-group fit is high and are less likely to monitor whether there are changes in person-group fit over time. Therefore, the association between objective and subjective person-group fit will be weaker for younger employees than for older employees.

Proposition 3c. The positive relationship between objective and subjective person-group fit is moderated by age such that the relationship will be stronger for older employees than for younger employees.

Age as a Moderator of the Relationship of P-E Fit to Occupational Strain and Well-Being

Feldman and Vogel (2009) noted that age not only has direct effects on P-E fit but also strengthens or weakens the effects of P-E fit on important work outcomes like in-role performance, citizenship behavior, and counterproductive behavior. In this section, we extend their argument by outlining how age may moderate the effects of both objective and subjective P-E fit on occupational strain and well-being.

As noted above, there is considerable evidence that poor objective P-E fit leads to greater psychosomatic complaints as individuals' job demands exceed their abilities. However, the extent to which individuals experience those psychosomatic complaints depends, at least in part, of how consciously aware they are of these mismatches. Here we suggest that age moderates the relationships of P-E fit with occupational strain and well-being because age impacts how individuals subjectively assess P-E fit.

Within-person changes in goal orientations along with age-related changes in work environments both account for this moderating effect (Propositions 4a and 4b). We expect that the overall relationship of person-group fit with well-being will be stronger (and more positive) for older employees than for younger employees because older employees derive more emotional gratification from intense social relationships (Carstensen et al., 1999). Moreover, we expect that the relationship of person-job fit to occupational strain will be stronger (and more negative) for older employees because they have fewer opportunities for occupational mobility and will feel stuck in jobs whose demands do not match their knowledge, skills, and abilities (Heckhausen, Wrosch, & Schulz, 2010; Zacher & Frese, 2009).

> **Proposition 4a.** The relationship of person-group fit with well-being will be moderated by age such that the relationship will be stronger (and more positive) for older employees than for younger employees.

> **Proposition 4b.** The relationship of person-job fit with occupational strain will be moderated by age such that the relationship will be stronger (and more negative) for older employees than for younger employees.

For similar reasons, in Propositions 4c and 4d, we posit that the relationship of supplementary fit with occupational well-being will be stronger (and more positive) for older employees because they value similarity to, and familiarity with, others in the workplace more highly than younger employees do (Kanfer & Ackerman, 2004). At the same time, we posit that the relationship of demands-abilities fit with occupational strain will be stronger (and more negative) for older employees than for younger employees – especially since organizations are less likely to invest in further training for older employees than for younger employees (Feldman & Vogel, 2009; Lazazzara, Karpinska, & Henkens, 2013). Thus, we predict:

> **Proposition 4c.** The relationship of supplementary fit with occupational well-being will be moderated by age such that the relationship will be stronger (and more positive) for older employees than for younger employees.

> **Proposition 4d.** The relationship of demands-abilities fit with occupational strain will be moderated by age such that the relationship will be stronger (and more negative) for older employees than for younger employees.

It should also be noted here that we expect that the interaction effects of age and P-E fit on occupational well-being and strain (discussed above) will be stronger for individuals with high work and career centrality. For example, older employees with low work and career centrality may prefer spending time with family and close friends rather than socializing with colleagues at work. As these older employees receive social support and affirmation from alternative sources, the association between person-group fit and well-being will be lower (Feldman et al., 2012). In addition, older employees with low work and career centrality will experience less occupational strain when their levels of person-job and demands-abilities fit are low because they attach much less importance to pursuing work success and career achievement.

> **Proposition 4e.** The interaction effect of age and P-E fit on occupational strain is moderated by work and career centrality such that the effect will be stronger for employees with high compared to low work and career centrality.

Direct Effects of Age on Occupational Strain and Well-Being

Independent of the P-E fit processes described above, age can also have direct effects on occupational strain and well-being (Proposition 5). We suggest these direct effects occur both because of psycho-physiological changes within individuals and because older employees experience changes in social status across the lifespan.

There is substantial evidence in the literature on general psychological well-being that middle-aged adults (i.e., between 35 and 50 years) experience lower levels of well-being than both younger and older adults (Blanchflower & Oswald, 2008; Ng & Feldman, 2010). Interestingly, the same pattern of results appears in both humans and great apes, suggesting that basic genetic factors play at least some role in explaining these trajectories of well-being over time (Weiss, King, Inoue-Murayama, Matsuzawa, & Oswald, 2012). Moreover, the "sandwich generation" often experiences greater occupational stress and lower levels of well-being because its work demands and its personal life demands are peaking at the same time (i.e., "the rush hour of life"; Allen & Shockley, 2012; Zacher et al., 2012).

> **Proposition 5a.** The relationships of age to occupational strain and well-being are likely to be curvilinear, with middle-aged employees experiencing greater occupational strain and poorer well-being compared to both younger and older employees.

Moreover, we expect that the relationships of age to occupational strain and well-being will be moderated by national culture. In most Western cultures, older employees suffer from negative age stereotypes and therefore experience lower social status at work (Ng & Feldman, 2012; Posthuma & Campion, 2009). Consequently, we expect that the relationship of age to occupational strain will be stronger in Western cultures than in Eastern cultures, where seniority and age are more highly valued. Thus, in Proposition 5b, we posit:

> **Proposition 5b.** The relationships of age to occupational strain and poor well-being will be positive in Western cultures and negative in Eastern cultures.

IMPLICATIONS FOR FUTURE RESEARCH AND PRACTICE

The aim of this final section is to highlight important directions for future research on age, P-E fit, occupational strain, and well-being. In addition, this final section provides several implications for the management of older employees.

Directions for Future Research

In the present chapter, we mainly focused on employees' complementary fit at different levels of the work environment (vocation, organization, group, and job). However, much more research is needed on supplementary fit across different levels of the work environment. Future research should investigate whether age-related changes have more (or less) pronounced effects on complementary or supplementary P-E fit and how age-related changes in complementary and supplementary fit differentially influence occupational strain and well-being. We expect that as employees age, their supplementary fit is likely to decrease at all levels of the environment as more young people enter their vocations, organization, and job. Moreover, because older employees value similarity and familiarity with others more than younger employees do (Carstensen et al., 1999), the effects of supplementary fit on occupational strain may become even stronger across the lifespan.

Second, in this chapter, we focused exclusively on chronological age (or calendar age) which is consistent with most previous research in this area (Schwall, 2012). The operationalization of age in this way has been most popular because many of the underlying rationales provided for the effects of aging derive from psychological, physiological, and physical within-person changes which occur across the lifespan. However, some researchers have argued that other definitions of age could explain additional variance in occupational strain and well-being (Cleveland, Shore, & Murphy, 1997; Pitt-Catsouphes, Matz-Costa, & James, 2012). For instance, subjective age (i.e., how old employees perceive themselves to be) might explain additional variance in subjective P-E fit above and beyond that of chronological age. Similarly, the relative age of employees compared to their coworkers or supervisors could be a relevant predictor of person-group and person-organization fit. Ng and Feldman (2013b) argue that several variables which are theoretically related to age (such as job tenure, organizational tenure, and career stage) might also affect relationships between age and P-E fit.

Third, most of the previous literature in this area implies that employees are relatively passive in managing or coping with the effects of P-E fit on occupational strain and well-being, and the present chapter has largely reviewed that literature. However, there is certainly evidence that employees not only react to poor P-E fit but also make active attempts to change work environments to their liking (Frese, Garst, & Fay, 2007; Zacher & Frese, 2011). Thus, another important direction for future research is examining when, how, and with which strategies employees establish initial P-E fit or re-establish P-E fit when it declines.

Along the same lines, more research is needed on whether the strategies employees use to monitor bad fit and re-establish good fit change across the lifespan. For instance, older employees might engage in more self-regulation strategies (e.g., selection, optimization, and compensation; Baltes & Baltes, 1990; Freund & Baltes, 2002) to establish fit than younger employees. Zacher and Frese (2011) note, for instance, that older employees in low-complexity jobs perceive more job opportunities when they use these self-regulation strategies. Another study in this area has shown that the negative relationship between age and work ability (i.e., a concept closely related to demands-abilities fit) was weaker when older employees had high levels of job control and used selection, optimization, and compensation strategies (Weigl, Müller, Hornung, Zacher, & Angerer, 2013). In contrast, younger employees might be more inclined to change vocations, organizations, or jobs when faced with work environments where organizational supplies are insufficient to meet individual needs.

Fourth, much of the previous research on aging has consisted of group-level studies that compare the work experiences of young, middle-aged, and older employees. This research is grounded in the static view of P-E fit, but much more longitudinal research is needed to understand dynamic P-E fit. Cross-sectional studies do not allow researchers to distinguish between effects due to aging and effects due to cohort effects. Unfortunately, of all the areas in applied psychology, studies of aging are the most difficult to conduct because the cycle times for data collection and publication are so long (Ng & Feldman, 2008). As at least a partial remedy in meeting this challenge, we encourage researchers to conduct shorter-term panel studies across such critical transition periods as career entry, career change, or career exit.

Finally, research on subjective P-E fit has far outpaced research on objective P-E fit. There are relatively few widely accepted measures of objective P-E fit and there is relatively little consensus about whether P-E fit should be measured in terms of congruence or discrepancy. To move empirical research on aging and occupational strain and well-being in the area of P-E fit ahead, much greater attention needs to be paid to operationalizing and measuring objective person-environment fit.

Implications for Practice

Our conceptual model has several potential implications for the management of older employees' P-E fit and occupational well-being. First, organizations should ensure that job analyses and performance evaluations are being used in the most effective ways for selecting, developing, and rewarding older employees. Modified job analyses and performance evaluation systems can help managers adapt work environments so that organizational demands are consistent with older employees' particular strengths and needs and that older employees have the relevant knowledge, skills, and abilities to perform their tasks. Moreover, modified job analyses and performance evaluation systems can be integrated into better career pathing for older employees so that their job responsibilities change as their sets of skills and needs change across the lifespan. For example, shift work is not associated with positive outcomes for any age group, but is particularly onerous for older employees.

Along the same lines, organizations can invest more heavily in human resource interventions (e.g., health promotion programs) to help older employees remain healthy and active both at work and at home. Another area in which organizations could invest more heavily is continuous training for older employees (Klein & Weaver, 2000). Moreover, in addition to more continuous training, some modifications may have to be made in the pace and delivery of that training (Kanfer & Ackerman, 2004). For instance, if one of the challenges for older employees is keeping up with new technology, on-line modules may not be the best way of bringing older employees up to speed.

More broadly, while supervisors are most likely to assess their subordinates' P-E fit in terms of demands-abilities fit, this limited perspective blinds managers to the numerous other ways in which older employees can contribute to organizations. It is highly unlikely (and arguably highly dysfunctional) to expect that individuals' abilities, needs, interests, and capabilities will not change across a career. By forcing older employees to compete with younger employees on only the criteria in which younger employees excel, managers lose the opportunity to take advantage of their unique contributions to the firm.

In addition, the literature on P-E fit supports the broader literature in career development (cf. Feldman & Ng, 2007) in rebutting the notion that there is only one acceptable way to manage a career. Rather than bemoan the fact that older employees are not as technically competent as their younger colleagues, organizations should rely more heavily on older employees in areas where they have competitive advantage: political savvy, implementation of new programs, mentoring younger employees, citizenship behaviors, and representing the organization to outsiders (Ng & Feldman, 2008; Zacher, Rosing, Henning, & Frese, 2011). Doing so not only makes greater use of older employees' human and social capital but also reduces older employees' occupational strain and enhances their well-being.

CONCLUSION

We hope that our conceptual model will provide a valuable agenda for future research on the complex relationships among employee age, P-E fit, occupational strain, and well-being. As the mean age of the workforce in industrial countries (as well as in some developing countries) continues to rise and middle-aged and older employees represent larger and larger segments of the workforce, organizations need to put more concerted effort into reducing negative age stereotypes and "benign neglect" of older employees. While organizations cannot stop the march of time, they can do much to stop negative assumptions regarding, attributions about, and evaluations of older employees.

REFERENCES

Adams, G., & Rau, B. (2004). Job seeking among retirees seeking bridge employment. *Personnel Psychology*, *57*(3), 719–744.

Allen, T. D., & Shockley, K. M. (2012). Older workers and work-family issues. In J. W. Hedge & W. C. Borman (Eds.), *The Oxford handbook of work and aging* (pp. 520–537). New York, NY: Oxford University Press.

Avery, D. R., McKay, P. F., & Wilson, D. C. (2007). Engaging the aging workforce: The relationship between perceived age similarity, satisfaction with coworkers, and employee engagement. *Journal of Applied Psychology*, *92*(6), 1542–1556.

Bäckman, L., & Dixon, R. A. (1992). Psychological compensation: A theoretical framework. *Psychological Bulletin*, *112*(2), 259–283.

Baltes, B. B., & Young, L. M. (2007). Aging and work/family issues. In K. S. Shultz & G. A. Adams (Eds.), *Aging and work in the 21st century* (pp. 251–275). Mahwah, NJ: Lawrence Erlbaum.

Baltes, P. B., & Baltes, M. M. (1990). Psychological perspectives on successful aging: The model of selective optimization with compensation. In P. B. Baltes & M. M. Baltes (Eds.), *Successful aging: Perspectives from the behavioral sciences* (pp. 1–34). New York, NY: Cambridge University Press.

Baltes, P. B., Staudinger, U. M., & Lindenberger, U. (1999). Lifespan psychology: Theory and application to intellectual functioning. *Annual Review of Psychology*, *50*, 471–507.

Blanchflower, D. G., & Oswald, A. J. (2008). Is well-being U-shaped over the life cycle? *Social Science & Medicine*, *66*(8), 1733–1749.

Caplan, R. D., Cobb, S., French, J. R. P., Van Harrison, R. V., & Pinneau, S. R. (1975). *Job demands and worker health: Main effects and occupational differences*. Ann Arbor, MI: Institute for Social Research.

Carstensen, L. L., Isaacowitz, D. M., & Charles, S. T. (1999). Taking time seriously: A theory of socioemotional selectivity. *American Psychologist*, *54*(3), 165–181.

Charles, S. T., & Carstensen, L. L. (2010). Social and emotional aging. *Annual Review of Psychology*, *61*, 383–409.

Cleveland, J. N., Shore, L. M., & Murphy, K. R. (1997). Person- and context-oriented perceptual age measures: Additional evidence of distinctiveness and usefulness. *Journal of Organizational Behavior*, *18*(3), 239–251.

de Jonge, J., & Dormann, C. (2006). Stressors, resources, and strain at work: A longitudinal test of the triple-match principle. *Journal of Applied Psychology*, *91*(5), 1359–1374.

Ebner, N. C., Freund, A. M., & Baltes, P. B. (2006). Developmental changes in personal goal orientation from young to late adulthood: From striving for gains to maintenance and prevention of losses. *Psychology and Aging*, *21*(4), 664–678.

Edwards, J. R. (1991). Person-job fit: A conceptual integration, literature review and methodological critique. In C. L. Cooper & I. T. Robertson (Eds.), *International review of industrial and organizational psychology* (Vol. 6, pp. 283–357). London: Wiley.

Edwards, J. R., Cable, D. M., Williamson, I. O., Lambert, L. S., & Shipp, A. J. (2006). The phenomenology of fit: Linking the person and environment to the subjective experience of person-environment fit. *Journal of Applied Psychology*, *91*(4), 802–827.

Edwards, J. R., Caplan, R. D., & Harrison, R. V. (1998). Person-environment fit theory: Conceptual foundations, empirical evidence, and directions for future research. In C. L. Cooper (Ed.), *Theories of organizational stress* (pp. 28–67). Oxford, UK: Oxford University Press.

Edwards, J. R., & Cooper, C. L. (1990). The person-environment fit approach to stress: Recurring problems and some suggested solutions. *Journal of Organizational Behavior*, *11*(4), 293–307.

Edwards, J. R., & Rothbard, N. P. (1999). Work and family stress and well-being: An examination of person-environment fit in the work and family domains. *Organizational Behavior and Human Decision Processes*, *77*(2), 85–129.

Edwards, J. R., & Shipp, A. J. (2007). The relationship between person-environment fit and outcomes: An integrative theoretical framework. In C. Ostroff & T. A. Judge (Eds.), *Perspectives on organizational fit* (pp. 209–258). San Francisco, CA: Jossey-Bass.

Farr, J. L., & Ringseis, E. L. (2002). The older worker in organizational context: Beyond the individual. In C. L. Cooper & I. T. Robertson (Eds.), *International review of industrial and organizational psychology* (Vol. 17, pp. 31–75). Chichester, UK: Wiley.

Feldman, D. C., & Ng, T. W. H. (2007). Careers: Mobility, embeddedness, and success. *Journal of Management*, *33*(3), 350–377.

Feldman, D. C., Ng, T. W. H., & Vogel, R. M. (2012). Off-the-job embeddedness: A reconceptualization and agenda for future research. In J. J. Martocchio, A. Joshi, & H. Liao (Eds.), *Research in personnel and human resources management* (Vol. 31, pp. 209–251). Research in Personnel and Human Resources Management. Bingley, UK: Emerald Group Publishing Limited.

Feldman, D. C., & Vogel, R. M. (2009). The aging process and person-environment fit. In S. G. Baugh & S. E. Sullivan (Eds.), *Research in careers* (pp. 1–25). Charlotte, NC: Information Age Press.

French, J. R. P., Caplan, R. D., & Van Harrison, R. (1982). *The mechanisms of job stress and strain*. Chichester, UK: Wiley.

Frese, M., Garst, H., & Fay, D. (2007). Making things happen: Reciprocal relationships between work characteristics and personal initiative in a four-wave longitudinal structural equation model. *Journal of Applied Psychology*, *92*(4), 1084–1102.

Freund, A. M., & Baltes, P. B. (2002). Life-management strategies of selection, optimization, and compensation: Measurement by self-report and construct validity. *Journal of Personality and Social Psychology*, *82*(4), 642–662.

Harrison, R. V. (1978). Person-environment fit and job stress. In C. L. Cooper & R. Payne (Eds.), *Stress at work* (pp. 175–205). New York, NY: Wiley.

Hassell, B. L., & Perrewe, P. L. (1995). An examination of beliefs about older workers: Do stereotypes still exist? *Journal of Organizational Behavior*, *16*(5), 457–468.

Heckhausen, J., Wrosch, C., & Schulz, R. (2010). A motivational theory of life-span development. *Psychological Review*, *117*(1), 32–60.

Hedge, J. W., & Borman, W. C. (2012). *The Oxford handbook of work and aging*. New York, NY: Oxford University Press.

Hurrell, J. J., & Lindström, K. (1992). Comparison of job demands, control, and psychosomatic complaints at different career stages of managers in Finland and the United States. *Scandinavian Journal of Work, Environment & Health*, *18*(Suppl. 2), 11–13.

Jansen, K. J., & Shipp, A. J. (2013). A review and agenda for incorporating time in fit research. In J. Billsberry & A. Kristof-Brown (Eds.), *Organizational fit: Key issues and new directions* (pp. 195–221). Chichester, UK: Wiley-Blackwell.

Kanfer, R., & Ackerman, P. L. (2004). Aging, adult development, and work motivation. *Academy of Management Review*, *29*(3), 440–458.

Kanfer, R., Beier, M. E., & Ackerman, P. L. (2013). Goals and motivation related to work in later adulthood: An organizing framework. *European Journal of Work and Organizational Psychology*, *22*(3), 253–264.

Keyes, C. L. M. (2007). Promoting and protecting mental health as flourishing: A complementary strategy for improving national mental health. *American Psychologist*, *62*(2), 95–108.

Klein, H. J., & Weaver, N. A. (2000). The effectiveness of an organizational-level orientation training program in the socialization of new hires. *Personnel Psychology*, *53*(1), 47–66.

Kooij, D. T. A. M., De Lange, A. H., Jansen, P. G. W., & Dikkers, J. S. E. (2013). Beyond chronological age: Examining perceived future time and subjective health as age-related mediators in relation to work-related motivations and well-being. *Work & Stress*, *27*(1), 88–105.

Kooij, D. T. A. M., De Lange, A. H., Jansen, P. G. W., Kanfer, R., & Dikkers, J. S. E. (2011). Age and work-related motives: Results of a meta-analysis. *Journal of Organizational Behavior*, *32*(2), 197–225.

Kristof, A. L. (1996). Person-organization fit: An integrative review of its conceptualizations, measurement and implications. *Personnel Psychology*, *49*(1), 1–49.

Kristof-Brown, A. L., & Billsberry, J. (2013). *Organizational fit: Key issues and new directions*. Chichester, UK: Wiley.

Kristof-Brown, A. L., Zimmerman, R. D., & Johnson, E. C. (2005). Consequences of individuals' fit at work: A meta-analysis of person-job, person-organization, person-group, and person-supervisor fit. *Personnel Psychology*, *58*(2), 281–342.

Lang, F. R., & Carstensen, L. L. (2002). Time counts: Future time perspective, goals, and social relationships. *Psychology and Aging*, *17*(1), 125–139.

Lawrence, B. S. (1988). New wrinkles in the theory of age: Demography, norms, and performance ratings. *Academy of Management Journal*, *31*(2), 309–337.

Lazazzara, A., Karpinska, K., & Henkens, K. (2013). What factors influence training opportunities for older workers? Three factorial surveys exploring the attitudes of HR professionals. *International Journal of Human Resource Management*, *24*(11), 2154–2172.

Lindström, K. (1988). Age-related differences in job characteristics and in their relation to job satisfaction. *Scandinavian Journal of Work, Environment & Health*, *14*(Suppl. 1), 24–26.

Maertens, J. A., Putter, S. E., Chen, P. Y., Diehl, M., & Huang, Y.-H. (2012). Physical capabilities and occupational health of older workers. In J. W. Hedge & W. C. Borman (Eds.), *The Oxford handbook of work and aging* (pp. 215–235). New York, NY: Oxford University Press.

Muchinsky, P. M., & Monahan, C. J. (1987). What is person-environment congruence? Supplementary versus complementary models of fit. *Journal of Vocational Behavior*, *31*(3), 268–277.

Ng, T. W. H., & Feldman, D. C. (2008). The relationship of age to ten dimensions of job performance. *Journal of Applied Psychology*, *93*(2), 392–423.

Ng, T. W. H., & Feldman, D. C. (2010). The relationship of age with job attitudes: A meta-analysis. *Personnel Psychology*, *63*, 667–718.

Ng, T. W. H., & Feldman, D. C. (2012). Evaluating six common stereotypes about older workers with meta-analytical data. *Personnel Psychology*, *65*(4), 821–858.

Ng, T. W. H., & Feldman, D. C. (2013a). Employee age and health. *Journal of Vocational Behavior*, *83*(3), 336–345.

Ng, T. W. H., & Feldman, D. C. (2013b). How do within-person changes due to aging affect job performance? *Journal of Vocational Behavior*, *83*(3), 305–314.

Noonan, A. E. (2005). "At this point now": Older workers' reflections on their current employment experiences. *International Journal of Aging and Human Development*, *61*(3), 211–241.

Ostroff, C., Shin, Y., & Feinberg, B. (2002). Skill acquisition and person-environment fit. In D. C. Feldman (Ed.), *Work careers: A developmental perspective* (pp. 63–90). San Francisco, CA: Jossey-Bass.

Paullay, I. M., Alliger, G. M., & Stone-Romero, E. F. (1994). Construct validation of two instruments designed to measure job involvement and work centrality. *Journal of Applied Psychology*, *79*(2), 224–228.

Perry, E. L., Dokko, G., & Golom, F. D. (2012). The aging worker and person–environment fit. In J. W. Hedge & W. C. Borman (Eds.), *The Oxford handbook of work and aging* (pp. 187–212). New York, NY: Oxford University Press.

Pitt-Catsouphes, M., Matz-Costa, C., & James, J. (2012). *Through a different looking glass: The prism of age*. Chestnut Hill, MA: Sloan Center on Aging & Work, Boston College.

Posthuma, R. A., & Campion, M. A. (2009). Age stereotypes in the workplace: Common stereo-types, moderators, and future research directions. *Journal of Management*, *35*(1), 158–188.

Rauschenbach, C., Krumm, S., Thielgen, M. M., & Hertel, G. (2013). Age and work-related stress: A review and meta-analysis. *Journal of Managerial Psychology*, *28*(7–8), 781–804.

Roberts, B. W., Walton, K. E., & Viechtbauer, W. (2006). Patterns of mean-level change in personality traits across the life course: A meta-analysis of longitudinal studies. *Psychological Bulletin*, *132*(1), 1–25.

Salthouse, T. (2012). Consequences of age-related cognitive declines. *Annual Review of Psychology*, *63*, 201–226.

Scheibe, S., & Carstensen, L. L. (2010). Emotional aging: Recent findings and future trends. *The Journals of Gerontology Series B: Psychological Sciences and Social Sciences*, *65*(2), 135–144.

Scheibe, S., & Zacher, H. (2013). A lifespan perspective on emotion regulation, stress, and well-being in the workplace. In P. L. Perrewé, C. C. Rosen, & J. Halbesleben (Eds.), *The role of emotion and emotion regulation in job stress and well being* (Vol. 11, pp. 167–197). Research in Occupational Stress and Well-Being. Bingley, UK: Emerald Group Publishing Limited.

Schmitt, A., Zacher, H., & Frese, M. (2012). The buffering effect of selection, optimization, and compensation strategy use on the relationship between problem solving demands and occupational well-being: A daily diary study. *Journal of Occupational Health Psychology*, *17*(2), 139–149.

Schwall, A. R. (2012). Defining age and using age-relevant constructs. In J. W. Hedge & W. C. Borman (Eds.), *The Oxford handbook of work and aging* (pp. 169–186). New York, NY: Oxford University Press.

Shipp, A. J., & Jansen, K. J. (2011). Reinterpreting time in fit theory: Crafting and recrafting narratives of fit in medias res. *Academy of Management Review*, *36*(1), 76–101.

Tsui, A. S., & O'Reilly, C. A. (1989). Beyond simple demographic effects: The importance of relational demography in superior-subordinate dyads. *Academy of Management Journal*, *32*(2), 402–423.

Tsui, A. S., Porter, L. W., & Egan, T. D. (2002). When both similarities and dissimilarities matter: Extending the concept of relational demography. *Human Relations*, *55*(8), 899–929.

von Hippel, C., Kalokerinos, E. K., & Henry, J. D. (2012). Stereotype threat among older employees: Relationships with job attitudes and turnover intentions. *Psychology and Aging*, *28*(1), 17–27.

Warr, P. B. (2001). Age and work behaviour: Physical attributes, cognitive abilities, knowledge, personality traits and motives. In C. L. Cooper & I. T. Robertson (Eds.), *International review of industrial and organizational psychology* (Vol. 16, pp. 1–36). Chichester, UK: Wiley.

Warr, P. B., Miles, A., & Platts, C. (2001). Age and personality in the British population between 16 and 64 years. *Journal of Occupational and Organizational Psychology*, *74*(2), 165–199.

Weigl, M., Müller, A., Hornung, S., Zacher, H., & Angerer, P. (2013). The moderating effects of job control and selection, optimization, and compensation strategies on the age-work ability relationship. *Journal of Organizational Behavior*, *34*(5), 607–628.

Weiss, A., King, J. E., Inoue-Murayama, M., Matsuzawa, T., & Oswald, A. J. (2012). Evidence for a midlife crisis in great apes consistent with the U-shape in human well-being. *Proceedings of the National Academy of Sciences*, *109*(49), 19949–19952.

White, A. T., & Spector, P. E. (1987). An investigation of age-related factors in the age-job satisfaction relationship. *Psychology and Aging*, *2*(3), 261–265.

World Health Organization. (2004). *Promoting mental health: Concepts, emerging evidence, practice*. Summary report. Geneva, Switzerland.

Zacher, H., & Frese, M. (2009). Remaining time and opportunities at work: Relationships between age, work characteristics, and occupational future time perspective. *Psychology and Aging*, *24*(2), 487–493.

Zacher, H., & Frese, M. (2011). Maintaining a focus on opportunities at work: The interplay between age, job complexity, and the use of selection, optimization, and compensation strategies. *Journal of Organizational Behavior*, *32*(2), 291–318.

Zacher, H., Jimmieson, N. L., & Winter, G. (2012). Eldercare demands, mental health, and work performance: The moderating role of satisfaction with eldercare tasks. *Journal of Occupational Health Psychology*, *17*(1), 52–64.

Zacher, H., Rosing, K., Henning, T., & Frese, M. (2011). Establishing the next generation at work: Leader generativity as a moderator of the relationships between leader age, leader-member exchange, and leadership success. *Psychology and Aging*, *26*(1), 241–252.

AGE, RESILIENCE, WELL-BEING, AND POSITIVE WORK OUTCOMES

Rachel King and Steve Jex

ABSTRACT

While well-being and resilience in the workplace continue to be important areas of research, the role age plays in well-being and resilience at work and associated positive work outcomes is often ignored. In most studies age is simply treated as a control variable. In this chapter, we outline the importance of considering age in well-being and resilience research by focusing on how age may impact both of these variables and drawing on research from both the organizational psychology and developmental psychology literature. Theoretical models of these relationships are put forth, and future research directions are discussed.

Keywords: Well-being; resilience; coping; occupational health psychology; positive work outcomes; age

While well-being and resilience in the workplace continue to be important areas of research, the role age plays in well-being and resilience at work and associated positive work outcomes is often ignored because it is typically treated as a control variable with little conceptual importance. In this

The Role of Demographics in Occupational Stress and Well Being
Research in Occupational Stress and Well Being, Volume 12, 113–133

ISSN: 1479-3555/doi:10.1108/S1479-355520140000012003

chapter we seek to outline the importance of considering age in this type of research by describing how age may impact both well-being and resilience in the workplace. We will draw on research from both the organizational psychology and developmental psychology literatures. By taking this interdisciplinary perspective, we hope to draw the attention of the occupational stress and well-being researcher to the importance of age in this field and relevant research that is being done in other fields.

We will begin the chapter by defining the current age demographics of the workforce and the unique challenges and opportunities this provides for researchers in Occupational Health Psychology (OHP). We will then discuss how the workforce is aging at a rapid rate with the pending retirement of the Baby Boomers in the United States and with the aging of the global population. We then will outline our theoretical model of the mechanisms by which age impacts well-being and resilience. We propose that age is an antecedent to high levels of well-being, which leads to positive work outcomes. We know from the developmental literature that subjective well-being (SWB) increases with age (Diener, Suh, Lucas, & Smith, 1999) which parallels the finding that job satisfaction, a component of well-being at work, increases with age (Ng & Feldman, 2010), theories such as discrepancy theory, downward social comparison (George, 2010), and the demands-control model (Karasek, 1979) will be examined to explain why older workers have higher levels of well-being at work, which in turn leads to positive outcomes such as increased organizational citizenship behaviors (OCB) and decreased turnover.

We also propose that coping, control, and sense of coherence are mediators between age and increased resilience, as older adults have had more life experiences, and as a result may have developed more coping resources to have at their disposal, which impacts positive outcomes such as post traumatic growth and lower levels of job stress.

AGE

Age is becoming more important to study within OHP because the global workforce is aging which provides unique challenges and opportunities for researchers. The number of people who are 65 or above in the U.S. workforce increased 101 percent between 1977 and 2007, whereas the overall workforce only increased 59 percent (U.S. Bureau of Labor Statistics, 2008). This trend is mirrored in the global population as well

(Kinsella & Phillips, 2005). In the United States this is at least partially due to the aging of the Baby Boomer cohort, and globally it is partially due similar population booms in other industrialized countries. Advances in health care have also contributed to the aging population in industrialized countries, and developing countries are beginning to follow suit (Kinsella & Phillips, 2005). Although the Baby Boomers are beginning to retire, many of them are waiting longer to do so than in previous generations.

There are a variety of reasons that aging workers are waiting longer to retire including both financial and personal reasons. For example, in the United States some of these financial reasons include changes in social security policy, or needing to continue to receive employer sponsored health care benefits (Rogowski & Karoly, 2000). Older workers are also delaying retirement for personal reasons. Some older workers are choosing to partially retire or engage in what is known as bridge employment. Bridge employment can take the form of fewer at hours at current job, or sometimes a part-time job with a new employer. This allows older workers to adapt to retirement more gradually and has been shown to have health benefits for those who choose a more gradual retirement (Cahill, Giandrea, & Quinn, 2012).

This gradual increase in the number of older workers has led OHP researchers to examine the impact of age on important outcomes such as employee health (Jex, Wang, & Zarubin, 2007), job satisfaction (Kacmar & Ferris, 1989), and job performance (Waldman & Avolio, 1986). This also has important implications for policy makers and public health as older workers may require additional accommodations or have more health care needs than younger workers.

Who is an Older Worker?

In any discussion of aging workers it is important to distinguish what exactly constitutes an "older worker." There has been disagreement in past research within industrial-organizational psychology as to when someone should be considered an older worker. Some researchers have used 40 and older as the definition of an older worker (Hansson, DeKoekkoek, Neece, & Patterson, 1997). This is primarily due to the Age Discrimination in Employment Act of 1967 which protects those 40 or older from employment discrimination in the United States. However, developmental psychologists often consider 65 as the beginning of old age, and research incorporating developmental theories into OHP research may not find the expected results if they include mostly middle age participants in their sample of older workers. Sixty-five was also once considered the appropriate age to retire, but more recently the retirement age has been shifting upward. Past research has used different minimum ages to distinguish older workers from younger workers, and future research should ensure that the rationale for choosing one cut-point over another is theoretically justified. Because this chapter incorporates developmental theories we will be defining an older worker as someone with a chronological age of 50 and older. This cut-point takes into consideration that many 65 year olds are no longer in the workforce, and past research has used this cut-point to define an older worker. Workers in this age group are also closer to retirement age and are more likely to spend time thinking about and planning their retirement as they get closer to being eligible to retire (Ekerdt, Kosloski, & DeViney, 2000). This is also in agreement with large, longitudinal panel studies of aging such as the Health and Retirement study (Hodes & Suzman, 2007). To fully understand the definition of an older worker we must also discuss the measurement of age.

Operationalization of Age

The most common operationalization of age is *chronological age*, which is quite simply time since birth measured in years. Chronological age is most commonly assessed by asking one's age in years or one's birthdate, which the researcher can use to calculate years or days since birth. While chronological age can be measured much more accurately than many constructs in our field, the value of chronological age is limited because it is only a proxy for other more substantive predictors such as experience and other changes one might experience through the lifespan. At the same time, it is certainly not a *perfect* proxy for these substantive changes associated with age. Therefore, chronological age may not be the most appropriate operationalization of age in all situations, and one must be cautious when drawing conclusions based on this measure.

Although the bulk of the research we will be reviewing in this chapter focuses on chronological age, it is important to recognize that age is also both a *psychological* and a *social* variable. Psychological age represents how old one *feels* and has been referred to in the literature by a number of different labels including subjective age (Berg, 2007) and identity age (Barak & Stern, 1986). Psychological age is important not only because it is part of a person's psychological identity, but it also impacts the way people present themselves to others in the workplace and in other social situations (Rioux & Mokounkolo, 2011). Thus, even when people are getting older chronologically, psychologically they may see themselves as much younger than their chronological age and project this to others in social situations.

If we view age as a social variable, this reflects the age-related perceptions that others may have of a particular individual (Kastenbaum, Derbin, Sabatini, & Artt, 1972). Often it is difficult to determine the chronological age of another person, but we typically try to do so based on their appearance and other cues (e.g., information they reveal to us). Social age is important primarily because it impacts the way other people are treated. As far as impacting well-being, we surmise that the congruence between a person's psychological age and their social age is an important issue. We will have more to say about this issue in the final section of the chapter.

Developmental Differences between Older and Younger Workers

To better understand how age impacts research, we must first understand the developmental effects of aging. Older workers differ developmentally from younger workers in several ways. One of the most frequently discussed developmental differences in the aging literature is the difference in cognitive ability between older and younger workers. Research has shown that older adults do have some difficulty with tasks that require retention of large amounts of information or rapid cognitive processing (Salthouse, 1993). Older workers tend to have less capacity in their working memory, or fluid intelligence, than their younger counterparts, but they have more knowledge, or crystalized intelligence (Park, 2000). Although there is a cognitive decline in working memory as people age, this is compensated for by a greater store of knowledge. For example, an older worker faced with a challenging task at work may choose to use his or her knowledge of previous times he or she has overcome a similar challenge and draw on a store of information about the job and the field, while a younger worker faced with the same problem will use his or her working memory to solve the same problem. The older worker does not show a decline in performance because he or she has a much greater store of knowledge than the younger worker. The older and younger workers solve the problem using different methodologies, but both are, on average, equally successful at solving problems and performing their jobs.

While changes in cognitive ability do not directly impact well-being they indirectly impact the well-being of older workers through perceptions of age discrimination. Both evidence for cognitive decline and stereotypes of older workers have led some to suggest that older workers perform their jobs less effectively than younger workers, but this is not supported by empirical evidence. Meta-analytic correlations suggest that job performance does not decrease with age (Waldman & Avolio, 1986), and thus older workers appear to be just as capable of performing their jobs as younger workers. However, some research has shown that when older workers have performance errors, younger raters are more likely to attribute the errors of older workers to age (Rupp, Vodanovich, & Credé, 2006) and suggest harsher sanctions. Because errors made by older workers are seen as stable and age related, younger coworkers and managers may be more likely to attribute errors to age, which can lead to age discrimination. This has important implications for the well-being of older workers because older workers who perceive that they are discriminated against based on their age tend to have lower levels of well-being (Garstka, Schmitt, Branscombe, & Hummert, 2004).

Research has also revealed differences in physical health between older and younger workers. Older workers tend to show declines in physiological functioning. One example of this is older workers are more likely to have functional limitations (Greenfield & Marks, 2007). They also experience slower metabolism, decreased muscle mass and bone density, and decreased lung capacity (Jex et al., 2007). These physiological changes can make it more difficult for older worker to engage in work that is physically demanding.

Because of these developmental differences, it is important to study this population in the workforce, as they have a different experience from younger workers. It is also important to understand how we as researchers can improve the lives of older workers by understanding how age impacts the workplace experience. We will focus specifically on the well-being and resilience of older workers in this chapter.

WELL-BEING

Well-being is a more recent area of study for both OHP and the field of psychology as a whole. Well-being can refer specifically to psychological well-being or it can be extended to include concepts such as physical well-being and social integration. We will begin by discussing psychological well-being and then move to physical well-being. Then we will outline the relationships between these types of well-being and age before moving into theoretical rationales for why these relationships exist.

There are two main ways of operationalizing psychological well-being depending on the research question being asked. SWB is often measured using a composite of positive and negative affect along with overall life satisfaction, and is considered a global evaluation of well-being. Experienced Well-being (EWB) is measured using Experience Sampling Methods or Day Reconstruction Methods and focuses on well-being at the moment of evaluation (Diener, 2000). EWB is an evaluation of well-being at the moment of assessment and usually measured longitudinally to examine fluctuations in well-being in relation to other variables.

There are benefits to both measurement techniques. EWB is subject to less error and allows researchers to examine more proximal outcomes, but it is time and resource intensive to collect this data. SWB is subject to more error, but is more global, less expensive, and can be measured at one time point. The type of well-being that is measured is often dependent on the hypotheses being examined.

It is also important to point out that psychological well-being can also be viewed as a construct that encompasses different domains of satisfaction. Some of the proposed domains include family, leisure, health, finances, and job satisfaction (Diener et al., 1999). Because job satisfaction is a frequently measured construct within the field of industrial-organizational psychology, we feel it is important to distinguish it from overall well-being for the purposes of this chapter. While job satisfaction can be conceptualized as a domain satisfaction, job satisfaction and SWB are distinct constructs with a reciprocal relationship (Judge & Watanabe, 1993). Engagement is another conceptualization of psychological well-being that we will briefly touch on in this chapter.

Physical well-being can be conceptualized as one's objective and subjective health. Objective measures of health can include information such as chronic health conditions, physiological measures, such as blood pressure and grip strength, and inventories of functional limitations. Functional limitations can be measured by asking about Instrumental Activities of Daily Living (IADL; Lawton & Brody, 1968); these are daily activities such as preparing meals, getting dressed, and paying bills. This provides a clear picture of the functional limitations associated with age.

Objective measures reflect the health of an individual with a great deal of accuracy; however, measures of subjective health have been shown to be more strongly correlated with other measures of well-being than objective health (Diener et al., 1999). Subjective health consists of self-rated health, and one's perception of one's health. Thus, it is important for researchers to capture how individuals perceive their health in addition to collecting physiological measures to obtain a more complete picture of physical well-being.

Age and Job Satisfaction

Job satisfaction is a component of domain satisfaction. Meta-analytic correlations have found that global job satisfaction is positively related with age (Ng & Feldman, 2010). This holds even in studies that have controlled for tenure (Kacmar & Ferris, 1989; Ng & Feldman, 2010). This indicates that older workers are more satisfied with their jobs than their younger counterparts for reasons other than just tenure.

There are many potential reasons for this positive relationship between age and job satisfaction. For example, older employees typically earn more than younger employees, and may be more likely to be in jobs that provide them with high levels of autonomy and flexibility. Of course another explanation, which is based on Social Information Processing Theory (Salancik & Pfeffer, 1978), is that higher satisfaction is way to justify a long commitment to a job or career.

The relationship between age and job satisfaction is a little less clear at the facet level of job satisfaction. Job satisfaction is frequently broken into facets to cover the different domains of work. One of the most commonly used measures of job satisfaction, the Job Descriptive Index (JDI; Smith, Kendall, & Hulin, 1969) breaks job satisfaction into *coworker satisfaction, work satisfaction, supervisor satisfaction, pay satisfaction,* and *promotion satisfaction*. Barnes-Farrell and Matthews (2007) found conflicting evidence for the direction of the relationship between the facets of job satisfaction and age in their review of the literature. More research is needed to determine the relationship and potential moderators of the relationship between the facets of job satisfaction and age.

Age and Engagement

Another form of well-being that has become a recent favorite among researchers and practitioners is engagement. Engagement is typically conceptualized as a higher order construct consisting of three sub dimensions *vigor*, *dedication*, and *absorption* (Bakker, Schaufeli, Leiter, & Taris, 2008; Schaufeli, Salanova, González-Romá, & Bakker, 2002). Vigor is typically described as the amount of energy one puts forth at work. Dedication describes one's enthusiasm for the work and the significance one places in the work. Finally, absorption deals with being fully engrossed in one's work. Engagement has a positive relationship with age; however, this relationship is somewhat weak (Schaufeli, Bakker, & Salanova, 2006). Most likely this is due to the fact that older employees may hold jobs that are higher level and thus provide many features that facilitate engagement. The relationship between engagement and age may be a small relationship, but it is an additional conceptualization of well-being that does increase with age.

Age and Subjective Well-Being

The relationship between age and well-being has been well established in the developmental literature, and is treated as a variable of interest rather than a control variable. We will be focusing in this chapter on contrasting older employees with younger employees in terms well-being as opposed to describing the process by which well-being changes over the course of one's life. We will also focus on SWB rather than EWB, as SWB is more commonly used in the OHP literature, and EWB is still an emerging area of research.

As was previously mentioned, SWB is a higher order construct composed of positive affect, negative affect, and life satisfaction. Affect consists of both positive and negative affects. These two components are independent of each other and both contribute to well-being (Diener & Emmons, 1984). Life satisfaction is a global assessment of one's satisfaction with life and also contributes to SWB (Diener, Emmons, Larsen, & Griffin, 1985).

SWB is higher in older adults (Diener et al., 1999), which parallels the finding that job satisfaction, a component of well-being at work, is also higher in older adults (Ng & Feldman, 2010). There is still some disagreement about why well-being increases with age, although multiple theories have been put forth. One potential mechanism, downward social comparison (Wills, 1981), proposes that when an individual experiences negative affect that individual can enhance his or her well-being by comparing themselves to a less fortunate referent other. In the case of older workers downward social comparison may take the form of comparing oneself to a coworker who did not attain as many careers goals, or a coworker who has recently lost a job.

Another potential mechanism is described by discrepancy theory (Campbell, Converse, & Rodgers, 1976). According to this theory, well-being is at its highest when the discrepancy between one's goals and one's achievements is small. Cheng (2004) examined this as a mechanism through which age impacts well-being and found that this accounted for much of the variance in the age – well-being relationship as older workers tend to have smaller discrepancies than their younger counterparts. This could be due to re-evaluating one's goals as time passes and revising them to be more proximal and attainable.

Additionally the demands-control model (Karasek, 1979) may be a mechanism through which age impacts well-being (Van der Doef & Maes, 1999). This model postulates that a mismatch between the level of job demands and decision latitude, or control, in a job will lead to strain in an employee; the most stressful jobs are those with high job demands and low control (e.g., "high strain jobs"). Jobs that are low on both demands and decision latitude are considered "passive jobs" and will not provide opportunities for growth or the development of new skills. However, jobs that are high on both demands and decision latitude, "active jobs," will challenge an employee and allow them to develop new skills and increase their well-being.

Because older workers on average have longer tenure and more senior positions than younger workers, we expect that they are more likely to be employed in active jobs, such as managerial positions, than younger workers who are still learning the ropes and may be in positions that are passive jobs or possibly high strain jobs. This may contribute to an increase in job satisfaction and SWB in older workers who have jobs that are not as strain inducing and allow them to have more control over their work despite having high levels of demand. These workers may also be more engaged because their jobs provide opportunities for them to experience absorption, vigor, and dedication.

One of the reasons there has been a recent interest in SWB within the OHP community is that it leads to positive outcomes for both the employee and the employer. We briefly mention two positive work outcomes, lower turnover and organizational citizenship behaviors as examples of potential positive outcomes although there are many other positive outcomes of SWB such as job satisfaction and higher levels of self-rated health (Diener et al., 1999).

Age and Physical Health

Subjective health is important to examine in older workers because it is related to psychological well-being, and captures additional variance in physical well-being. Objective health is also a major concern in relation to older workers; older adults are more prone to chronic conditions and functional limitations that can lead to avoidable hospitalizations (Wolff, Starfield, & Anderson, 2002) than younger adults. The number of older adults with functional limitations is increasing, and they are living longer (Greenfield & Marks, 2007). There are many physiological functions that deteriorate with age. On average, as people age they cannot metabolize carbohydrates as well as younger people, they have less bone density, their level of cognitive functionality decreases, and it becomes more difficult for them to perform daily tasks (Rowe & Kahn, 1987). As people age they are generally able to do fewer of these tasks and their mobility decreases, although most individuals will have left the workforce before losing the ability to perform most of the these tasks.

The deterioration of physical health is what Rowe and Kahn (1987) refer to as usual aging. In contrast, they defined successful aging as being characterized by a below average level of physiological deterioration and above average levels of autonomy and functionality. A person who is aging successfully will be at a lower risk for disease, will have a high level of mobility and cognitive function, and can be classified as having a high level of physical well-being.

Subjective Well-Being and Positive Workplace Outcomes

Past research has proposed a link between well-being and various positive workplace outcomes such as lower turnover (Wright & Bonett, 2007) and OCB, which are extra role behaviors by the employee that benefit either the organization or an individual within the organization (Griffeth, Hom, & Gaertner, 2000; Smith, Organ, & Near, 1983). Because previous research has established the relationship between age and well-being, and the relationship between well-being and these positive work outcomes, we expect that age impact these outcomes through the mechanism of well-being. Specifically, we expect that older workers will have higher well-being, which will in turn lead to positive outcomes. Our model situates well-being as a mediator of the relationship between age and these outcomes. The proposed model is illustrated in Fig. 1.

By examining age as an antecedent to well-being and, indirectly, as an antecedent to positive work outcomes, we can begin to highlight the importance of taking age into consideration and not treating as an insignificant

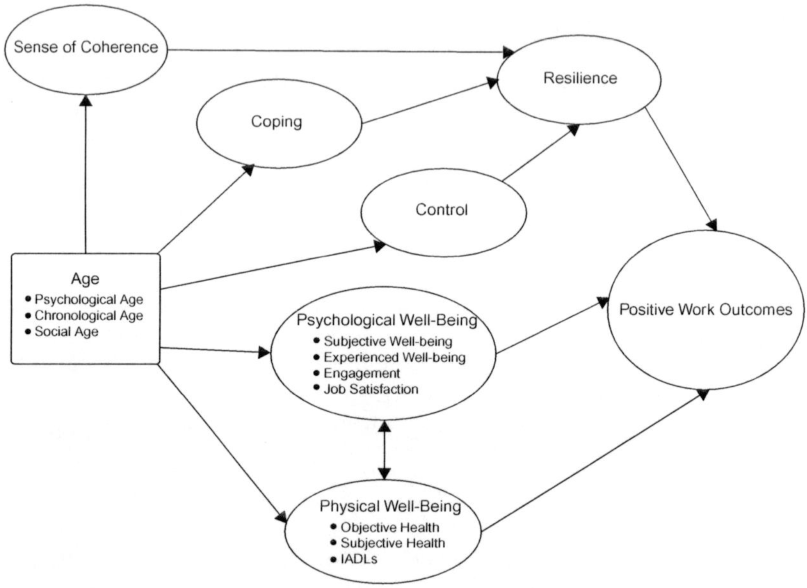

Fig. 1. Proposed Relationships among Constructs.

demographic variable. In the next section, we will focus on the impact of age on resilience in the workplace.

RESILIENCE

Resilience represents one's capacity to successfully cope with stressors in the work or non-work environment (Jex, Kain, & Park, 2013). Those who are highly resilient seemed to be unaffected or even thrive in the face of stressors, while those who are less resilient exhibit symptoms of strain. Although being resilient can protect one from a variety of stressors, research in this area has focused on traumatic stressors such as the death of a loved one (Bonanno, 2004) or being exposed to combat during military operations (Schaubroeck, Riolli, Peng, & Spain, 2011).

Research on resilience has tended to focus on two broad categories of predictors: (1) individual differences and (2) situational predictors. The primary individual difference variable that has been shown to predict resilience is hardiness (Kobasa, 1979), which is a personality trait characterized by a heightened sense of perceived control, a high level of commitment, and a view that stressors are challenges rather than threats. More recently resilience researchers have begun to focus on a concept called Trait Psychological Capital (Luthans, Avolio, Avey, & Norman, 2007), which is a conglomeration of the traits of optimism, hope, and ego resilience. Research on situational predictors of resilience has focused heavily on socially supportive environments (Cohen & Wills, 1985), as well as organizational interventions to train resilience (Reivich, Seligman, & McBride, 2011).

Since resilience has both trait and situational predictors, this suggests that although there is likely to be some stability in a person's resilience over time, it can also change. For example, a person may possess the psychological traits associated with resilience, yet at some point in their lives lose some of the supportive relationships that may contribute to resilience. From a methodological point of view, this suggests that there is some value in examining *changes* in resilience over a person's lifetime, even though some predictors of resilience will remain relatively stable.

For the most part, age has largely been ignored as a *predictor* of resilience although studies have investigated differences in resilience *within* older aged cohorts (e.g., Felton, 2000; McEwen, 2003). Jex et al. (2007) suggest that many of the cognitive and physical changes associated with aging tend to make older employees *less* resilient in the face of certain types of stress such as physical demands, increases in the pace of work, and increases in the speed of processing necessary to complete the work.

It is also possible, however, that with increased aging comes *increased* resilience in the face other types of stressors that are encountered in the workplace. The reason for this, we believe, is that as people age they acquire a wide variety of work-related experiences; some of these are satisfying and some of them are experienced as stressful. This heighted experience serves older employees in two ways. First, since older employees know the work-related experiences that have led to satisfaction they will be more likely to seek out those experiences and self-select into work environments that provide them.

Secondly, stressful experiences can also be helpful in the development of resilience in older employees. As pointed out by Britt and Jex (2015), stressors in the workplace lead to employee strain, but at the same time also help employees develop resources that facilitate resilience. According to Conservation of Resources (COR) Theory (Hobfoll, 1989), people's ability to successfully cope with stressful situations depends on their ability to develop or acquire the emotional and behavioral resources to do so. While stressful experiences are certainly "resource depleting" in the sense that they require the expenditure of resources in order to successfully cope, that are also potentially "resource enhancing" because they provide people with the opportunity to learn successful ways to cope.

Since older employees have likely experienced a greater variety of stressors, and experienced them over a long period of time, they have had the opportunity to try out different coping responses and see which of these are most effective. From a COR Theory perspective, what we are arguing is that for many older workers the sum total of their working experiences has left them with a "positive balance" when it comes to the resources needed to cope with stressors in the work environment. Those older employees who may have a negative resource balance, or who are less successful in their coping efforts, may possibly self-select out of the workforce through early retirement or simply reduce their commitment to work.

In addition to facilitating effective coping responses, experiencing stressors over a long period of time may also increase older employees' sense of control when they experience similar stressors in the present timeframe. According to Fox and Spector (2006), a sense of control impacts the stress process in two ways. First, a heightened sense of control makes it less likely that conditions in the work environment will be perceived as stressors. For example, if one has an impending deadline yet feels they can rearrange their work so they can meet this impending deadline, it will not be perceived as a stressor. Secondly, a heightened sense of control attenuates stressor–strain relationships. For example, if one perceives a high level of role ambiguity in their job, yet feels as though they have a high level of control over their work, they will be able to take steps to clarify job responsibility and thus will be less likely to exhibit strain responses.

A final mechanism by which resilience may increase with age is suggested by Antonovsky's (1979) Sense of Coherence (SOC) Theory. According to SOC Theory, coping with stress is enhanced by three interrelated sets of beliefs. First is the belief that what happens in people's lives has some structure, order, and predictability; in other words, things in life make sense. Second is the belief that one has the resources and capabilities to meet the challenges one may face in life. Third is the belief that the demands one faces in life are challenges that one is able to overcome. According to Antonovsky, when a person has these three sets of beliefs this represents a high SOC, which ultimately facilitates coping with the stressors one may face in their lives. Although Antonovsky proposed that SOC developed during adolescence, and stabilizes during early adulthood, there is very little evidence supporting or refuting this proposition.

Thus, we propose that for some individuals there may be an increased SOC with increased age. Specifically, as many people get older they may look back and recognize that things in life have ultimately worked out as they had hoped which increases their perceptions that there is some order and predictability in the world. To the extent that they have successfully coped with the stressors in their lives, this increases both the perception that they can successfully cope in the future, as well as the view that stressors are challenges, which they can overcome. We hasten add, however, that little empirical work has examine changes in SOC over the lifespan so what we are proposing certainly needs to tested in future research.

In essence what we are arguing is that older employees have a greater potential to develop three of the most important resources that are needed to achieve a high level of well-being and resilience; coping responses, perceptions of control and a sense of coherence about things that happen in their lives. As an example, if an older employee experiences interpersonal conflict with a fellow employee, the fact that he or she has likely experienced this stressor numerous times in the past gives this person a greater sense of control over this situation. Furthermore, if he or she has been able to successfully resolve conflict in the past, this provides coping resources that can be brought to bear on the present situation. A high SOC may result in the view that conflict is a normal part of life, as well as similar beliefs regarding the ability to cope with this potential stressor. What we are arguing, in essence, is that perceptions of control, coping, and SOC mediate the relationship between age and resilience (see Fig. 1).

METHODOLOGICAL CONSIDERATIONS

Studying age as a predictor can present methodological challenges for a variety of reasons. As we previously discussed, there are a variety of ways to operationalize age and some research participants may differ on the relationship between their chronological age and their psychological or social age. This can also vary by field or organization, and can be especially problematic in stereotypically younger jobs due to prototype matching.

Prototype matching (Perry & Finkelstein, 1999) is the idea that jobs should be filled by individuals who fit the prototype for the job. For example, an entry-level job is seen as being appropriately filled by a young adult just beginning his or her career. Likewise, an upper level management position is seen as being most appropriate for a middle-aged employee with experience. Because jobs in technology industries, for example, are prototyped as younger jobs (Kanter, 1994), even a manager who is in a position that is appropriate for his or her age may still experience more discrimination due to his or her industry than a manager in an industry that is not seen as a young industry. This can present a measurement problem if one is studying chronological age in a situation where social age and prototype matching play strong roles in how age is perceived.

It is also important for researchers to examine age-related findings longitudinally. When studying age cross-sectionally it is difficult to parse variance due to cohort from variance due to age. By looking at the impact of age using longitudinal designs it is possible to examine changes in well-being and resilience within person across time to better understand the impact of age apart from the impact of cohort. However, attrition is an important issue to consider when conducting longitudinal studies of aging. The oldest workers are the most likely to drop out of a study, and workers with poor health or lower job satisfaction are more likely to retire early. Health can also be a barrier data collection, as some individuals who struggle with daily activities may have difficulty completing a survey or interview.

Some older workers may be making the decision to retire and leave the workforce because working is no longer providing them with enhanced well-being and positive outcomes (Wang & Shultz, 2010), or they may have already begun to pull away from work in anticipation of retirement making it difficult to collect data from them. If we as researchers are only able to sample the older workers who are most satisfied with their jobs and have the highest level of well-being, we may be finding inaccurate results. Additionally, older workers are harder to collect data on as student samples contain very few older workers, if any, and even data collection within an organization may lead to an imbalance in the number of older and younger workers sampled, depending on the demographics of the organization.

In addition to longitudinal and sampling concerns, researchers should also ensure that they are clear on how they are operationalizing well-being in their research. The term "well-being," as we have previously discussed, is used to describe a variety of related constructs that all have slightly different relationships with important outcomes. It is important for researchers to use the correct operationalization of well-being for their research question.

FUTURE DIRECTIONS FOR RESEARCH

Researchers can begin to more fully acknowledge the role of age and the importance of examining it in the context of well-being and resilience in the workplace simply by treating it as a substantive variable of interest instead of merely a control variable. Because age is a proxy for so many important variables, such as changes in health and cognitive processes it is important to include this variable in research. Furthermore, even when adding these changes into one's model, age still accounts for additional variance as it captures developmental changes and additional nuances. Instead of controlling for age, researchers should begin to hypothesize why age and the consequences of aging will impact their variables of interest, and include this among their findings instead of relegating age as something to be controlled for, unless the relationship between age and the variables in question has already been established. With any discussion of control variables it is important to acknowledge that variables should not be controlled for in an effort to "purify" the data (Spector & Brannick, 2011). Therefore, if the relationship among age and the other variables in a model has not been established, researchers should take the time to build hypotheses based on theory and include age in their model.

A second important recommendation for future research on age and well-being is to broaden the operationalization of age. As we point out earlier in the chapter, age is not only a chronological variable but a psychological and social one as well. It would be interesting, for example, to investigate the convergence between an older employee's psychological age and the way that their age is perceived by their coworkers (e.g., social age). We suspect strong convergence between psychological and social age would enhance well-being, while poor convergence (e.g., an employee feels younger than he or she is perceived by others) would reduce it.

Another ripe area for future research would be to examine the mechanisms that mediate the relationship between age and resilience. As we pointed out in the previous section, resilience is a key to older employees being able to thrive and maintain their well-being in the face of stressors so it is important to understand how age may enhance or detract from it. We proposed that increased age may lead to a heightened sense of control over stressors, as well as the development of effective coping responses. It is certainly possible, however, that other mediating mechanisms may exist as well and thus future research is needed to explore this issue.

Future research should also examine organizational moderators of the relationship between age and well-being. For example, examining how the level of age discrimination within an organization could potentially moderate the relationship between age and well-being. Perceived age discrimination is an individual's perceptions of age discrimination across situations. It is correlated with lower well-being in older adults (Garstka et al., 2004). It is also correlated with lower affective commitment to the organization (Snape & Redman, 2006). This suggests that older workers who feel discriminated against feel less of an obligation to stay with their organization, which could increase turnover costs for the organization. In light of this, does working for an organization with a culture of age discrimination result in a negative relationship between age and well-being? More generally, does working for an organization that values the contributions of older employees result in a positive relationship between age and well-being? By examining moderators such as these, researchers can help shed some light on how age plays a role in this field as well as design interventions that could potentially increase the well-being of older workers.

Finally, it is important to expand our understanding of the impact of age on important outcomes such as motivation and OCB through the mechanism of SWB. This will help researchers better understand the importance of incorporating age into models not only within the field of OHP, but also within the broader fields of I/O psychology and organizational behavior as well. As the global population continues to age, it will become crucial for all types of organizational researchers to better understand the impact of age so that we can prepare for the aging of the workforce and improve the health and well-being of older workers.

REFERENCES

Antonovsky, A. (1979). *Health, stress, and coping*. San Francisco, CA: Jossey-Bass.

Bakker, A. B., Schaufeli, W. B., Leiter, M. P., & Taris, T. W. (2008). Work engagement: An emerging concept in occupational health psychology. *Work & Stress*, *22*(3), 187–200.

Barak, B., & Stern, B. (1986). Subjective age correlates: A research note. *Gerontologist*, *26*, 571–578.

Barnes-Farrell, J. L., & Matthews, R. A. (2007). Age and work attitudes. In K. S. Shultz & G. A. Adams (Eds.), *Aging and work in the 21st century* (pp. 139–162). Mahwah, NJ: Lawrence Erlbaum.

Berg, J. A. (2007). Subjective age identity during the transition to adulthood: Psychological and sociological perspectives. *Social Thought and Research*, *28*, 145–163.

Bonanno, G. (2004). Loss, trauma, and human resilience. *American Psychologist*, *59*, 20–28.

Britt, T. D., & Jex, S. M. (2015). *Thriving under stress: Harnessing the demands of the modern workplace*. New York, NY: Oxford University Press.

Cahill, K. E., Giandrea, M. D., & Quinn, J. F. (2012). Bridge employment. In M. Wang (Ed.), *The oxford handbook of retirement* (pp. 293–310). New York, NY: Oxford University Press.

Campbell, A., Converse, P. E., & Rodgers, W. L. (1976). *The quality of American life: Perceptions, evaluations, and satisfactions* (Vol. 3508). New York, NY: Russell Sage Foundation.

Cheng, S. T. (2004). Age and subjective well-being revisited: A discrepancy perspective. *Psychology and Aging*, *19*(3), 409–415.

Cohen, S., & Wills, T. A. (1985). Stress, social support, and the buffering hypothesis. *Psychological Bulletin*, *98*, 310–357.

Diener, E. (2000). Subjective well-being: The science of happiness and a proposal for a national index. *American Psychologist*, *55*(1), 34–43.

Diener, E., Emmons, R., Larsen, R., & Griffin, S. (1985). The satisfaction with life scale. *Journal of Personality Assessment*, *49*(1), 71–75.

Diener, E., & Emmons, R. A. (1984). The independence of positive and negative affect. *Journal of Personality and Social Psychology*, *47*(5), 1105–1117.

Diener, E., Suh, E. M., Lucas, R. E., & Smith, H. L. (1999). Subjective well-being: Three decades of progress. *Psychological Bulletin*, *125*(2), 276–302.

Ekerdt, D. J., Kosloski, K., & DeViney, S. (2000). The normative anticipation of retirement by older workers. *Research on Aging*, *22*(1), 3–22.

Felton, B. (2000). Resilience in a multicultural sample of community-dwelling women older than age 85. *Clinical Nursing Research*, *9*, 102–123.

Fox, S., & Spector, P. E. (2006). The many roles of control in a stressor-emotion theory of counterproductive work behavior. In P. L. Perrewé & D. C. Ganster (Eds.), *Employee health, coping and methodologies* (Vol. 5, pp. 171–201). Research in Occupational Stress and Well Being. Bingley, UK: Emerald Group Publishing Limited.

Garstka, T. A., Schmitt, M. T., Branscombe, N. R., & Hummert, M. L. (2004). How young and older adults differ in their responses to perceived age discrimination. *Psychology and Aging*, *19*(2), 326–335.

George, L. K. (2010). Still happy after all these years: Research frontiers on subjective well-being in later life. *The Journals of Gerontology Series B: Psychological Sciences and Social Sciences*, *65*(3), 331–339.

Greenfield, E. A., & Marks, N. F. (2007). Continuous participation in voluntary groups as a protective factor for the psychological well-being of adults who develop functional limitations: Evidence from the national survey of families and households. *Journals of Gerontology: Series B: Psychological Sciences and Social Sciences*, *62B*(1), 560–568.

Griffeth, R. W., Hom, P. W., & Gaertner, S. (2000). A meta-analysis of antecedents and correlates of employee turnover: Update, moderator tests, and research implications for the next millennium. *Journal of Management*, *26*(3), 463–488.

Hansson, R. O., DeKoekkoek, P. D., Neece, W. M., & Patterson, D. W. (1997). Successful aging at work: Annual review, 1992–1996: The older worker and transitions to retirement. *Journal of Vocational Behavior*, *51*(2), 202–233.

Hobfoll, S. E. (1989). Conservation of resources: A new attempt at conceptualizing stress. *American Psychologist*, *44*, 513–524.

Hodes, R. J., & Suzman, R. (2007). *Growing older in America: The health and retirement study*. Bethesda, MD: National Institute on Aging, National Institute of Health, US Department of Health and Human Services.

Jex, S. M., Kain, J., & Park, Y. (2013). Situational factors and resilience: Social support, organizational issues. In R. R. Sinclair & T. W. Britt (Eds.), *Building psychological resilience in military personnel: Theory and practice* (pp. 67–84). Washington, DC: American Psychological Association.

Jex, S. M., Wang, M., & Zarubin, A. (2007). Aging and occupational health. In K. S. Shultz & G. A. Adams (Eds.), *Aging and work in the 21st century* (pp. 199–224). New York, NY: Psychology Press.

Judge, T. A., & Watanabe, S. (1993). Another look at the job satisfaction-life satisfaction relationship. *Journal of Applied Psychology*, *78*(6), 939–948.

Kacmar, K. M., & Ferris, G. R. (1989). Theoretical and methodological considerations in the age-job satisfaction relationship. *Journal of Applied Psychology*, *74*(2), 201–207.

Kanter, R. M. (1994). U.S. competitiveness and the aging workforce: Toward organizational and institutional change. In J. A. Auerback & J. C. Welsch (Eds.), *Aging and competition: Rebuilding the U.S. workforce* (pp. 7–32). Washington, DC: National Planning Association.

Karasek, R. A. (1979). Job demands, job decision latitude, and mental strain: Implications for job redesign. *Administrative Science Quarterly*, *24*, 285–308.

Kastenbaum, R., Derbin, V., Sabatini, P., & Artt, S. (1972). "The ages of me". Toward personal and interpersonal definitions of functional age. *International Journal of Aging and Human Development*, *3*, 197–202.

Kinsella, K. G., & Phillips, D. R. (2005). *Global aging: The challenge of success* (Vol. 60, No. 1). Washington, DC: Population Reference Bureau.

Kobasa, S. C. (1979). Stressful life events, personality, and health: An inquiry into hardiness. *Journal of Personality and Social Psychology*, *37*(1), 1–11.

Lawton, M. P., & Brody, E. M. (1968). Assessment of older people: Self-maintaining and instrumental activities of daily living. *The Gerontologist*, *9*(3), 179–186.

Luthans, F., Avolio, B. J., Avey, J. B., & Norman, S. M. (2007). Positive psychological capital: Measurement and relationship with performance and satisfaction. *Personnel Psychology*, *60*, 541–572.

McEwen, B. S. (2003). Interacting mediators of allostasis and allostatic load: Toward an understanding of resilience in aging. *Metabolism*, *52*, 10–16.

Ng, T. W., & Feldman, D. C. (2010). The relationships of age with job attitudes: A meta-analysis. *Personnel Psychology*, *63*(3), 667–718.

Park, D. C. (2000). The basic mechanisms accounting for age-related decline in cognitive function. In D. C. Park & N. Schwarz (Eds.), *Cognitive aging: A primer* (pp. 3–22). Philadelphia, PA: Psychology Press.

Perry, E. L., & Finkelstein, L. M. (1999). Toward a broader view of age discrimination in employment-related decisions: A joint consideration of organizational factors and cognitive processes. *Human Resource Management Review*, *9*, 21–49.

Reivich, K. J., Seligman, M. E. P., & McBride, S. (2011). Master resilience training in the U.S. Army. *American Psychologist*, *66*, 25–34.

Rioux, L., & Mokounkolo, R. (2011). Investigation of subjective age in the work context: Study of a sample of French workers. *Personnel Review*, *42*, 372–395.

Rogowski, J., & Karoly, L. (2000). Health insurance and retirement behavior: Evidence from the health and retirement survey. *Journal of Health Economics*, *19*(4), 529–539.

Rowe, J. W., & Kahn, R. L. (1987). Human aging: Usual and successful. *Science*, *237*(4811), 143–149.

Rupp, D. E., Vodanovich, S. J., & Credé, M. (2006). Age bias in the workplace: The impact of ageism and causal attributions. *Journal of Applied Social Psychology*, *36*(6), 1337–1364.

Salancik, G. R., & Pfeffer, J. (1978). A social information processing approach to job attitudes and task design. *Administrative Science Quarterly*, *23*(2), 224–253.

Salthouse, T. A. (1993). Speed mediation of adult age differences in cognition. *Developmental Psychology*, *29*(4), 722–738.

Schaubroeck, J. M., Riolli, L. T., Peng, A. C., & Spain, E. S. (2011). Resilience to traumatic exposure among soldiers developed in combat. *Journal of Occupational Health Psychology*, *16*, 18–37.

Schaufeli, W. B., Bakker, A. B., & Salanova, M. (2006). The measurement of work engagement with a short questionnaire a cross-national study. *Educational and Psychological Measurement*, *66*(4), 701–716.

Schaufeli, W. B., Salanova, M., González-Romá, V., & Bakker, A. B. (2002). The measurement of engagement and burnout: A two sample confirmatory factor analytic approach. *Journal of Happiness Studies*, *3*(1), 71–92.

Smith, C. A., Organ, D. W., & Near, J. P. (1983). Organizational citizenship behavior: Its nature and antecedents. *Journal of Applied Psychology*, *68*(4), 653–663.

Smith, P. C., Kendall, L. M., & Hulin, C. L. (1969). *The measurement of satisfaction in work and retirement: A strategy for the study of attitudes*. Skokie, IL: Rand-McNally.

Snape, E., & Redman, T. (2006). Too old or too young? The impact of perceived age discrimination. *Human Resource Management Journal*, *13*(1), 78–89.

Spector, P. E., & Brannick, M. T. (2011). Methodological urban legends: The misuse of statistical control variables. *Organizational Research Methods*, *14*(2), 287–305.

U.S. Bureau of Labor Statistics. (2008). *Older workers: BLS spotlight on statistics*. Retrieved from http://www.bls.gov/ooh/About/Projections-Overview.htm. Accessed on December 5, 2012.

Van der Doef, M., & Maes, S. (1999). The job demand-control (-support) model and psychological well-being: A review of 20 years of empirical research. *Work & Stress*, *13*(2), 87–114.

Waldman, D. A., & Avolio, B. J. (1986). A meta-analysis of age differences in job performance. *Journal of Applied Psychology*, *71*(1), 33.

Wang, M., & Shultz, K. S. (2010). Employee retirement: A review and recommendations for future investigation. *Journal of Management*, *36*(1), 172–206.

Wills, T. A. (1981). Downward comparison principles in social psychology. *Psychological Bulletin*, *90*(2), 245–271.

Wolff, J. L., Starfield, B., & Anderson, G. (2002). Prevalence, expenditures, and complications of multiple chronic conditions in the elderly. *Archives of Internal Medicine*, *162*(20), 2269.

Wright, T. A., & Bonett, D. G. (2007). Job satisfaction and psychological well-being as nonadditive predictors of workplace turnover. *Journal of Management*, *33*(2), 141–160.

RELIGION AND SPIRITUALITY AS FACTORS THAT INFLUENCE OCCUPATIONAL STRESS AND WELL-BEING

Christopher J. L. Cunningham

ABSTRACT

This chapter explores religion and spirituality as a form and source of demographic differences relevant to the study of occupational stress and well-being. The purpose of the chapter is to provide a resource and starting point to occupational health and stress researchers who may be interested in religion/spirituality. A review of critical religion/spirituality concepts is provided, along with a discussion of how religion/spirituality can be integrated into common occupational stress theories and reconciled with commonly studied variables within this domain. A series of future research directions involving religion/spirituality and occupational health and stress are ultimately presented.

Keywords: Religion; spirituality; occupational stress; occupational health; demographic differences

The Role of Demographics in Occupational Stress and Well Being
Research in Occupational Stress and Well Being, Volume 12, 135–172

ISSN: 1479-3555/doi:10.1108/S1479-355520140000012004

"Important as stress and coping are, they do not make an all-embracing philosophy of life. We do more than cope". (Pargament, 1997, p. 14)

INTRODUCTION

The opening quote captures an underlying sentiment found in most occupational stress research, that work creates stress and workers must cope with stress or suffer the consequences. I find this perspective to be restrictive and have written this chapter to discuss how the complex, but immensely relevant construct domain of religion/spirituality could help occupational stress researchers to more fully consider the person and context that we so desperately seek to understand. Of all the demographic variables discussed in the present volume, it can be argued that none lend themselves as directly to occupational stress-related theory development and practical application as a person's religious or spiritual beliefs, values, and practices. The content I present in this chapter is limited in scope to provide a high-level, yet hopefully sufficient overview of the many ways in which religion/spirituality may be incorporated into future occupational stress research.

The roadmap for this chapter is as follows: I begin with important background and context regarding occupational stress, well-being, and demographic differences. I then describe the religion/spirituality construct and content domain in terms of its relevance to a more comprehensive study of occupational stress and well-being. Following this, emphasis shifts to demonstrating how religion/spirituality can be incorporated into dominant theories of occupational stress and reconciled with existing empirical support for their relevance in the occupational stress domain. I conclude this chapter with a discussion of methodological and measurement issues, as well as future research directions for researchers who might be interested in considering religion/spirituality in their own future occupational stress-related work.

Background and Context

Readers of this volume most likely already have some understanding of the phenomenon known as *occupational stress* and its complex relationship with outcomes such as general well-being. To ensure some degree of contextual clarity, though, it is worth briefly defining these key elements before shifting into the core focus of this chapter.

Stress and Well-Being

Occupational stress develops within the work environment as a result of work-related stressors. More generally, *stress* is conceptualized and defined using several perspectives: it can be seen as a stimulus that triggers a reaction, it can be a form of response unto itself, it can be the result of a person–environment transaction, or the result of a real or perceived discrepancy between what a person wants/desires and what that person's environment can provide (Sonnentag & Frese, 2012). As is evident when considering these various perspectives, most applied psychological research on this topic tends to view stress as a response or reaction to other stimuli. In this way, stress represents a person's experience of arousal and/or anxiety in response to a stimuli that a person perceives as stress-inducing (i.e., some form of *stressor* stimuli). Over time, if a person's stress response to stressors is uninterrupted or chronic, *strains* may develop. This is where well-being comes in, as one of the primary outcomes of interest among occupational health researchers.

Well-being is a "messy" construct. There is some agreement that well-being is broad, likely multidimensional or multifaceted, and representative of something more generalized than good physical health (e.g., Cunningham, De La Rosa, & Jex, 2008). As attention has increasingly turned to the concept of well-being among workers, there has been a noticeable shift from what initially was more of a medically minded approach to defining, conceptualizing, and measuring well-being to something that is perhaps most accurately referenced as a holistic wellness model, which frames well-being as multidisciplinary associated with a person's general ability to handle and adapt to whatever life brings (Hoffmann & Tetrick, 2003; Warr, 2005, 2013).

Within the occupational stress and health arena, well-being is commonly included in research because it is such a generalizable outcome that transcends the work domain. The general hypothesis in such studies usually revolves in some way around the notion that workers who are experiencing more stress (quantitative) or worse stress (qualitative) are those who also are experiencing less positive well-being. Thus, well-being (typically self-reported) serves as a (and perhaps *the*) common operationalized form of psychological and physical strain.

With this brief background in mind, it is important to remember that stress and well-being are not mutually exclusive aspects of life. In other words, occupational stress researchers would do well to remember that stress is not always a bad thing, nor is it something to be eradicated from the workplace (e.g., Sulsky & Smith, 2005). Research has repeatedly shown that it is not always the case that high levels of occupational stress lead to problems such as low performance or well-being, nor is it true that low levels of occupational stress are automatically associated with positive outcomes such as high performance or well-being (Jackson, Firtko, & Edenborough, 2007; LePine, LePine, & Jackson, 2004; Moore, Vine, Wilson, & Freeman, 2012; Podsakoff, LePine, & LePine, 2007; Webster, Beehr, & Love, 2011).

It is the case, however, that occupational stress is as much a daily reality in most of our workplaces as the desks at which we often sit. Given this constant, though, what makes occupational stress so fascinating is that different people in the same work environment can experience the same potentially stress-inducing stimuli (i.e., stressors) in very different ways. This is particularly likely when considering psychological and social stressors (e.g., workload, incivility, role ambiguity) within the work environment, which impact the person via perceptual and cognitive processes, in contrast to physical stressors (e.g., noise, heat, noxious fumes), which impact the person through direct contact or exposure. Researchers who work to explain the differential impact of occupational stressors on workers often resort to what has become a stock explanation for this phenomenon, that various individual differences allow some people to be more or less stress-reactive, resilient, or adaptive than others. While some individual differences like personality traits are commonly studied for their influence on occupational stress processes (e.g., Conard & Matthews, 2008; Grant & Langan-Fox, 2007), there is an entire other set of individual difference variables that typically is ignored.

Demographic Differences

This missing set of individual differences includes characteristics that are broadly descriptive of large groups of people and often ignored by occupational stress researchers. Chapters in this volume delve into many of these demographic variables that are relevant to the study of occupational stress and can help researchers to more comprehensively study and understand how and why different people respond differently to stress. Most chapters address demographic characteristics that are typically included in stress and well-being research as statistical covariates, deployed to better isolate the variables that researchers are more interested in understanding (i.e., employee perceptions of stress and well-being).

Unfortunately, this common practice of using demographic differences to enhance statistical control of unknown factors creates a major challenge to and shortcoming of research in this area. This is primarily the case when such variables are included without a clear theoretical or empirical justification (for a more thorough treatment of these issues, see Edwards, 2008; Spector & Brannick, 2011). While including demographic information in our statistical models may partially improve the realism of and context around the more narrowly defined stress and well-being phenomena, a more complete consideration of these differences could help this field move beyond existing and restricted theories and studies of isolated constructs and toward a more comprehensive and holistic understanding of how and why people function as they do.

It is difficult to incorporate demographic differences into existing stress and well-being related theories, because many such characteristics essentially describe a feature that a person or group of people either does or does not possess (e.g., male vs. female sex, majority vs. minority group membership, urban vs. rural geographic location). This type of information does not lend itself to strong theorizing or deep thinking about the potential impact such variables may have, nor does it appeal to researchers who are interested in ultimately developing interventions that could, for example, reduce the impact of occupational stress on employee well-being.

Not all demographic variables are like this, however; some reflect underlying differences that are rich and central to daily functioning. Such variables do not have to be measured and studied only as nominal classifications, but instead can be studied in terms of their degree of influence, intensity, strength, frequency, etc. In this chapter I discuss one demographic characteristic that fits within this latter classification; it also happens to be a demographic characteristic that is not commonly considered in occupational stress and well-being research: religion and spirituality.

The limited consideration of religion/spirituality within the occupational stress field of study and practice constitutes a major omission. This demographic and individual difference serves as both a form of demographic expression and a source of direct influence on group and person-level cognitions and behaviors. It is beyond the scope of this chapter to discuss the many reasons that religion/spirituality has not factored more prominently in studies of occupational stress. This situation is characteristic of the longstanding general separation between psychology and religion that has existed since the early days of psychological research (Pargament, 1997). Unfortunately, ignoring religion and spirituality when studying stress and well-being virtually guarantees that our understanding of these phenomena will be deficient. As noted by Pargament (1997), "[a]ny understanding of the human response to extraordinary moments remains incomplete without an appreciation of religion" (p. 4). Posed somewhat differently, "[h]ow can we grasp human resilience if we neglect some of the most common ways people deal with major life stressors" (Pargament, Mahoney, Exline, Jones, & Shafranske, 2013, p. 10)?

Throughout this chapter, I use *religion/spirituality* or *religion and spirituality* when referring this form of demographic difference, unless citing research that is more specifically focused on one aspect or the other of this complex domain. This follows Pargament et al.'s (2013) recommendation that religion and spirituality be identified jointly when discussing concepts that are likely to be associated with both aspects of a person's search for the sacred (p. 17). In the spirit of inclusiveness, I have also tried to avoid emphasizing any one form of religion/spirituality or set of religious/spiritual principles too strongly. Instead, my focus is on providing a conceptual and theoretical overview of how spirituality is likely to influence many other variables that we often study when trying to understand the development and consequences of work-related stress. Thus, my primary objective in this chapter is to provide a resource and starting point to researchers who are open to considering issues of religion/spirituality either as focal constructs or as demographic covariates in studies of other stress–outcome relationships.

RELIGION/SPIRITUALITY AS FORM AND SOURCE OF DIFFERENCE

As a construct domain, religion/spirituality provide diverse options for researchers seeking to describe and understand stress, well-being, and related phenomena. Indicators of personal experiences with religions/spirituality can be descriptive and functional, as they are deeply connected to the basic human need for managing the aspects of life that are ambiguous and uncontrollable. The psychological, philosophical, and behavioral aspects of religion/spirituality make this form of demographic difference incredibly valuable for future consideration in occupational stress research. It has even been suggested that religion/spirituality, more than any other background or demographic characteristic may be the key to understanding how people think and act, particularly among Americans (Gallup, 1999), but also quite likely among individuals in other countries and cultures.

A critical feature of religion/spirituality that makes it different from many of the other demographic variables discussed in this volume is that while most common demographic factors (e.g., age, sex, ethnicity) are wholly or mostly determined by factors beyond the control of the person, religious/spiritual beliefs and practices are largely self-selected and open to revision and modification. Even within religions in which one's membership is determined by birth (i.e., descent) rather than personal choice to opt-in (i.e., ascent; e.g., Cohen, Gorvine, & Gorvine, 2013), peoples' adherence to values and actual behaviors is influenced by personal choice. In this way, religious/spiritual involvements have the potential to create and influence a person's (a) environments and situations, (b) personal routines and habits, and (c) general perspective on life. This volitional aspect of religion/spirituality makes this demographic characteristic both a form and source of demographic and individual difference. Because of this, there are many possible ways in which a person's religion/spirituality can be expected to play a role in determining not only how a person experiences stress within the workplace, but also how such stress impacts that person's well-being.

Pargament et al. (2013) offer perhaps the most generalizable definitions of religion and spirituality, emphasizing that while spirituality can be seen as "the search for the sacred" (p. 14), religion is "the search for significance that occurs within the context of established institutions that are designed to facilitate spirituality" (p. 15). Within this definitional framework, it is neither possible, nor productive to separate religion and spirituality into separate constructs when considering religion/spirituality as meaningful variables in a more developed approach to understanding occupational stress and its effects. Instead, researchers interested in considering religion/spirituality need to approach the development of their research with an open mind and more holistic view on factors that impact human cognition, perception, and behaviors.

As will become apparent through the remainder of this chapter, religion/spirituality constitute a construct domain that is vast. Because of this, the potential value associated with including religion/spirituality in future studies of occupational stress is tremendous. One reason for this is that focusing on religion/spirituality may provide a mechanism by which elements of culture can be clearly and meaningfully incorporated into stress and well-being research and theory. For additional perspective regarding why occupational stress researchers should consider working with the complexity that can be religion/spirituality, recent statistics show that extremely large proportions of the population see themselves as connected, at least to some degree, with some form of religion/spirituality. For example, close to 84% of Americans report an affiliation with some form of organized religion (Pew Research Center, 2008) and 65% of Americans and 84% of people worldwide see religion as an "important part of their daily lives" (Crabtree, 2010). Such figures are obviously general, but provide a high-level and likely conservative estimate of the potential influence religion/spirituality on large proportions of workers worldwide. As such, religion/spirituality represent a demographic difference that can be expected to be at least as influential as most other demographic factors that are more commonly considered.

THEORETICAL CONNECTIONS TO OCCUPATIONAL STRESS

To many people (at least in the Western world), religion/spirituality is intensely personal; many individuals monitor and in some cases hide their religious/spiritual beliefs and values from general public display. This stands in contrast with most peoples' work experiences, which are typically very public. This is perhaps one reason why religion/spirituality has been so commonly ignored by occupational stress researchers (but see recent work by Arnetz et al., 2013 as well as work by researchers cited throughout this chapter for notable exceptions).

Perhaps the first path to integrating religion/spirituality into occupational stress research is through alignment with and expansion of dominant stress-related theories. At a general level, the potential linkages between religion/spirituality, stress, and well-being are intuitive and commonsensical, at least for those who have some personal experience with or knowledge of religion/spirituality. For example, religion/spirituality can help people to come to terms with the most difficult parts of the human experience. As noted by Pargament (1997), "every religion offers a way to come to terms with tragedy, suffering, and the most significant issues in life" (p. 3). Religion and spirituality are also relevant when the goal is to understand how people perceive and respond to the world around them. Soenke, Landau, and Greenberg (2013) further suggest that, "[a] primary function of religiousness is to buffer the individual against anxiety" and that "… motivated adherence to religion shapes people's attitudes and behaviors regarding a range of domains" (p. 105).

To facilitate the consideration of religion/spirituality in future occupational stress research, I present in this section a summary of several dominant models of the occupational stress process that occupational stress researchers rely upon to frame and structure their research. Readers are also encouraged to consider ways in which religion/spirituality could be used to enhance many other excellent and widely leveraged theories of stress and well-being that cannot be discussed fully within the confines of this chapter. I selected the following subset of theories for inclusion here because each can easily accommodate religious and spiritual elements. In the following subsections, then, I demonstrate how each of these theories provides fertile ground for seeding religion/spirituality into future studies of occupational stress.

Religion/Spirituality and Conservation of Resources Theory

As described by Hobfoll and colleagues over the last few decades (e.g., Hobfoll, 1989; Hobfoll & Freedy, 1993; Hobfoll, Lilly, & Jackson, 1992), Conservation of Resources (COR) theory explains stress as that which is experienced when someone perceives a threat to or actually loses critical psychological and social resources that they otherwise possess. As traditionally presented, resources can include a wide variety of psychological, social, and material elements that have utility to us as we adapt and respond to the world around us. The COR theory itself is general enough that a very large number of psychological, social, and material factors within a person's life can function and be identified as "resources."

This particular theoretical framework provides an ideal pathway for incorporating religion/spirituality into occupational stress research. One reason for this is that the tenets of COR theory clearly illustrate several direct connections that are possible between religion/spirituality as a resource itself and as a context or mechanism that can influence and build upon individuals' other psychological and social resources. Among the different types of resources identified within COR theory, the personal characteristics and conditions subcategories are especially relevant when religion/spirituality is considered. As a brief illustration, the practice of religion/spirituality, either alone or through some form of organized religion, can help people to develop and build a variety of psychological (e.g., home, controllability, relative place in world) and social resources (e.g., support, family, friends, community). Such resources transcend just the work environment, but yet are likely to impact our ability to function within a work environment as in all other domains of life.

Some preliminary research supports this possibility. Patel and Cunningham (2012) found that one's degree of involvement in a religion, in this case Hinduism, is associated with an increased in perceived psychological and social resources through one's religious involvements. Within a work context, Gervais (2014) found that being active within one's religion may buffer or protect workers against strains that might otherwise result from stress experiences with one's work. As more occupational stress and health researchers consider religion/spirituality in their theory and research developments the case will continue to build for how a person's religion/spirituality may itself serve as a form and source of critical psychological and social resources.

Incorporating religion/spirituality into our studies of occupational stress within a COR framework also raises the interesting possibility of better understanding and potentially further developing one or more aspects of this theory. As one example, there is some evidence that a threat to resources associated with one's religion/spirituality (e.g., hope, sense of self-worth, faith) may strengthen one's beliefs in their religious/spiritual traditions (e.g., McGregor, Haji, Nash, & Teper, 2008). These findings raise an interesting possibility that may conflict slightly with the COR principle that resource loss or the threat of resource loss is especially distressing (e.g., Wells, Hobfoll, & Lavin, 1999). Instead, it may be that when resources associated with one's religion/spirituality are threatened, people become more aware of these resources and the value and perceived strength of these resources may increase (cf. Pargament, 1997). In this type of situation, instead of resource loss being associated with stress, the increased strength and conviction associated with a person's religious/spirituality beliefs (a resource in its own right) may be strengthened, not unlike steel being tempered by fire.

From a COR theory perspective, then, religion/spirituality provide an entire domain of potential forms and sources of resource gain. There is also the possibility that involvement with religious/spiritual practices and groups could contribute to resource loss or drain. The concept of an entire class of religious/spiritual resources also arises as a potentially relevant and worthwhile extension of existing resource theories (e.g., Pargament, 1997). There is a great deal of work to be done to better understand the influence of religion/spirituality on a person's actual and perceived resources, but given the wide impact of COR theory, such work is likely to yield valuable insights.

Religion/Spirituality and Effort-Recovery Theory

The Effort-Recovery theory (Meijman & Mulder, 1998) frames occupational stress as what results when one is unable to recover sufficiently from their physiological and psychological efforts to manage workload (although the core elements of this theory may also apply to other forms of work-related stressors). Workers' efforts to meet work-related demands are made within a broader context in which workers have a degree of subjective and objective decision latitude over their effortful response to workload. When workers are able to control when and how much effort is expended in addressing work stressors, and when workers can engage in regular periods of recovery, the effortful response to workload does not have lasting negative impact on the person. Recovery, therefore, allows workers to return to levels of functioning in-line with their pre-exposure state. However, when effort in response to stressors is expended for an extended period of time, and/or when workers' decision latitude is extremely limited, strains are likely to develop. Such strains may include decrements to workers overall work potential (i.e., ability to perform the job) and physical and psychological health (i.e., fatigue, burnout, reduced well-being).

There are several components to the Effort-Recovery theory that provide possible integration points for occupational stress researchers interested in religion/spirituality. For example, personal effort in response to work stressors arises out of energetical processes (Meijman & Mulder, 1998), which are influenced by psychological states and general dispositions within the person. One element closely linked to these energetical processes is the possible discrepancy that may exist between a worker's actual state and required state on the job. It is possible that religion/spirituality may modify the likelihood and/or severity of this type of discrepancy, given the influence of religion/spirituality on our perceptions of controllability and suffering (e.g., Pargament, 1997).

For example, workers who adhere to religion-inspired values of hard-work, diligence, and find through religion/spirituality the ability to minimize the suffering associated with perceived stressors may be more likely to perceive a smaller discrepancy between their actual and required states. Alternatively, those who are inspired through their religious/spiritual beliefs to strive for perfection in their actions may tend to perceive their actual as significantly less than the required state, as means of motivation through discrepancy maximization. There is also a possible connection point involving subjective and objective forms of decision latitude. Religion/spirituality may strongly impact individuals' general perspectives on things that are and are not controllable in daily life (including work environments). The implication here is that there may be value in considering how religion/spirituality influences workers' subjective perceptions of decision latitude.

Along these lines, Meijman and Mulder (1998) note that "[a]s long as control is possible, thereby preventing the task demands from exceeding the possibilities of self-regulation, the effort will remain within limits acceptable to the individual and will not necessarily elicit a tension reaction" (p. 24). When such control is not available or possible, workers may have to provide more effort and expend more resources (making linkages with COR theory possible) than they have to offer. "Being confronted with such a situation or just anticipating it, generates the typical reaction pattern … which may be characterized as a tension or stress reaction" (p. 24). Here again, though we have an opportunity to incorporate religion/spirituality, in that practices and beliefs associated with this may help individual avoid anticipatory stress reactions, as well as avoidance of situations that are likely to comprise one's ethics or create interpersonal conflicts (which could also lead to these situations).

Religion/Spirituality and Attention Restoration Theory

A third theoretical perspective that could support the inclusion of religion/spirituality in occupational stress research is Attention Restoration Theory (ART; Kaplan, 1995; Kaplan & Kaplan, 1989). This theory shares much in common with the two preceding theories, but focuses on a critical resource, voluntary or directed attention, and how it can be restored or replenished once fatigued (Kaplan, 2001). As cited by Kaplan (1995), directed attention is an extension of James' (1892) concept of voluntary attention. Within a work context, it takes a great deal of physical and psychological effort to focus our attention on the tasks at hand. In contrast, when we are communing with nature, the attention we direct at our surroundings is involuntarily pulled from us, rather than requiring additional effort. This notion of voluntary/directed versus involuntary/pulled attention is closely aligned with more general concepts of resource drain and resource gain during periods of recovery. Within ART, the concept of involuntary attention is also referred to as fascination.

Although widely referenced in the occupational stress literature, the ART perspective provides another excellent starting point for stress researchers seeking ways to integrate religion/spirituality into their work. Whereas many theories within the occupational stress literature focus most on ways in which stress develops and takes its toll on the body and mind, ART is more oriented toward how people can be restored. On a high-level (and tailored to the work context), such restorative experiences come through periods of fascination either with process (e.g., engagement in some activity) or content (e.g., observation of natural phenomenon). These experiences can be optimized when they align with a person's interests, occur outside of the work environment, and can involuntarily engage our attention for an extended period of time without requiring effort to avoid boredom (Berman, Jonides, & Kaplan, 2008; Kaplan, 1995).

The core elements of ART, however, also provide another possible tie-in for researchers interested in applications of religions/spirituality within the study of occupational stress and recovery. Kaplan (2001) notes that "[n]atural environments are not the only contexts that permit such effortless attention …" (p. 508), but they are especially potent in this regard. One has only to read works by Muir (e.g., "The mountains of California"; "My first summer in the Sierra") or Whitman (e.g., "Leaves of grass") to understand the direct linkage between nature and the highest and strongest forms of spirituality. Very similar sentiments, though, are also expressed by many authors more directly affiliated with a wide variety of religious/spiritual traditions (e.g., The Dalai Lama, Thich Nhat Hanh, Thomas Merton, Thomas Aquinas). This being the case, it is not only nature that can provide opportunities for fascination. Aside from incorporating spirituality directly into nature-based experiences, the ART also lends itself to studies of the impact of involvement in structured religious services, which also can easily meet the criteria for restorative experiences. This being the case, I encourage researchers interested in religion/spirituality to more fully study this theory and consider integrating it into future occupational stress and recovery research.

Opportunities for New Theory Development

As illustrated in the preceding subsections, it is easily possible to integrate religion/spirituality into occupational stress and well-being research, even when leveraging a theoretical framework that already guides research in this area. As research along these lines develops, however, it may also be worthwhile to consider further developing and/or extending these and other theories so that they are more inclusive of demographic difference factors (including religion/spirituality), that operate both outside and within the person and which may impact multiple aspects of the stress experience.

More complete consideration of religious and spiritual traditions may also serve to open up our theories and models to alternative, more holistic, and better conceptualized conceptualizations of the reason for the sometimes positive and sometimes negative effects of stress on workers. As a starting point, consider that within many religious/spiritual traditions, stress experiences serve the purpose of improving our ability to see all of what is, the good, bad, suffering, joy, etc. Researchers interested in pursuing this type of theory development can find considerable guidance in the readings and traditions associated with specific religions and forms of spirituality. As noted by Pargament (1997), "stressful periods represent a crossroads, a point at which the individual may have to choose among paths that lead in very different directions" (p. 5). For many people, religion/spirituality provides guidance and support to people as they navigate these crossroads. Researchers interested in pursuing this line of development are also encouraged to revisit work on stress appraisal and coping by Lazarus and colleagues (e.g., Folkman, Lazarus, Dunkel-Schetter, DeLongis, & Gruen, 1986; Folkman, Lazarus, Gruen, & DeLongis, 1986; Lazarus, 1993).

EMPIRICAL CONNECTIONS TO OCCUPATIONAL STRESS

Incorporating religion/spirituality into existing occupational stress theories is one way of facilitating its consideration in future research. A related strategy is to integrate religion/spirituality through its shared connections with other individual differences that are already present in the occupational stress literature. In this section I review some of these existing linkages, providing some preliminary and high-level construct validation and "starter references" for researchers who may be interested in religion/spirituality, but unsure of where to begin when developing their research ideas, hypotheses, and designs.

Before turning to existing evidence of relationships that have been identified between religion/spirituality-related variables and other individual differences, it is also important to note that religion/spirituality are not simply proxies for other, more commonly studied personality traits or characteristics. The evidence for this assertion is widespread, and perhaps best presented by Piedmont and Wilkins (2013), who summarize the inconsistent evidence base to the contrary and emphasize that while relationships between religion/spirituality and basic personality traits (e.g., the traits of the Five Factor Model of personality) have been identified, these relationships are typically only small to moderate in strength. With this in mind, it is increasingly common for occupational stress researchers to consider personality characteristics; it may also be worthwhile to expand this consideration to other forms of demographic difference, including variables associated with religion/spirituality.

Potentially Positive Relationships

It is widely asserted that religion/spirituality is associated with positive psychological functioning. This has been shown in terms of relationships between involvement in religious/spiritual practices and a variety of outcomes (e.g., hope, sense of purpose, generalized self-efficacy; French & Joseph, 1999; George, Ellison, & Larson, 2002; George, Larson, Koenig, & McCullough, 2000). The following subsections delve into several more specific areas of study that are linked with these types of positive outcomes, yet also relevant to the study of occupational stress.

Religion/Spirituality and Sense of Control

Control over work and life events is generally seen as critically important to workers' psychological well-being. Many constructs have been developed to facilitate the quantification and study of individual differences in general perceptions of control over life events, including sense of coherence (Antonovsky, 1993), locus of control (Grotz, Hapke, Lampert, & Baumeister, 2011; Luszczynska & Schwarzer, 2005; Masters & Wallston, 2005; Wallston, 1997), and core self-evaluations (Judge, Erez, Bono, & Thoresen, 2002, 2003). Personal perceptions of control may operate in tandem with personal mindsets regarding the experience of stress itself (e.g., whether it is enhancing or debilitating; Crum, Salovey, & Achor, 2013).

A question worth considering here, however, is whether particular aspects of a person's life can contribute to healthy versus unhealthy perceptions and mindsets. Here is a potential tie-in for religion/spirituality. On a more theoretical level, Pargament (1997) highlights the concept of a continuum that extends between psychology and religion, from a science focused on control and explanation to a belief and appreciation of what cannot be controlled (p. 8). This difference may be manifested and observable in those persons who do not hold religious/spiritual beliefs compared to those who do. As noted and described rather colloquially by Sapolsky (1998), people who believe in a god or gods (i.e., people who have religious/spiritual beliefs) benefit from the:

> stress-reducing advantages of attribution – it may not be clear what the deity is up to, but you at least know who is responsible … if it is an intervening deity with discernible rules, it provides the comfort of both attribution and predictive information … if it is a deity who does all the above, *and* will respond to your personal and specific entreaties … there is an added and wonderfully stress-reducing element of control introduced. (p. 317, italics in original)

Empirically, there is also some evidence that religion/spirituality may protect a related and valuable resource that is our perception of control. Kay, Whitson, Gaucher, and Galinsky (2009) considered this possibility and found that when our sense of personal control is threatened or lost, people may benefit from forms of what they refer to as "compensatory control." Such compensatory control can be activated by considering various stimuli, including belief in a God that controls even the most seemingly random events that might happen in a person's life.

Religion/Spirituality and Self-Regulation

Building on the perception or sense of control, there is also a large and growing body of literature pertaining to our abilities to self-regulate and direct our control and influence toward specific goals or targets. By definition, self-control is demonstrated when people guide consciously and with effort toward some goal. The resource required to maintain and demonstrate self-control is typically referred to as self-regulation (e.g., Ackerman, Goldstein, Shapiro, & Bargh, 2009), which itself can be understood as a muscle that can be fatigued with use, but replenished with rest and nourishment (e.g., Muraven & Baumeister, 2000; see also Rachlin, 2000 for a broader treatment of self-control). A considerable amount of research has demonstrated that use or depletion of self-control reduces that person's subsequent ability to successfully utilize the same type of resource (Baumeister, Bratslavsky, Muraven, & Tice, 1998; Baumeister, Vohs, & Tice, 2007; Muraven & Baumeister, 2000; Muraven, Tice, & Baumeister, 1998).

Occupational stress research has periodically touched on the self-control realm over the decades, most recently through related streams of research involving recovery from work-related stress. In this most recent iteration, self-control is typically hypothesized to be influenced by a person's available resources, including self-regulation (as already noted) and more generalized attentional control (e.g., Cunningham, 2007). The growing literature on recovery from occupational stress and the literature on regaining spent self-regulatory resources has clearly shown that these attentional and cognitive resources can be restored (e.g., Korpela, Hartig, Kaiser, & Fuhrer, 2001; Sonnentag, 2001; Trougakos & Hideg, 2009).

As discussed earlier in this chapter, several of the dominant theories that guide occupational stress research incorporate the notion of recovery of spent resources. Here, as with those theories, there are many possible integration opportunities with relevant research conducted from a religion/spirituality perspective. Perhaps most immediately in line with the dominant research on self-regulation and self-control is the notion that within many religious/spiritual traditions, great emphasis is placed on practicing discipline and adhering to some form of moral code. Such activities can serve as a form of self-regulatory exercise, and may function as means of improving and strengthening one's self-regulatory muscles.

Some research has explored these possibilities, paving the way for further investigation. For example, McCullough and Carter (2013) suggest that religion, "fosters the development and exercise of self-control and self-regulation, which lead to beneficial outcomes in a variety of behavioral and psychological domains" (p. 123). Their rationale for this assertion is that religion has evolved to present-day forms out of a need to help us wait, tolerate, and cooperate better in social groupings than was the case before humans replaced their primary focus on hunting-gathering for a more sedentary and agricultural (now white-collar) lifestyle. One need not agree with an evolutionary rationale to support the role of religion/spirituality in this manner, as there is additional evidence demonstrating the link between self-control and religiosity (see also McCullough & Willoughby, 2009). Along these lines, Laurin, Kay, and Fitzsimons (2012) also found that simply reminding people of God was enough to modify goal pursuit behaviors and increase individuals' resistance to temptation, which might otherwise derail a person's progress toward goal attainment.

Thus, although the literature directly examining the role of religion/spirituality in determining work-related self-regulation and self-control is limited, there is reason to believe that additional efforts along these lines are warranted. The existing research may not fully clarify causal priority among these constructs, but it does suggest that religion/spirituality is one of perhaps several causal factors influencing a person's self-regulatory capabilities (McCullough & Carter, 2013).

Social and Spiritual Support

Within the occupational stress field there has long been a fascination with the construct of social support, primarily because of its negative association with strain (e.g., Beehr, Jex, Stacy, & Murray, 2000) and potential buffering effect on the relationship between stress and strain (e.g., Etzion, 1984). Occupational stress research that incorporates constructs aligned with social support represents another area in which it may prove fruitful to incorporate a religious/spiritual perspective. For example, research has shown that people who participate in religious activities report larger social support systems and networks that are also perceived as favorable or positive in their nature (Koenig, McCullough, & Larson, 2001). In other words, involvement with a religion's activities may be a source of high-quality or high-value social support. This is particularly important in light of recent research suggesting that not all social support is equally beneficial when it comes to protecting or helping a worker who is experiencing occupational stress (Beehr, Bowling, & Bennett, 2010; Halbesleben, 2006).

Down a different path, there is some evidence that religious involvement may also yield alternative forms of support with health-protective benefits. As one example, Maton (1989) found that support that is perceived to come from God (i.e., spiritual support) was associated with well-being among bereaved parents and emotional adjustment among college freshmen. Although these examples are not specifically aligned with the work environment, Maton's study does raise the possibility that additional research into the protective effects of support may strengthened with the inclusion of elements of religion/spirituality.

Religion/Spirituality and Coping

There is a vast literature on the ways in which people cope with stress. Discussing this separate arena of research is beyond the scope of the present chapter. Nevertheless, because coping can be directed at both the stress experience and the stressor that triggers a stress response, it is important to note another area in which consideration of religion/spirituality might prove valuable. It is generally understood that people with strong and deeply held religious/spiritual beliefs may have a different perspective on many common daily events that might be perceived as hassles and stressors by those who do not have similarly strong religious/spiritual beliefs and who might therefore view certain events as extremely difficult to manage or understand (cf. Bade & Cook, 2008; Cacioppo & Brandon, 2002; Fehring, Miller, & Shaw, 1997; Koenig et al., 2001). Aside from influencing perceptions and emotions, religious/spiritual involvements may also help people to build sources of social and spiritual support, which themselves can be helpful to individuals when they need to cope with stress in their work and nonwork lives (e.g., George et al., 2002; Holahan & Moos, 1987; Maton, 1989).

Occupational stress researchers are likely familiar with traditional psychological perspectives on coping. From a religion/spirituality perspective, however, many other elements emerge. There is a growing literature focused on religious coping, using models that link religious involvement to more effective response to stress when it arises. As noted by Pargament (1997), "… religion adds a unique dimension to the coping process, one that cannot be described simply as good or bad … religion has the potential to help people through their hardest times and it also has the potential to make bad matters worse" (p. 10).

Exactly what constitutes religious coping is a topic that is actively discussed (e.g., Gall et al., 2005). For example, some studies within this area have demonstrated that when facing decreased perceptions of control, people often cope via believing in the existence of a God that is controlling (Kay, Gaucher, McGregor, & Nash, 2010; Kay, Gaucher, Napier, Callan, & Laurin, 2008). Other researchers have focused on how people form a sense of meaning through their religions, when coping with stress (Gall et al., 2005; Park, 2005; Park & Folkman, 1997). Still others have focused on specific religious/spiritual practices such as prayer, as a means of coping with stress (Ai et al., 2010; Bade & Cook, 2008; Ganzevoort, 1998; Hood, Morris, & Watson, 1989). Although most of the work on religious coping has been within Christian populations, there is a growing body of literature pertaining to other religions, including Judaism (Rosmarin, Pargament, Krumrei, & Flannelly, 2009), Islam (e.g., Aflakseir & Coleman, 2011; Khan & Watson, 2006) and across a variety of life domains (Tix & Frazier, 1998).

Religion/Spirituality and Recovery

Perhaps one of the greatest avenues for religious/spiritual expansion within the occupational stress arena is that pertaining to one's recovery from stress exposure. Recovery is generally defined as a process of restoration and within the occupational stress world, recovery is typically linked to replenishment of resources (Meijman & Mulder, 1998; Sonnentag, 2001; van Hooff, Geurts, Beckers, & Kompier, 2011). Interestingly, most formal religions and spiritual belief systems incorporate some degree of rest and recovery as central components to their teachings (e.g., Christian and Jewish traditions of a day of rest or Sabbath, respectively).

There is also some evidence that specific religion/spiritual practices may provide restorative benefits to people. In particular, prayer, meditation, and active mindfulness also present potential mechanisms by which religion/spirituality can positively impact individual's recovery from work stress and well-being. As noted by Hood (2013) it has long been asserted that prayer may have physical and neurobiological effects similar to those associated with Yoga and other forms of meditative activities. In many ways, these assertions have been borne out in the developing literature on the effects of prayer; for a detailed summary of this literature, interested readers are directed to Ladd and Spilka's (2013) handbook chapter. There is also a significant and growing body of literature supporting the link between meditative practices and increased ability to concentrate, be mindful, achieve relaxation, and generally improve well-being (e.g., Hanh, 1987; Shapiro, Astin, Bishop, & Cordova, 2005; Wang et al., 2010; Wolever et al., 2012).

Potentially Negative Relationships

As noted by Pargament (1997), Abu-Raiya (2013), and others, our connections with religion/spirituality are often associated with positive outcomes, but this is not always the case. Instead, religion and spirituality are multivalent, meaning that our religious/spiritual experiences and involvements can lead to negative outcomes as well as positive ones. Although the bulk of material presented in this chapter highlights the potentially positive role that involvement with religion/spiritual practices can have on a person's ability to manage occupational stress, this overview of potential empirical connections with occupational stress would be incomplete without some discussion of the darker side of religion/spirituality. The literature pertaining to this topic is not as broad or developed as the more positively oriented religion/spirituality literature. Nevertheless, there are several areas in which religious/spiritual beliefs, experiences, and practices could be expected to potentially contribute to one's risk of experiencing stress within the work environment or damage one's ability to effectively cope with such stress when it is experienced.

Most of these areas are associated in some way with a tendency for religious/spiritual involvement to sometimes have a polarizing effect on individuals and groups. For example, there is some evidence that those who hold fundamental religious/spiritual beliefs and authoritarian attitudes (a common combination), may be more disposed to treat members of other minority groups (or simply different religious/spiritual beliefs) with prejudice (Altemeyer, 2003; Laythe, Finkel, Bringle, & Kirkpatrick, 2002). In a similar way, the more individuals identify with a specific religion or set of spiritual beliefs, the more likely they are to feel closely connected to those who share those beliefs and more separated from those who do not (e.g., Kalkan, Layman, & Uslaner, 2009). It may, therefore, be valuable for occupational stress researchers to consider the occupational health implications of relationships between religious/spiritual involvement, identification, beliefs, and practices, and phenomena such as interpersonal intolerance, inter-group conflict, and excessive conformity. Researchers interested in pursuing studies along these lines would do well to remember early work on Social Identity Theory (e.g., Ashforth & Mael, 1989) as well as work within the religion/spirituality research realm pertaining to religious identification. Related to the above issues is the risk that public aspects or displays of religion/spirituality within a work environment (e.g., observance of prayer rituals, religious fasting, norms for dress or mixed-gender interactions) could lead to acts of incivility or outright discrimination among coworkers. Although this type of behavior would fall under the broader occupational stress category of incivility, little to no research has considered incivility that is motivated by differences within a workforce that are due to religion/spirituality.

There is also the possibility that some aspects of religion/spirituality that are typically beneficial to personal health and well-being might be detrimental in certain contexts. For example, McCullough and Carter (2013) note that, "religion is well-suited to motivate any behavior that is predicated on self-control and self-regulation" (p. 132). As an example, the positive influence of religion/spirituality on self-control can also have negative consequences, leading to heightened aggression (e.g., Bushman, Ridge, Das, Key, & Busath, 2007) and prejudice (e.g., Hunsberger & Jackson, 2005). As one additional example along these lines, there is some preliminary work by Pargament, Smith, Koenig, and Perez (1998) demonstrating the possible negative impact of religion-focused coping.

Finally, aside from linkages between religion/spirituality and the other occupational stress and health related concepts summarized above, there is a growing literature on more severe forms of religiously motivated violence and conflict. Readers who are interested in these topics are directed to a series of volumes on this subject by Ellens (2004) and a more theoretical discussion by Fox (2002). Although such violence and conflict may be more severe than what is typically observed in work environments, if and when such violence occurs, the occupational health implications would be severe.

METHODOLOGICAL MATTERS AND FUTURE DIRECTIONS

The content I have presented in this chapter provides an overview and introduction to religion/spirituality as an important form and source of demographic difference that should be considered in occupational stress and well-being research. Given the scope of this chapter, this was necessarily a high-level overview, but throughout the various sections of this chapter, readers will find a large number of critical references and a solid foundation upon which future occupational stress-related studies can be developed to incorporate religious and spiritual constructs, concepts, and theoretical elements. In this final section, I turn attention to a few more methodologically focused issues, which should hopefully make it even easier for interested occupational health and stress researchers to seriously consider incorporating religion and spirituality into their future work.

Methodological Matters

In addition to understanding relevant existing empirical results and theoretical orientations, researchers interested in religion/spirituality as constructs for inclusion in future occupational stress studies face several methodological challenges. In this section, I provide guidance to facilitate the incorporation of religion/spirituality into occupational stress research.

Design Considerations

Occupational stress and well-being are incredibly complex constructs themselves. Incorporating aspects of individuals' religion/spirituality creates potential research nightmares, given that these constructs are themselves at least as complex as stress and well-being. Because of the inherent complexity faced by researchers who pursue studies along these lines, a primary design-related recommendation is that a variety of methods be used when developing studies that incorporate these various elements (cf. Hood, 2013). To be more specific, occupational stress research that incorporates religion/spirituality should be mixed method in its design and approach, including a combination of quantitative and qualitative data gathering and interpretation techniques (Cameron, 2011; Creswell, 2004; Johnson, Onwuegbuzie, & Turner, 2007; O'Cathain, 2009; Tashakkori & Creswell, 2008).

In addition to designing studies to yield the richest and most complete data possible, researchers interested in these topics are also advised to remember that religion/spirituality and their related constructs are necessarily multidimensional, multilevel, and multivalent. The multidimensionality of religion/spirituality may seem obvious, given the many different forms of religious belief and practice that exist even within a single form of religion (e.g., Christianity). Despite this, it is important for researchers to remember that focusing too explicitly on isolated components or elements within a specific religious or spiritual tradition may result in an incomplete understanding of the role that a given form of religion/spirituality may play. This challenge is well-described by Abu-Raiya (2013) in his discussion of the multidimensionality of Islam when he notes that, "Islam might mean different things to different people, and some people might adhere to some of its elements but not to others" (p. 683). This same caution can easily apply to the study of any religious/spiritual tradition, and the implication is that researchers need to consider these construct domains broadly and holistically, rather than in terms of a few isolated, generic items that will fail to "capture the depth, richness, and multifaceted nature of Islam" (p. 683) or any other religion.

From a design perspective, the multilevel reality of religion/spirituality raises the possibility that data should be gathered longitudinal for within-person development studies and across levels of a person's engagement with religion/spirituality, for studies that attempt to discuss cross-level influences of a person's religious beliefs, practices, and more formal faith communities, etc. This is particularly the case when researchers are interested in how religion/spirituality may influence stressor perception processes or the development and maintenance of well-being (e.g., Abu-Raiya, 2013).

The multivalence of religion/spirituality is associated with the power of religion/spirituality to wield positive and negative influence on a person, particularly in terms of work-related stress and general well-being (Pargament et al., 2013). This complexity, however, is also what makes the inclusion of religion/spirituality into studies of occupational stress and well-being so appropriate. Thankfully for occupational stress researchers, the workplace constitutes a definable environment or context within which the impact of a person's religious and spiritual beliefs and practices can potentially be studied. Occupational health and stress researchers have a legitimate opportunity to contribute to the developing understanding of religion/spirituality's effects on human cognition and behavior. A primary reason for this is that these effects can differ dramatically across contexts

(Pargament et al.), but occupational health and stress researchers have the ability to focus their research within well-defined work environments. As illustrated in the preceding sections of this chapter, however, even within a defined context of a work environment, the impacts of religion/spirituality may be positive or negative. This may mean that initial occupational stress studies incorporating religion/spirituality should consider competing hypotheses about the positive and negative consequences of religion/spirituality within specific work environments, at least until our knowledge base grows to a point where more specific hypotheses can be formed.

Measurement Considerations

In addition to the design-related concerns already discussed, researchers interested in occupational stress and religion/spirituality will face challenges when it is time to operationalize religious/spiritual constructs and determine the most appropriate measurement strategies. As typically studied, religion/spirituality are examined as a demographic descriptor, a cultural reflection of a person's philosophy and religious/spiritual group membership, and as an individual difference variable (Piedmont & Wilkins, 2013). Researchers interested in religion/spirituality do not typically measure these high-level constructs directly. Instead, and as with most other human behaviors, it is assessed in terms of peoples' involvement with spirituality (e.g., intensity, duration, frequency – often evaluated in terms of faith commitments or belief in specific teachings or forms of religious practice), the degree to which people identify with or form their identity around their religion/spirituality, and relatedly the impact of religion/spirituality on a person's underlying values.

It should be noted that although religion/spirituality are complicated constructs and content domains, they are not necessarily any more "messy" than working with the complex and multifaceted stress and health constructs and content domains that readers of this volume have worked with for decades. Studying complicated phenomena has not prevented us from learning a great deal (and also generating even more questions). I emphasize this point to encourage occupational health and stress researchers to consider religion/spirituality seriously in their future studies. I have already noted the critical importance of incorporating mixed method design elements into research that includes religion/spirituality. Most occupational stress researchers, however, are far more comfortable with measures that facilitate the quantification of perceptions, attitudes, intentions, behaviors, etc. regarding the constructs that are at the heart of our studies.

Interested readers looking for a more thorough treatment of various ways in which religion/spirituality might be incorporated into psychological research designs to address occupational stress and well-being topics may find some helpful grounding and perspective in Hood (2013). To provide some starting point for researchers who are considering religion/spirituality in their future occupational stress research, I also strongly recommend a detailed treatment of the measurement-related challenges by Hill and Edwards (2013). Within the same handbook that includes these two chapters, I also recommend Abu-Raiya's (2013) discussion of reasons for avoiding single-item measures or indicators of religious/spiritual phenomenon, as this approach to measuring any variable associated with religion/spirituality fails to capture any richness or depth associated with these multidimensional constructs.

Finally, to help interested researchers find a starting point when it is time to operationalize religious and spiritual constructs for inclusion in future studies, I have summarized in Table 1 a variety of measureable variables that could facilitate this process. This content comes primarily from a much more detailed summary provided by Hill and Edwards (2013), but I have also supplemented it with some additional material from other researchers who work in this area.

Future Directions

The unifying thread to the chapters in this volume is a focus on demographic differences that may help to explain individual responses to workplace stressors and their consequences. These chapters summarize and present a picture of what has been, what is, and what can be in terms of critical demographic and individual differences research pertaining to occupational stress and well-being. The present chapter was written to focus on religion/spirituality as one such demographic difference. There would be limited reason for writing such a chapter if there were not clear and compelling future directions for researchers to take if/when they are ready to consider religion/spirituality as a critical player in the development of occupational stress and its consequences. In this final section of the chapter, I present several examples of future directions that may be worthwhile starting points for a more integrated and holistic approach to occupational stress research that includes a consideration of religion/spirituality.

Most of these ideas walk the line between present-day and traditional psychology and a more holistic, and integrated perspective on the study of

Table 1. Summary of Religion/Spirituality-Related Variables Relevant to Occupational Health and Stress Research.

General Measurement Focus	Examples of What Is Assessed
General religiousness/ spirituality	• Spiritual transcendence (Piedmont, 1999) • Mysticism (Hood, 1975) • Spiritual well-being (Paloutzian & Ellison, 1991) • Religious involvement (Hilty, Morgan, & Burns, 1984)
Beliefs and religious preferences	• Religious orthodoxy (Fullerton & Hunsberger, 1982; Hunsberger, 1989)
Religious/spiritual commitment	• Level of religious/spiritual commitment (Worthington et al., 2003) • Strength of faith (Plante & Boccaccini, 1997)
Attachment to God	• Strength of bond/connection with God (Beck & McDonald, 2004; Rowatt & Kirkpatrick, 2002)
God concept/image	• Descriptive concepts of God (Benson & Spilka, 1973) • Awareness of God (Hall & Edwards, 2002)
Religious/spiritual private practices	• Personal religious practices such as prayer, meditation, worship attendance (Connors, Tonigan, & Miller, 1996)
Religious motivation	• Religious orientation (Gorsuch & McPherson, 1989; Koenig, Parkerson, & Meador, 1997) • Degree and type of fundamentalism (Altemeyer & Hunsberger, 2004; Williamson, Hood, Ahmad, Sadiq, & Hill, 2010)
Religion as source of meaning	• Purpose in life/sense of meaning (Antonovsky, 1993)
Religious support	• Degree of support through religious involvement (Fiala, Bjorck, & Gorsuch, 2002) • Spiritual support (Genia, 1997) • Religious social support (Krause, 2008)
Spiritual experiences	• Interactions/involvement with the transcendent (Underwood & Teresi, 2002)
Religious coping	• Spiritual connection, support seeking, religious forgiveness (Pargament et al., 1998) • Religion problem solving (Pargament et al., 1988)
Religious struggle/strain	• Religious beliefs about suffering (Hale-Smith, Park, & Edmondson, 2012) • Religious comfort/strain (Exline, Yali, & Sanderson, 2000) • Attitudes toward God (Wood et al., 2010)

Source: Adapted from Hill and Edwards (2013).

human functioning, one that incorporates the psychological and the spiritual. In many ways, this is an application of what has been referred to as integral psychology, or an effort to "endeavor to honor and embrace every legitimate aspect of human consciousness" (Wilber, 2000, p. 2).

Considering More of the Person and Context

One important future direction that is facilitated by a consideration of religion/spirituality involves more complete consideration of people in contexts. There is a tendency within occupational stress research, as in many other areas of psychology, to focus so intensely on isolated constructs that we end up creating myopic research questions and designs. The risk from such research is that we then end up over-reaching or extrapolating too far from the data we actually collect in our attempts to answer the questions we really want to answer. For example, De Lange, Taris, Kompier, Houtman, and Bongers (2004) conducted what was, by many standards, a strong study of occupational factors that may influence mental health, due primarily to its longitudinal nature and the "big" nature of the questions they addressed. A limitation of this study and so many others in the occupational stress literature, however, is that mental health is not only impacted by one's work demands, work environment, or coworkers. If researchers open their minds and research models to consider other relevant domains such as religion/spirituality, we have an opportunity to move away from a tendency to over-simplify and over-focus and toward a more contextualized understanding of how work, as a part of life, may impact well-being.

Considering Non-Western Cultures

There is a need to better understand the functioning of occupational stress and well-being within persons of all cultures (e.g., Burke, 2010). This need, however, is not being well-addressed by the standard theories and measures employed by researchers in this field. This is indicated by major gaps in the existing literature regarding critical demographic variables (one of the reasons for the present volume). This limitation is mirrored within the existing research on religion and spirituality. Indeed, most of what has been written about these topics comes from research done in Western, industrialized countries in which Christianity in its many forms is the dominant religious orientation (Hood, Spilka, Hunsberger, & Gorsuch, 1996). Although there have been some forays into other religions and cultures (e.g., see the special section on Islam and Mental health in Research in the Social Scientific Study of Religion), there is still a great deal left to understand about how stress, well-being, and religion/spirituality function independently and jointly in other cultures.

More specifically, there is a need to consider how different forms of religion/spirituality and occupational stress influence worker well-being in non-Western environments. Before this is possible, though, there will need to be theory and measurement development that is broad, universal, and yet focused and culture-specific elements before researchers can really begin to understand the influence of religion/spirituality in these contexts. Researchers who ultimately pursue this path are advised to pay careful attention to the way in which they approach their cross-cultural research, particularly with respect to the religious/spiritual components. As noted by Ghorbani, Shamohammadi, Watson, and Cunningham (2009), attempts to understand the influence of religion/spirituality within other cultures that have not been studied can either be etic (outside in) or emic (inside out) in their focus. A third alternative is to take what Ghorbani and colleagues refer to as a dialogical model and interested readers are encouraged to read more in-depth on this subject, even though it falls beyond the scope of this chapter (for starters, see Ghorbani, Watson, Krauss, Bing, & Davison, 2004).

Considering Meaning

A third future occupational health and stress research direction that is potentially meaningfully informed with inclusion of religion/spirituality involves developing a more complete understanding of the importance of work itself. Along these lines, most religious and spiritual traditions have quite a bit to say about work and its function within our lives. As one example, within Catholic tradition and teaching, work provides an opportunity to act and treat others with dignity in the image of God; similar sentiments are expressed within most other religious traditions. The psychological literature also has periodically addressed this issue of our search for meaning within work (Morse & Weiss, 1955; Vecchio, 1980). Maybe it is time to reconcile these different perspectives to create a truly powerful research agenda (e.g., Davidson & Caddell, 1994; Weiss & Rupp, 2011).

Considering Alternative Occupations

As a fourth and final example of worthwhile future directions for occupational health and stress research that considers religion and spirituality, we should also not ignore what is perhaps the lowest hanging fruit: researching the occupational health, stress, and well-being of those who provide religious and spiritual services and support to others. These individuals often work under extremely stressful conditions and deserve the attention of occupational health researchers as much as workers in any other occupation (perhaps more so, given the potential multiplier effect that can be had by ensuring adequate health and well-being among those who provide so much support to so many others every day). One starting point for research along these lines is to consider preliminary work on a context-specific measure of occupational stressors by Birk, Rayburn, and Richmond (2001). Similarly, extension of traditional occupational stress and well-being theories and models into these alternative occupations may also provide relatively immediate value as the bridge is built between these two broad areas of inquiry.

CONCLUSION

For readers who actually wade through the entire chapter up to this point, I apologize if I managed to offend or bother anyone by failing to reference more specific religious or spiritual traditions, practices, or beliefs. I probably tried to summarize too much information about a construct domain that is typically viewed by applied researchers as too much to handle. This really was the purpose behind writing this chapter, however, to confront this perspective and to facilitate a more comprehensive and scientific understanding of occupational stress and well-being through the consideration of one of the most critical demographic differences affecting humankind. It is my sincere hope that more occupational health and stress researchers will seriously consider the role that religion/spirituality can play and that those who are interested may benefit from my attempt at providing an accessible discussion and demonstration of how this form and source of demographic difference can play nice with many of the theories and variables already common to the study of occupational stress and health.

ACKNOWLEDGMENTS

Sincere thanks are owed to my colleagues Paul Watson and Ralph Hood for their support, encouragement, and review of elements of this work. I also sincerely appreciate the efforts of my graduate assistant at the time of writing this chapter, Craig Holton, for helping to locate critical resources that support various elements in this chapter.

REFERENCES

Abu-Raiya, H. (2013). The psychology of Islam: Current empirically based knowledge, potential challenges, and directions for future research. In K. I. Pargament, J. J. Exline, & J. W. Jones (Eds.), *APA handbook of psychology, religion, and spirituality: Context, theory, and research* (Vol. 1, pp. 681–695). Washington, DC: APA.

Ackerman, J. M., Goldstein, N. J., Shapiro, J. R., & Bargh, J. A. (2009). You wear me out: The vicarious depletion of self-control. *Psychological Science*, *20*(3), 326–332. doi:10.1111/j.1467-9280.2009.02290.x

Aflakseir, A., & Coleman, P. G. (2011). Initial development of the Iranian religious coping scale. *Journal of Muslim Mental Health*, *6*(1). Retrieved from http://quod.lib.umich.edu/j/jmmh/10381607.0006.104?view=text;rgn=main

Ai, A. L., Ladd, K. L., Peterson, C., Cook, C. A., Shearer, M., & Koenig, H. G. (2010). Long-term adjustment after surviving open heart surgery: The effect of using prayer for coping replicated in a prospective design. *Gerontologist*, *50*(6), 798–809. doi:10.1093/geront/gnq046

Altemeyer, B. (2003). Research: Why do religious fundamentalists tend to be prejudiced? *International Journal for the Psychology of Religion*, *13*(1), 17–28. doi:10.1207/s15327582ijpr1301_03

Altemeyer, B., & Hunsberger, B. (2004). Research: A revised religious fundamentalism scale: The short and sweet of it. *International Journal for the Psychology of Religion*, *14*(1), 47–54.

Antonovsky, A. (1993). The structure and properties of the sense of coherence scale. *Social Science & Medicine*, *36*(6), 725–733.

Arnetz, B. B., Ventimiglia, M., Beech, P., DeMarinis, V., Lökk, J., & Arnetz, J. E. (2013). Spiritual values and practices in the workplace and employee stress and mental well-being. *Journal of Management, Spirituality & Religion*, *10*(3), 271–281. doi:10.1080/14766086.2013.801027

Ashforth, B. E., & Mael, F. (1989). Social identity theory and the organization. *Academy of Management Review*, *14*(1), 20–39. doi:10.2307/258189

Bade, M. K., & Cook, S. W. (2008). Functions of Christian prayer in the coping process. *Journal for the Scientific Study of Religion*, *47*(1), 123–133. doi:10.1111/j.1468-5906.2008.00396.x

Baumeister, R. F., Bratslavsky, E., Muraven, M., & Tice, D. M. (1998). Ego depletion: Is the active self a limited resource? *Journal of Personality and Social Psychology*, *74*(5), 1252–1265.

Baumeister, R. F., Vohs, K. D., & Tice, D. M. (2007). The strength model of self-control. *Current Directions in Psychological Science*, *16*(6), 351–355. doi:10.1111/j.1467-8721.2007.00534.x

Beck, R., & McDonald, A. (2004). Attachment to God: The attachment to God inventory, tests of working model. *Journal of Psychology and Theology*, *32*(2), 92–103.

Beehr, T. A., Bowling, N. A., & Bennett, M. M. (2010). Occupational stress and failures of social support: When helping hurts. *Journal of Occupational Health Psychology*, *15*(1), 45–59. doi:10.1037/a0018234

Beehr, T. A., Jex, S. M., Stacy, B. A., & Murray, M. A. (2000). Work stressors and coworker support as predictors of individual strain and job performance. *Journal of Organizational Behavior*, *21*, 391–405.

Benson, P., & Spilka, B. (1973). God image as a function of self-esteem and locus of control. *Journal for the Scientific Study of Religion*, *12*(3), 297–310. doi:10.2307/1384430

Berman, M. G., Jonides, J., & Kaplan, S. (2008). The cognitive benefits of interacting with nature. *Psychological Science*, *19*(12), 1207–1212. doi:10.1111/j.1467-9280.2008.02225.x

Birk, J. M., Rayburn, C. A., & Richmond, L. J. (2001). Religious occupations and stress questionnaire (ROS): Instrument development. *Counseling and Values*, *45*, 136–144.

Burke, R. J. (2010). Workplace stress and well-being across cultures: Research and practice. *Cross Cultural Management: An International Journal*, *17*(1), 5–9. doi:10.1108/13527601011016871

Bushman, B. J., Ridge, R. D., Das, E., Key, C. W., & Busath, G. L. (2007). When God sanctions killing effect of scriptural violence on aggression. *Psychological Science*, *18*(3), 204–207.

Cacioppo, J. T., & Brandon, M. E. (2002). Religious involvement and health: Complex determinism. *Psychological Inquiry*, *13*(3), 204–206.

Cameron, R. (2011). Mixed methods research: The five Ps framework. *The Electronic Journal of Business Research Methods*, *9*(2), 96–108.

Cohen, A. B., Gorvine, B. J., & Gorvine, H. (2013). The religion, spirituality, and psychology of Jews. In K. I. Pargament, J. J. Exline, & J. W. Jones (Eds.), *APA handbook of psychology, religion, and spirituality: Context, theory, and research* (Vol. 1, pp. 665–679). Washington, DC: APA.

Conard, M. A., & Matthews, R. A. (2008). Modeling the stress process: Personality eclipses dysfunctional cognitions and workload in predicting stress. *Personality and Individual Differences*, *44*(1), 171–181. doi:10.1016/j.paid.2007.07.023

Connors, G. J., Tonigan, J. S., & Miller, W. R. (1996). A measure of religious background and behavior for use in behavior change research. *Psychology of Addictive Behaviors*, *10*(2), 90.

Crabtree, S. (2010). *Religiosity highest in world's poorest nations*. Retrieved from http://www.gallup.com/poll/142727/religiosity-highest-world-poorest-nations.aspx. Accessed on January 18, 2014.

Creswell, J. W. (2004). Designing a mixed methods study in primary care. *The Annals of Family Medicine*, *2*(1), 7–12. doi:10.1370/afm.104

Crum, A. J., Salovey, P., & Achor, S. (2013). Rethinking stress: The role of mindsets in determining the stress response. *Journal of Personality and Social Psychology*, *104*(4), 716–733. doi:10.1037/a0031201

Cunningham, C. J. L. (2007). *Need for recovery and ineffective self-management*. Ph.D. dissertation, Bowling Green State University, Bowling Green, OH.

Cunningham, C. J. L., De La Rosa, G. M., & Jex, S. M. (2008). The dynamic influence of individual characteristics on employee well-being: A review of the theory, research, and future directions. In K. Naswall, J. Hellgren, & M. Sverke (Eds.), *The individual in the changing working life* (pp. 258–283). Cambridge: Cambridge University Press.

Davidson, J. C., & Caddell, D. P. (1994). Religion and the meaning of work. *Journal for the Scientific Study of Religion*, *33*(2), 135–147. doi:10.2307/1386600

De Lange, A. H., Taris, T. W., Kompier, M. A. J., Houtman, I. L. D., & Bongers, P. M. (2004). The relationships between work characteristics and mental health: Examining normal, reversed and reciprocal relationships in a 4-wave study. *Work & Stress*, *18*(2), 149–166. doi:10.1080/02678370412331270860

Edwards, J. R. (2008). To prosper, organizational psychology should … overcome methodological barriers to progress. *Journal of Organizational Behavior*, *29*(4), 469–491. doi:10.1002/job.529

Ellens, J. H. (Ed.). (2004). *The destructive power of religion: Violence in Judaism, Christianity, and Islam*. Westport, CT: Praeger Publishers.

Etzion, D. (1984). Moderating effect of social support on the stress-burnout relationship. *Journal of Applied Psychology*, *69*(4), 615–622.

Exline, J. J., Yali, A. M., & Sanderson, W. C. (2000). Guilt, discord, and alienation: The role of religious strain in depression and suicidality. *Journal of Clinical Psychology*, *56*(12), 1481–1496.

Fehring, R. J., Miller, J. F., & Shaw, C. (1997). Spiritual well-being, religiosity, hope, depression, and other mood states in elderly people coping with cancer. *Oncology Nursing Forum*, *24*(4), 663–671.

Fiala, W. E., Bjorck, J. P., & Gorsuch, R. (2002). The religious support scale: Construction, validation, and cross-validation. *American Journal of Community Psychology*, *30*(6), 761–786.

Folkman, S., Lazarus, R. S., Dunkel-Schetter, C., DeLongis, A., & Gruen, R. J. (1986). Dynamics of a stressful encounter: Cognitive appraisal, coping, and encounter outcomes. *Journal of Personality and Social Psychology*, *50*(5), 992–1003.

Folkman, S., Lazarus, R. S., Gruen, R. J., & DeLongis, A. (1986). Appraisal, coping, health status, and psychological symptoms. *Journal of Personality and Social Psychology*, *50*(3), 571–579.

Fox, J. (2002). *Ethnoreligious conflict in the late twentieth century: A general theory*. New York, NY: Lexington Books.

French, S., & Joseph, S. (1999). Religiosity and its association with happiness, purpose in life, and self-actualisation. *Mental Health, Religion & Culture*, *2*(2), 117–120. doi:10.1080/13674679908406340

Fullerton, J. T., & Hunsberger, B. (1982). A unidimensional measure of Christian orthodoxy. *Journal for the Scientific Study of Religion*, *21*(4), 317–326. doi:10.2307/1385521

Gall, T. L., Charbonneau, C., Clarke, N. H., Grant, K., Joseph, A., & Shouldice, L. (2005). Understanding the nature and role of spirituality in relation to coping and health: A conceptual framework. *Psychologie Canadienne. [Canadian Psychology.]*, *46*(2), 88–104. doi:10.1037/H0087008

Gallup, G., Jr. (1999). *Easter draws Americans back to church*. Retrieved from http://www.gallup.com/poll/3958/Easter-Draws-Americans-Back-Church.aspx%20retrieved%201/17/14. Accessed on January 14, 2014.

James, W. (1892). *Psychology: The briefer course*. New York, NY: Holt.

Ganzevoort, R. R. (1998). Religious coping reconsidered, Part one: An integrated approach. *Journal of Psychology and Theology*, *26*(3), 260–275.

Genia, V. (1997). The spiritual experience index: Revision and reformulation. *Review of Religious Research*, *38*(4), 344–361. doi:10.2307/3512195

George, L. K., Ellison, C. G., & Larson, D. B. (2002). Explaining the relationships between religious involvement and health. *Psychological Inquiry*, *13*(3), 190–200. doi:10.1207/S15327965pli1303_04

George, L. K., Larson, D. B., Koenig, H. G., & McCullough, M. E. (2000). Spirituality and health: What we know, what we need to know. *Journal of Social and Clinical Psychology*, *19*(1), 102–116. doi:10.1521/jscp.2000.19.1.102

Gervais, R. (2014). Religiosity and its influence on coping and well-being. Paper presented at the annual conference of the British Psychological Society's Division of Occupational Psychology, Brighton, UK.

Ghorbani, N., Shamohammadi, K., Watson, P. J., & Cunningham, C. J. L. (2009). Post-critical beliefs in Iran: Predicting religious and psychological functioning. *Research in the Social Scientific Study of Religion*, *20*, 151–194.

Ghorbani, N., Watson, P. J., Krauss, S. W., Bing, M. N., & Davison, H. K. (2004). Social science as dialogue: Narcissism, individualist and collectivist values, and religious interest in Iran and the United States. *Current Psychology*, *23*(2), 111–123. doi:10.1007/Bf02903072

Gorsuch, R. L., & McPherson, S. E. (1989). Intrinsic/extrinsic measurement: I/E-revised and single-item scales. *Journal for the Scientific Study of Religion*, *28*(3), 348–354. doi:10.2307/1386745

Grant, S., & Langan-Fox, J. (2007). Personality and the occupational stressor-strain relationship: The role of the big five. *Journal of Occupational Health Psychology*, *12*(1), 20–33. doi:10.1037/1076-8998.12.1.20

Grotz, M., Hapke, U., Lampert, T., & Baumeister, H. (2011). Health locus of control and health behaviour: Results from a nationally representative survey. *Psychology, Health & Medicine*, *16*(2), 129–140. doi:10.1080/13548506.2010.521570

Halbesleben, J. R. (2006). Sources of social support and burnout: A meta-analytic test of the conservation of resources model. *Journal of Applied Psychology*, *91*(5), 1134–1145. doi:10.1037/0021-9010.91.5.1134

Hale-Smith, A., Park, C. L., & Edmondson, D. (2012). Measuring beliefs about suffering: Development of the views of suffering scale. *Psychological Assessment*, *24*(4), 855–866. doi:10.1037/a0027399

Hall, T. W., & Edwards, K. J. (2002). The spiritual assessment inventory: A theistic model and measure for assessing spiritual development. *Journal for the Scientific Study of Religion*, *41*(2), 341–357.

Hanh, T. N. (1987). *The miracle of mindfulness: A manual on meditation*. Boston, MA: Beacon Press.

Hill, P. C., & Edwards, E. (2013). Measurement in the psychology of religiousness and spirituality: Existing measures and new frontiers. In K. I. Pargament, J. J. Exline, & J. W. Jones (Eds.), *APA handbook of psychology, religion, and spirituality: Context, theory, and research* (Vol. 1, pp. 51–77). Washington, DC: APA.

Hilty, D. M., Morgan, R. L., & Burns, J. E. (1984). King and Hunt revisited: Dimensions of religious involvement. *Journal for the Scientific Study of Religion*, *23*(3), 252–266. doi:10.2307/1386040

Hobfoll, S. E. (1989). Conservation of resources – A new attempt at conceptualizing stress. *American Psychologist*, *44*(3), 513–524. doi:10.1037/0003-066x.44.3.513

Hobfoll, S. E., & Freedy, J. (1993). Conservation of resources a general stress theory applied to burnout. In W. B. Schaufeli, C. Maslach, & T. Marek (Eds.), *Professional burnout: Recent developments in theory and research* (pp. 115–133). Philadelphia, PA: Taylor & Francis.

Hobfoll, S. E., Lilly, R. S., & Jackson, A. P. (1992). Conservation of social resources and the self. In H. Veiel & U. Baumann (Eds.), *The meaning and measurement of social support* (pp. 125–141). Washington, DC: Hemisphere.

Hoffmann, D. A., & Tetrick, L. E. (2003). The etiology of the concept of health: Implications for "organizing" individual and organizational health. In D. A. Hofmann & L. E.

Tetrick (Eds.), *Health and safety in organizations: A multi-level perspective* (pp. 1–28). San Francisco, CA: Jossey-Bass.

Holahan, C. J., & Moos, R. H. (1987). Personal and contextual determinants of coping strategies. *Journal of Personality and Social Psychology*, *52*(5), 946–955.

Hood, R. W., Jr. (1975). The construction and preliminary validation of a measure of reported mystical experience. *Journal for the Scientific Study of Religion*, *14*(1), 29–41. doi:10.2307/1384454

Hood, R. W., Jr. (2013). Methodological diversity in the psychology of religion and spirituality. In K. I. Pargament, J. J. Exline, & J. W. Jones (Eds.), *APA handbook of psychology, religion, and spirituality: Context, theory, and research* (Vol. 1, pp. 79–102). Washington, DC: APA.

Hood, R. W., Jr., Morris, R. J., & Watson, P. J. (1989). Prayer experience and religious orientation. *Review of Religious Research*, *31*(1), 39–45. doi:10.2307/3511022

Hood, R. W., Jr., Spilka, B., Hunsberger, B., & Gorsuch, R. (1996). *The psychology of religion: An empirical approach* (2nd ed.). New York, NY: Guilford.

Hunsberger, B. (1989). A short version of the Christian orthodoxy scale. *Journal for the Scientific Study of Religion*, *28*(3), 360–365. doi:10.2307/1386747

Hunsberger, B., & Jackson, L. M. (2005). Religion, meaning, and prejudice. *Journal of Social Issues*, *61*(4), 807–826.

Jackson, D., Firtko, A., & Edenborough, M. (2007). Personal resilience as a strategy for surviving and thriving in the face of workplace adversity: A literature review. *Journal of Advanced Nursing*, *60*(1), 1–9. doi:10.1111/j.1365-2648.2007.04412.x

Johnson, R. B., Onwuegbuzie, A. J., & Turner, L. A. (2007). Toward a definition of mixed methods research. *Journal of Mixed Methods Research*, *1*(2), 112–133. doi:10.1177/1558689806298224

Judge, T. A., Erez, A., Bono, J. E., & Thoresen, C. J. (2002). Are measures of self-esteem, neuroticism, locus of control, and generalized self-efficacy indicators of a common core construct? *Journal of Personality and Social Psychology*, *83*(3), 693–710. doi:10.1037//0022-3514.83.3.693

Judge, T. A., Erez, A., Bono, J. E., & Thoresen, C. J. (2003). The core self-evaluations scale: Development of a measure. *Personnel Psychology*, *56*, 303–331.

Kalkan, K. O., Layman, G. C., & Uslaner, E. M. (2009). "Bands of others"? Attitudes toward Muslims in contemporary American society. *The Journal of Politics*, *71*(3), 847. doi:10.1017/s0022381609090756

Kaplan, R. (2001). The nature of the view from home: Psychological benefits. *Environment and Behavior*, *33*(4), 507–542. doi:10.1177/00139160121973115

Kaplan, R., & Kaplan, S. (1989). *The experience of nature: A psychological perspective*. Cambridge: Cambridge University Press.

Kaplan, S. (1995). The restorative benefits of nature – Toward an integrative framework. *Journal of Environmental Psychology*, *15*(3), 169–182. doi:10.1016/0272-4944(95)90001-2

Kay, A. C., Gaucher, D., McGregor, I., & Nash, K. (2010). Religious belief as compensatory control. *Personality and Social Psychology Review*, *14*(1), 37–48. doi:10.1177/1088868309353750

Kay, A. C., Gaucher, D., Napier, J. L., Callan, M. J., & Laurin, K. (2008). God and the government: Testing a compensatory control mechanism for the support of external systems. *Journal of Personality and Social Psychology*, *95*(1), 18–35. doi:10.1037/0022-3514.95.1.18

Kay, A. C., Whitson, J. A., Gaucher, D., & Galinsky, A. D. (2009). Compensatory control: Achieving order through the mind, our institutions, and the heavens. *Current Directions in Psychological Science*, *18*(5), 264–268.

Khan, Z. H., & Watson, P. J. (2006). Construction of the Pakistani religious coping practices scale: Correlations with religious coping, religious orientation, and reactions to stress among Muslim university students. *International Journal for the Psychology of Religion*, *16*, 101–112.

Koenig, H., Parkerson, G. R., Jr., & Meador, K. G. (1997). Religion index for psychiatric research. *American Journal of Psychiatry*, *154*(6), 885–886.

Koenig, H. G., McCullough, M. E., & Larson, D. B. (2001). *Handbook of religion and health*. New York, NY: Oxford University Press.

Korpela, K. M., Hartig, T., Kaiser, F. G., & Fuhrer, U. (2001). Restorative experience and self-regulation in favorite places. *Environment and Behavior*, *33*(4), 572–589. doi:10.1177/00139160121973133

Krause, N. (2008). The social foundation of religious meaning in life. *Research on Aging*, *30*(4), 395–427.

Ladd, K. L., & Spilka, B. (2013). Prayer: A review of the empirical literature. In K. I. Pargament, J. J. Exline, & J. W. Jones (Eds.), *APA handbook of psychology, religion, and spirituality: Context, theory, and research* (Vol. 1, pp. 293–310). Washington, DC: APA.

Laurin, K., Kay, A. C., & Fitzsimons, G. M. (2012). Divergent effects of activating thoughts of God on self-regulation. *Journal of Personality and Social Psychology*, *102*(1), 4–21. doi:10.1037/a0025971

Laythe, B., Finkel, D. G., Bringle, R. G., & Kirkpatrick, L. A. (2002). Religious fundamentalism as a predictor of prejudice: A two-component model. *Journal for the Scientific Study of Religion*, *41*(4), 623–635. doi:10.1111/1468-5906.00142

Lazarus, R. S. (1993). From psychological stress to the emotions: A history of changing outlooks. *Annual Review of Psychology*, *44*, 1–21. doi:10.1146/annurev.ps.44.020193.000245

LePine, J. A., LePine, M. A., & Jackson, C. L. (2004). Challenge and hindrance stress: Relationships with exhaustion, motivation to learn, and learning performance. *Journal of Applied Psychology*, *89*(5), 883–891. doi:10.1037/0021-9010.89.5.883

Luszczynska, A., & Schwarzer, R. (2005). Multidimensional health locus of control: Comments on the construct and its measurement. *Journal of Health Psychology*, *10*(5), 633–642. doi:10.1177/1359105305055307

Masters, K. S., & Wallston, K. A. (2005). Canonical correlation reveals important relations between health locus of control, coping, affect and values. *Journal of Health Psychology*, *10*(5), 719–735. doi:10.1177/1359105305055332

Maton, K. I. (1989). The stress-buffering role of spiritual support, cross-sectional and prospective investigations. *Journal for the Scientific Study of Religion*, *28*(3), 310–323. doi: 10.2307/1386742

McCullough, M. E., & Carter, E. C. (2013). Religion, self-control, and self-regulation: How and why are they related? In K. I. Pargament, J. J. Exline, & J. W. Jones (Eds.), *APA handbook of psychology, religion, and spirituality: Context, theory, and research* (Vol. 1, pp. 123–138). Washington, DC: APA.

McCullough, M. E., & Willoughby, B. L. (2009). Religion, self-regulation, and self-control: Associations, explanations, and implications. *Psychological Bulletin*, *135*(1), 69–93. doi:10.1037/a0014213

McGregor, I., Haji, R., Nash, K. A., & Teper, R. (2008). Religious zeal and the uncertain self. *Basic and Applied Social Psychology*, *30*(2), 183–188. doi:10.1080/01973530802209251

Meijman, T. F., & Mulder, G. (1998). Psychological aspects of workload. In P. J. D. Drength & H. Thierry (Eds.), *Handbook of work and organizational psychology* (Vol. 2, pp. 5–33). Hove, UK: Psychology Press.

Moore, L. J., Vine, S. J., Wilson, M. R., & Freeman, P. (2012). The effect of challenge and threat states on performance: An examination of potential mechanisms. *Psychophysiology*, *49*(10), 1417–1425. doi:10.1111/j.1469-8986.2012.01449.x

Morse, N. C., & Weiss, R. S. (1955). The function and meaning of work and the job. *American Sociological Review*, *20*(2), 191–198.

Muraven, M., & Baumeister, R. F. (2000). Self-regulation and depletion of limited resources: Does self-control resemble a muscle? *Psychological Bulletin*, *126*(2), 247–259.

Muraven, M., Tice, D. M., & Baumeister, R. F. (1998). Self-control as limited resource: Regulatory depletion patterns. *Journal of Personality and Social Psychology*, *74*(3), 774–789. doi:10.1037/0022-3514.74.3.774

O'Cathain, A. (2009). Editorial: Mixed methods research in the health sciences: A quiet revolution. *Journal of Mixed Methods Research*, *3*(1), 3–6. doi:10.1177/1558689808326272

Paloutzian, R. F., & Ellison, C. W. (1991). *Manual for the spiritual well-being scale*. Nyack, NY: Life Advance.

Pargament, K. I. (1997). *The psychology of religion and coping: Theory, research, practice*. New York, NY: The Guilford Press.

Pargament, K. I., Kennell, J., Hathaway, W., Grevengoed, N., Newman, J., & Jones, W. (1988). Religion and the problem-solving process: Three styles of coping. *Journal for the Scientific Study of Religion*, *27*, 90–104.

Pargament, K. I., Mahoney, A., Exline, J. J., Jones, J. W., & Shafranske, E. P. (2013). Envisioning an integrative paradigm for the psychology of religion and spirituality. In K. I. Pargament, J. J. Exline, & J. W. Jones (Eds.), *APA handbook of psychology, religion, and spirituality: Context, theory, and research* (Vol. 1, pp. 3–19). Washington, DC: APA.

Pargament, K. I., Smith, B. W., Koenig, H. G., & Perez, L. (1998). Patterns of positive and negative religious coping with major life stressors. *Journal for the Scientific Study of Religion*, *37*(4), 710–724. doi:10.2307/1388152

Park, C. L. (2005). Religion as a meaning-making framework in coping with life stress. *Journal of Social Issues*, *61*(4), 707–729. doi:10.1111/j.1540-4560.2005.00428.x

Park, C. L., & Folkman, S. (1997). Meaning in the context of stress and coping. *Review of General Psychology*, *1*(2), 115–144.

Patel, S. P., & Cunningham, C. J. L. (2012). Religion, resources, and work-family balance. *Mental Health, Religion & Culture*, *15*(4), 389–401. doi:10.1080/13674676.2011.577765

Pew Research Center. (2008). U.S. religious landscape survey. Retrieved January 13, 2014 from http://religions.pewforum.org/

Piedmont, R. L. (1999). Does spirituality represent the sixth factor of personality? Spiritual transcendence and the five-factor model. *Journal of Personality*, *67*(6), 985–1013.

Piedmont, R. L., & Wilkins, T. A. (2013). Spirituality, religiousness, and personality: Theoretical foundations and empirical applications. In K. I. Pargament, J. J. Exline, & J. W. Jones (Eds.), *APA handbook of psychology, religion, and spirituality: Context, theory, and research* (Vol. 1, pp. 173–186). Washington, DC: APA.

Plante, T. G., & Boccaccini, M. T. (1997). The Santa Clara strength of religious faith questionnaire. *Pastoral Psychology*, *45*(5), 375–387.

Podsakoff, N. P., LePine, J. A., & LePine, M. A. (2007). Differential challenge stressor-hindrance stressor relationships with job attitudes, turnover intentions, turnover, and withdrawal behavior: A meta-analysis. *Journal of Applied Psychology*, *92*(2), 438–454. doi:10.1037/0021-9010.92.2.438

Rachlin, H. (2000). *The science of self-control*. Cambridge, MA: Harvard University Press.

Rosmarin, D. H., Pargament, K. I., Krumrei, E. J., & Flannelly, K. J. (2009). Religious coping among Jews: Development and initial validation of the JCOPE. *Journal of Clinical Psychology*, *65*(7), 670–683.

Rowatt, W., & Kirkpatrick, L. A. (2002). Two dimensions of attachment to God and their relation to affect, religiosity, and personality constructs. *Journal for the Scientific Study of Religion*, *41*(4), 637–651.

Sapolsky, R. M. (1998). *Why zebras don't get ulcers: An updated guide to stress, stress-related diseases, and coping*. New York, NY: W. H. Freeman and Company.

Shapiro, S. L., Astin, J. A., Bishop, S. R., & Cordova, M. (2005). Mindfulness-based stress reduction for health care professionals: Results from a randomized trial. *International Journal of Stress Management*, *12*(2), 164–176. doi:10.1037/1072-5245.12.2.164

Soenke, M., Landau, M. J., & Greenberg, J. (2013). Sacred armor: Religion's role as a buffer against the anxieties of life and the fear of death. In K. I. Pargament, J. J. Exline, & J. W. Jones (Eds.), *APA handbook of psychology, religion, and spirituality: Context, theory, and research* (Vol. 1, pp. 105–122). Washington, DC: APA.

Sonnentag, S. (2001). Work, recovery activities, and individual well-being: A diary study. *Journal of Occupational Health Psychology*, *6*(3), 196–210.

Sonnentag, S., & Frese, M. (2012). Stress in organizations. In I. B. Weiner, N. W. Schmitt, & S. Highhouse (Eds.), *Handbook of psychology* (2nd ed., Vol. 12, pp. 560–592). Hoboken, NJ: Wiley.

Spector, P. E., & Brannick, M. T. (2011). Methodological urban legends: The misuse of statistical control variables. *Organizational Research Methods*, *14*(2), 287–305. doi:10.1177/1094428110369842

Sulsky, L., & Smith, C. (2005). *Work stress*. Belmont, CA: Thomson Wadsworth.

Tashakkori, A., & Creswell, J. W. (2008). Editorial: Mixed methodology across disciplines. *Journal of Mixed Methods Research*, *2*(1), 3–6. doi:10.1177/1558689807309913

Tix, A. P., & Frazier, P. A. (1998). The use of religious coping during stressful life events: Main effects, moderation, and mediation. *Journal of Consulting and Clinical Psychology*, *66*(2), 411–422. doi:10.1037/0022-006x.66.2.411

Trougakos, J. P., & Hideg, I. (2009). Momentary work recovery: The role of within-day work breaks. In S. Sonnentag, P. L. Perrewé, & D. C. Ganster (Eds.), *Current perspectives on job-stress recovery* (Vol. 7, 37–84). Research in Occupational Stress and Well Being. Bingley, UK: Emerald Group Publishing Limited. doi:10.1108/s1479-3555(2009)0000007005

Underwood, L. G., & Teresi, J. A. (2002). The daily spiritual experience scale: Development, theoretical description, reliability, exploratory factor analysis, and preliminary construct validity using health-related data. *Annals of Behavioral Medicine*, *24*(1), 22–33.

van Hooff, M. L. M., Geurts, S. A. E., Beckers, D. G. J., & Kompier, M. A. J. (2011). Daily recovery from work: The role of activities, effort and pleasure. *Work & Stress*, *25*(1), 55–74. doi:10.1080/02678373.2011.570941

Vecchio, R. P. (1980). The function and meaning of work and the job: Morse and Weiss (1955) revisited. *Academy of Management Journal*, *23*(2), 361–367.

Wallston, K. A. (1997). Perceived control and health behaviour. In A. Baum, C. McManus, S. Newman, J. Weinman, & R. West (Eds.), *Cambridge handbook of psychology, health and medicine* (Vol. 1, pp. 151–154). Cambridge, UK: Cambridge University Press.

Wang, C., Bannuru, R., Ramel, J., Kupelnick, B., Scott, T., & Schmid, C. H. (2010). Tai Chi on psychological well-being: Systematic review and meta-analysis. *BMC Complementary and Alternative Medicine*, *10*, 23. doi:10.1186/1472-6882-10-23

Warr, P. (2005). Work, well-being, and mental health. In J. Barling, E. K. Kelloway, & M. R. Frone (Eds.), *Handbook of work stress* (pp. 547–573). Thousand Oaks, CA: Sage.

Warr, P. (2013). How to think about and measure psychological well-being. In R. R. Sinclair, M. Wang, & L. E. Tetrick (Eds.), *Research methods in occupational health psychology: Measurement, design, and data analysis* (pp. 76–90). New York, NY: Routledge.

Webster, J. R., Beehr, T. A., & Love, K. (2011). Extending the challenge-hindrance model of occupational stress: The role of appraisal. *Journal of Vocational Behavior*, *79*(2), 505–516. doi:10.1016/j.jvb.2011.02.001

Weiss, H. M., & Rupp, D. E. (2011). Experiencing work: An essay on a person-centric work psychology. *Industrial and Organizational Psychology*, *4*(1), 83–97.

Wells, J. D., Hobfoll, S. E., & Lavin, J. (1999). When it rains, it pours: The greater impact of resource loss compared to gain on psychological distress. *Personality and Social Psychology Bulletin*, *25*(9), 1172–1182. doi:10.1177/01461672992512010

Wilber, K. (2000). *Integral psychology: Consciousness, spirit, psychology, therapy*. Boston, MA: Shambhala.

Williamson, P. W., Hood, R. W., Jr., Ahmad, A., Sadiq, M., & Hill, P. C. (2010). The intratextual fundamentalism scale: Cross-cultural application, validity evidence, and relationship with religious orientation and the Big 5 factor markers. *Mental Health, Religion & Culture*, *13*(7–8), 721–747.

Wolever, R. Q., Bobinet, K. J., McCabe, K., Mackenzie, E. R., Fekete, E., Kusnick, C. A., & Baime, M. (2012). Effective and viable mind-body stress reduction in the workplace: A randomized controlled trial. *Journal of Occupational Health Psychology*, *17*(2), 246–258. doi:10.1037/a0027278

Wood, B. T., Worthington, E. L., Jr., Exline, J. J., Yali, A. M., Aten, J. D., & McMinn, M. R. (2010). Development, refinement, and psychometric properties of the attitudes toward God scale (ATGS-9). *Psychology of Religion and Spirituality*, *2*(3), 148.

Worthington, E. L., Jr., Wade, N. G., Hight, T. L., Ripley, J. S., McCullough, M. E., Berry, J. W., … O'Connor, L. (2003). The religious commitment inventory–10: Development, refinement, and validation of a brief scale for research and counseling. *Journal of Counseling Psychology*, *50*(1), 84.

ANTECEDENTS, OUTCOMES, PREVENTION AND COPING STRATEGIES FOR LESBIAN, GAY, AND BISEXUAL WORKPLACE STRESS

Isaac Sabat, Alex Lindsey and Eden King

ABSTRACT

Lesbian, gay, and bisexual (LGB) individuals experience institutionalized prejudice within society and in their working lives. This prejudice increases the stress that these individuals experience within the workplace. Thus, in this chapter, we outline the mechanisms of LGB-workplace stress, detailing the antecedents, outcomes, and strategies to remediate this form of stress. We first outline theoretical conceptualizations of workplace stress before explaining how sexual orientation minorities experience additional workplace stressors due to their specific, stigmatized identities. Then, we explain how the stressors of formal discrimination, interpersonal discrimination, stigma consciousness, internalized heterosexism, concealment, and social isolation each contribute to workplace stress and ultimately health and workplace outcomes. Finally, we discuss several strategies that organizations, stigmatized individuals,

The Role of Demographics in Occupational Stress and Well Being
Research in Occupational Stress and Well Being, Volume 12, 173–198

ISSN: 1479-3555/doi:10.1108/S1479-355520140000012005

and allies can engage in to prevent and cope with each of these LGB-related workplace stressors. In so doing, this chapter encourages researchers and practitioners to continue to develop more comprehensive and effective strategies to combat the negative outcomes experienced by these and all other stigmatized employees, thereby promoting more healthy and inclusive organizations.

Keywords: Sexual orientation; LGB; minority; stress; health; workplace

Despite recently improving attitudes (Hicks & Lee, 2006), sexual orientation minorities (individuals who identify as lesbian, gay, or bisexual [LGB]) continue to report experiencing prejudice and hostility within society and their places of work (Badgett, Lau, Sears, & Ho, 2007; Herek, 2009). Compared to heterosexual individuals, sexual orientation minority employees are less likely to be hired and promoted (Badgett et al., 2007) and are more likely to have negative interpersonal experiences in the workplace (Badgett et al., 2007; Hebl, Foster, Mannix, & Dovidio, 2002). Importantly, this pervasive workplace discrimination adversely affects the workplace outcomes of these individuals, including increased stress and decreased feelings of wellbeing. Thus, the current chapter examines the processes associated with sexual orientation minority employees' experiences of workplace stress. We begin by outlining theoretical conceptualizations of workplace stress. Then, we identify the stressors commonly experienced by sexual orientation minority employees and explain how these stressors differentially impact workplace stress. Next, we describe the health and organizational outcomes associated with this form of stress. Finally, we draw upon work from organizational diversity research to suggest several prevention and coping strategies to counteract these stressors. Thus, the current chapter provides a comprehensive framework through which practitioners and researchers can better understand how the demographic characteristic of sexual orientation impacts stress in the workplace.

OCCUPATIONAL STRESS

Stress is a negative physiological response to an event that cognitively taxes an individual beyond what they are able to endure (Dohrenwend, 2000).

These events, often referred to as stressors, can produce a variety of negative psychological and physical health outcomes (see Cohen, Kessler, & Gordon, 1995 for reviews). Stressors have been shown to be related to depression, heart disease, and decreased immune functioning (Cohen, Janicki-Deverts, & Miller, 2007). These stressors can therefore have a major impact on an organization's bottom line. Workplace stressors have been shown to relate to increased absenteeism (Jacobson et al., 1996), increased turnover intentions, and decreased job commitment, motivation, and job satisfaction (Podsakoff, LePine, & LePine, 2007). Thus, organizations and organizational researchers have become more and more interested in decreasing the prevalence and impact of workplace stressors (Bevan, 2010).

There are a number of ways to conceptualize the stressors that produce stress in the workplace. For the purposes of this chapter, we will be differentiating stressors that are socially derived from those that are individually derived (Meyer, 2003). Socially derived stressors are those that are caused by situations within an environment that are outside of a person's control (Meyer, 2003). These stress-inducing situations can involve major negative life changes or smaller, long-lasting negative experiences (Kanner, Coyne, Schaefer, & Lazarus, 1981). Examples of social stressors within the workplace include having to work in a hostile work environment or expecting to be laid off when a company encounters economic instability.

Stressors may also be considered individual stressors if they involve ambiguously stressful situations that some individuals appraise as harmful whereas others do not. Within these ambiguously stressful situations, a large degree of individual variability will emerge as individuals must cognitively assess whether they have the mental capacities to cope with the stressors that they experience (Lazarus, 1991; Lazarus & Folkman, 1984) Within the workplace, these individualized stressors can include feeling personally hurt by a criticism that may or may not have been intentionally harmful or trying to hide family-related difficulties from coworkers.

Although all employees are susceptible to experiencing both forms of stressors within the workplace, stigmatized minority members will likely experience a greater number of social stressors and therefore a greater number of individual stressors in organizations as a result of their minority status. We examine both external events and individual reactions to these events in order to fully understand the mechanisms of stress that sexual orientation minorities encounter within their working lives.

LGB Stress

The Minority Stress Model (Meyer, 1995) postulates that individuals with stigmatized social characteristics are likely to endure heightened levels of stress within their daily lives as a result of their stigmatized, minority status. This model is based on social and psychological research on the negative outcomes of prejudice and stigma on the lives of these minority groups (e.g., Allport, 1954; Crocker, Major, & Steele, 1998; Goffman, 1963). According to this model, institutionalized discrimination toward specific minority groups leads to an ascribed inferior status toward those groups, causing minority group members to be subjected to direct and indirect negative life events (Brooks, 1981; Meyer, 1995). According to Meyer (1995, 2003), LGB individuals commonly experience a specific set of stressors as a result of their stigmatized sexual orientation. These stressors, which involve both social and individual forms, include experiencing prejudiced events, fears, and expectations of experiencing prejudice, internalization of homophobia, and concealing one's sexual orientation. Our focus is on workplace-related stress, which requires that we contextualize Meyer's model within the characteristics and concerns of the workplace. In so doing, we refine Meyer's model in two specific ways. First, we identify workplace social isolation as an additional LGB-related workplace stressor. Second, we distinguish between formal and interpersonal discrimination and explain how both independently relate to LGB-workplace stress. Below we describe the stressors of formal discrimination, interpersonal discrimination, stigma consciousness, internalized heterosexism, concealing, and social isolation, and explain how each of these stressors independently and interactively produce workplace stress (see Fig. 1).

Formal Discrimination

Meyer (1995, 2003) identifies prejudiced events as one of the antecedents of LGB-related stress. Heterosexist prejudice, defined as "an ideological system that denies, denigrates, and stigmatizes any non-heterosexual form of behavior, identity, relationship, or community" (Herek, 1992, p. 89), is still widely prevalent in American society. Within the workplace, this form of prejudice often manifests itself in formal job discrimination, or the discrimination of individuals with regard to formal job outcomes, such as selection, retention, promotion, or termination based primarily on one's sexual orientation (Badgett et al., 2007).

Formal discrimination against LGB employees has been widely documented. A review of studies (Badgett et al., 2007) demonstrates that 8–17% of

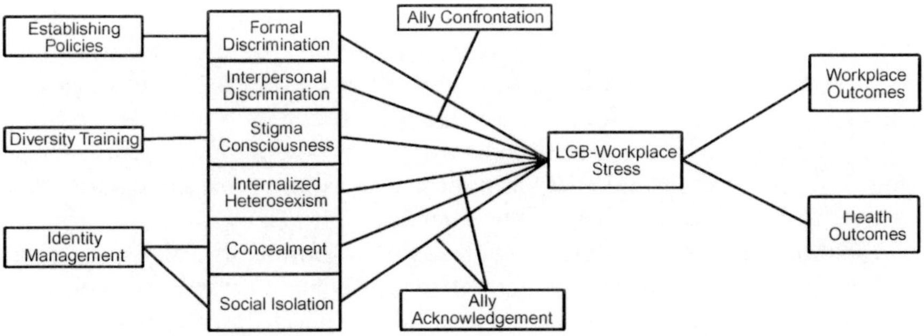

Fig. 1. Model of Prevention and Coping Strategies for LGB-Workplace Stress.

sexual orientation minorities report being unfairly fired or not hired as a result of their sexual orientations. 10–28% of these individuals indicated that they received unfair promotion decisions due to their stigmatized sexual orientations. The 2008 General Social Survey (GSS) indicated that 42% of a nationally representative sample of LGB individuals reported experiencing formal workplace discrimination within their working lives (Pizer, Sears, Mallory, & Hunter, 2012). Unlike several other minority groups (e.g., ethnic minorities and religious minorities), LGB employees are not currently federally protected from workplace discrimination, and only 21 states ban this form of discrimination (Employment Non-Discrimination Act, 2014). Thus, they often have no legal recourse against these formal discriminatory acts.

Importantly, these acts of discrimination have been shown to produce a high level of work-related stress for sexual orientation minorities for several reasons. First, this form of discrimination is most likely to be carried out by organizational leaders. Thus, this type of discrimination is likely to signal to the targets that the organization as a whole is unsupportive of them and that it has a hostile or negative diversity culture. Indeed, organizational leaders have a great deal of influence regarding the culture of their organizations (Schein, 1985). Second, this power difference is likely to make the targets feel helpless in dealing with the incident and less capable of coping with the resulting stress. The stress that they experience from these incidents may be compounded by the fact that this form of discrimination is not legally protected in most states, and thus, there is often little that targets can officially do to prevent it. Third and finally, these acts have the potential to harm an individual's livelihood. If an individual is either unable to obtain employment or terminated unfairly due to their minority sexual orientation, they will feel stress as a result of being unable to support themselves and their families financially. These job and life outcomes are social stressors that produce a great deal of stress within virtually any individual who experiences them. Indeed, survey studies have demonstrated that experiencing formal discrimination is predictive of workplace stress (Mays, Coleman, & Jackson, 1996; Pizer et al., 2012).

Despite the lack of federally protective legislation, several states, cities, and municipalities have implemented or are beginning to implement laws to prohibit this form of discrimination, and a majority of Americans support such federal protection (Gallup, 2006; Krehely, 2011). Thus, although formal discrimination persists, legal and societal pressure against formal, overt acts of discrimination serve as countervailing forces. Accordingly, the nature of workplace discrimination is changing to become more implicit or subtle or nature (Ruggs, Martinez, & Hebl, 2011).

Interpersonal Discrimination

Interpersonal discrimination involves the negative treatment of stigmatized individuals in the workplace in ways that are not directly tied to workplace outcomes. Examples of this form of discrimination involve social interactions that are brief, unfriendly, and infrequent with sexual orientation minority employees compared to social interactions with heterosexual employees (see Hebl et al., 2002). Studies have found that sexual orientation minorities experience a great deal of interpersonal discrimination within their places of work (Badgett et al., 2007). Interpersonal discrimination is becoming increasingly more common in American workplaces, as it continues to replace traditional methods of formal discrimination. These trends highlight the fact that heterosexist prejudice still continues to exist, but because of increasing pressure for individuals and organizations to appear egalitarian, this prejudice is now "leaking out" in more subtle ways. The difficulty with interpersonal discrimination is that it is difficult to create policies or laws that regulate these interpersonal acts (Sue et al., 2007). Indeed, one cannot simply claim that one was treated unfairly or discriminated against simply because a coworker was unfriendly toward them.

Although one may think that this change in the nature of discrimination from formal to interpersonal should be hailed as an accomplishment, recent evidence suggest that both forms can be destructive and psychologically damaging, but for different reasons. There are several reasons why this might be the case. First, interpersonal discrimination is much more ambiguous in nature. Therefore, it requires more cognitive effort to attend to signs that one is being discriminated against. Whereas overt, formal acts of discrimination may be easier to ignore due to the fact that they clearly stem from prejudice toward one's stigmatizing characteristics, it may be more difficult to decipher the true root causes of interpersonal negativity as a result of interpersonal discrimination (Noh, Kaspar, & Wickrama, 2007). Because LGB employees are often unaware of who has information regarding their stigmatized sexual orientations, they may find it especially difficult to distinguish the root causes of this negativity. Thus, LGB targets may be more likely to internalize these behaviors and feel as though they have done something to deserve this negative, differential treatment. Thus, interpersonal discrimination can be more cognitively taxing to stigmatized individuals, thereby producing high amounts of workplace stress.

Second, interpersonal discrimination often manifests itself through decreases in the quality of social interactions. Thus, individuals experiencing interpersonal discrimination are likely to feel as though they do not fit in to the organizational social hierarchies. Consequently, interpersonal discrimination can lead to feelings of social isolation, which we will discuss in more detail later.

Third and finally, interpersonal discrimination can lead to high levels of workplace stress due to the fact that this form of discrimination is a more chronic and pervasive form of discrimination compared to formal discrimination. While employees are rarely facing the possibility of formal discrimination through selection, evaluation, and termination decisions, they are frequently engaged in social interactions or communications with other employees. Thus, interpersonal discrimination has the potential to be a chronic and long lasting form of subtle negativity that pervades one's working life. Stress researchers have noted that minor but long-lasting stressors can be more harmful than singular, major life events (Kanner et al., 1981). Thus, interpersonal discrimination can be just as stressful if not more stressful than blatant acts of prejudice that are tied to one's employment outcomes.

Studies have corroborated these findings, showing that interpersonal discrimination does lead to high levels of workplace stress (Deitch et al., 2003). A meta-analysis comparing interpersonal and formal discrimination found that interpersonal discrimination was at least as damaging as formal discrimination, if not more so (Jones, Peddie, Gilrane, King, & Gray, 2013). More work is needed to experimentally test which form of discrimination produces higher levels of workplace stress. However, as interpersonal discrimination becomes much more prevalent in today's society in comparison to formal discrimination, it is likely that interpersonal discrimination is more of a problem for modern organizations. Thus, researchers should expend greater efforts in developing and testing strategies to combat interpersonal forms of workplace discrimination in addition to previous efforts focused on combating formal discrimination.

Stigma Consciousness

As a result of directly experienced heterosexist prejudice and institutionalized societal heterosexism, LGB individuals may become vigilant in their social interactions with coworkers and employers. This vigilance regarding one's stigma has been labeled stigma consciousness, or "the extent to which people focus on their stereotyped status" (Pinel & Paulin, 2005, p. 1). Stigma consciousness is considered an LGB work-related stressor due to the fact that it can be cognitively taxing to constantly monitor one's interactions. Individuals with high levels of stigma consciousness are constantly aware of their stigmatized status and frequently expect to be subjected to discriminatory actions (Pinel, 1999). Even in the absence of discrimination, stigma consciousness can produce workplace stress in LGB minorities due to the fact that they are constantly fearful and expecting to be subject to discrimination. Additionally, this stressor may cause individuals to assume they are being discriminated against even in instances where they are not. For instance, women who were higher in stigma consciousness were more likely to interpret negative performance ratings from a man as being derived from discrimination (Pinel, 2004). Thus, stigma consciousness is a predominantly individual stressor.

Importantly, because stigma consciousness relates to heightened levels of perceived discrimination, this stressor should also relate to workplace stress. Indeed, studies have found that having higher levels of stigma consciousness relates to higher levels of psychological distress (Berghe, Dewaele, Cox, & Vincke, 2010). Thus, organizations should employ strategies to minimize the levels of stigma consciousness among their sexual orientation minority employees.

Internalized Heterosexism

Internalized heterosexism – previously referred to as internalized homophobia (Maylon, 1982) or internalized homonegativity (Mayfield, 2001) – is when sexual orientation minorities direct negatively held beliefs inward toward the self, leading to a devaluation of one's sexual minority identity (Meyer & Dean, 1998; Williamson, 2000). Experiencing heterosexism or expecting to experience heterosexism can in some cases lead to a situation where individuals view their own stigmas with a sense of shame and negativity. Thus, internalized heterosexism is considered an LGB workplace stressor.

This stressor can cause a state of internal conflict between one's identity and one's attitudes toward one's identity. This internalization of a deviant identity is likely to produce severe levels of stress throughout one's life. Although internalized heterosexism is most likely to affect LGB individuals at the earlier stages of the "coming out" process, it is unlikely that this stressor ever completely ceases to affect these individuals (Cass, 1984; Coleman, 1982; Meyer, 1995). Especially given that LGB individuals continuously experience societal negativity and discrimination, it is likely that internalized heterosexism continues to have an impact on their health and wellbeing throughout all stages of their development, including their working lives (Gonsiorek, 1988; Maylon, 1982; Meyer, 1995).

A meta-analysis showed that internalized heterosexism is related to distress and anxiety (Newcomb & Mustanski, 2010) for sexual orientation minority individuals. Thus, organizational researchers and practitioners should do what is in their power to promote positivity and acceptance regarding all sexual orientation identities within the workplace.

Concealing

LGB individuals have the ability to conceal their stigmatized identities. This allows these individuals to avoid experiencing acts of formal discrimination at work, and thus, can be a beneficial strategy overall in workplace environments that are hostile toward sexual orientation minorities. Additionally, individuals who conceal their identities do not have to worry about whether their identities will be perceived negatively by others, and thus, they do not have to worry about experiencing stress associated with interpersonal discrimination (Clair, Beatty, & MacLean, 2005). Although it may seem as though concealing reduces the likelihood that sexual orientation minorities experience LGB workplace stress, this is simply not the case (Pachankis, 2007). The act of concealing may still produce high levels of workplace stress but for a different set of reasons.

First, individuals who conceal create fewer opportunities for contact with other sexual orientation minorities within their organizations, and they are not able to obtain resources from the organization such as social support and organizational attention. For instance, an organization may assume that there are no sexual orientation minority employees if all sexual minorities within that organization conceal their sexual identities. Thus, this organization may decide not to implement policies that could have otherwise supported and protected these individuals. Second, individuals who reveal their identities are more likely to receive social support from allies and other sexual orientation minorities within their organization. Revealing one's LGB-identity may also spur others to reveal their minority sexual orientations, thus forming a social network of similar and/or supportive individuals within the workforce. Thus, all in all, concealing one's minority sexual identity reduces opportunities for social contact, which reduces one's ability to gain resources to cope with LGB workplace stressors.

Second, concealing produces workplace stress due to the fact that these individuals have to constantly monitor their concealed identities, which can be highly cognitively taxing. Individuals who are not "out" must worry about whether "to display or not to display, to tell or not to tell, to let on or not to let on, to lie or not to lie, and in each case, to whom, how, when, and where" (Goffman, 1963, p. 42), which requires a tremendous amount of cognitive effort. Indeed, it is difficult to keep track of what information about one's stigmatized identity is known to others, especially when there is a large amount of variability in the amount and type of information that one decides to conceal from each interaction partner. It may also be the case that individuals are "closeted" within the workplace but "out" within their non-work domains. This has the potential to produce concealment disconnects, which lead to greater levels of stress if LGB individuals are concealing differentially across life domains (Ragins, 2008).

Third, coworkers may obtain information about an individual's stigmatized identity through alternate, indirect means, such as gossip, stereotypical cues, or physical identifiers (Ambady, Hallahan, & Conner, 1999; Colgan, Creegan, McKearney, & Wright, 2007; Jernigan & Mistree, 2009). In these scenarios, the concealer may appear inauthentic or untrustworthy if they are caught lying or withholding information about their identity. Survey studies have shown that gay or lesbian individuals were rated more negatively if others knew they were concealing (Oswald, 2007) or if others gained this information from a third party (Ward & Brenner, 2006). Thus, individuals who conceal their identities in the workplace must worry about what sources and amounts of prior information their interaction partners have regarding their identities.

Fourth and finally, individuals who conceal may experience stress due to internal feelings of inauthenticity (Clair et al., 2005; Goffman, 1963). According to Smart and Wegner, "concealing a stigma leads to an inner turmoil that is remarkable for its intensity and its capacity for absorbing an individual's mental life" (2000, p. 221). Furthermore, Self-Verification Theory (Swann, 1983) states that individuals are highly motivated to reach consistency between others' views of them and their views of themselves. Thus, sexual orientation minority individuals who decide to conceal their identities are helping to perpetuate inauthentic personas to their coworkers. On a very basic level, this is an example of a fundamental cognitive dissonance between one's internalized self and the self that is manifest at work (see Festinger, 1962). Wegner and Lane (1995) also discuss the impact that perpetuating secret identities can have on psychological and physical health outcomes. Some research has highlighted that those who consider their minority sexual orientation identities to be a central part of their self-concepts are more likely to disclose (Griffith & Hebl, 2002), highlighting the importance of having authentic selves in workplace contexts.

As demonstrated, there are several potential reasons why concealing one's stigmatized sexual identity can produce workplace stress. Studies have even shown that the stress associated with concealing in the workplace is more detrimental than the disclosure itself (Clair et al., 2005; Ragins & Cornwell, 2001). Thus, especially in the absence of social stressors, LGB targets could disclose their sexual orientation within organizations in order to reduce this individual stressor of concealment. More work is needed to understand how to promote these positive disclosures within a workplace setting.

Social Isolation

Social isolation, or the lack of social support and connections, is a determinant of LGB stress that may be of particular importance in a workplace domain. LGB employees are likely to experience social isolation in the workplace for several reasons. First, LGB employees make up a very small percentage of the population, with estimates of LGB employees ranging from 4% to 17% (Gonsiorek & Weinrich, 1991; Powers, 1996). According to the seminal piece by Kanter (1977), belonging to a social category that is underrepresented in the workplace is a direct determinant of social isolation. A major tenant of Meyer's (1995) LGB stress theory is that sexual orientation minorities experience negative psychological outcomes as a result of being in environments where they are almost always minorities. Second, unlike other social contexts, LGB employees have little choice regarding with whom they interact. Because a large number of individuals in this country hold heterosexist beliefs (Gallup, 2006, 2012), it is likely that sexual orientation minorities have to work in environments surrounded by individuals who do not support them. Third and finally, because sexual orientation minorities have the ability to – and often do – conceal their stigmatized identities within the workplace, other LGB individuals will perceive the organization as being even less diverse in terms of sexuality than it really is. Thus, it is likely to be quite difficult for these individuals to make friends with coworkers who share their same sexual orientation. For these and other reasons, sexual orientation minorities are likely to experience fewer opportunities for social connections and increased social isolation within their places of work.

Importantly, social isolation is likely to produce workplace stress. Some theories have postulated that social stress is purely a result of the conflict between an individual and their society (e.g., Lazarus & Folkman, 1984). Individuals who experience social isolation within the workplace are likely to perceive a mismatch between themselves and their organizations' social networks, thereby eliciting social stress. Studies have shown that social isolation does in fact impact physiological health and stress responses (Grant, Hamer, & Steptoe, 2009; House, Landis, & Umberson, 1988), and a recent meta-analysis showed that social support (the opposite of social isolation) moderated the relationship between experienced discrimination against LGB individuals and stress (Pascoe & Richman, 2009). Thus, social isolation is a significant individual-level workplace stressor that affects many LGB employees and targets and allies should do what is in their power to remediate this source of stress.

Interactive Effects

Although each of the aforementioned LGB workplace stressors are theorized to have main effects on the stress levels of LGB minority employees, it is important to note that these stressors may also interact to produce stress. For instance, experiencing a greater number of social stressors (such as formal discriminatory treatment) can increase the number of experienced individual stressors (such as stigma consciousness and concealing). Additionally, concealing behaviors can increase the negative effects associated with social isolation, as individuals who conceal must hide a part of their identities from others and therefore cannot fully connect with others who may share similar characteristics. Lastly, the stressor of social isolation may enhance the negative effects of all other LGB stressors. Indeed, social support has been shown to act as an important buffering mechanism between stressful events and harmful stress-related outcomes.

It is important to understand how these stressors can independently and interactively produce workplace stress among this stigmatized population. Below, we outline the many potential health and workplace outcomes associated with LGB-workplace stress.

OUTCOMES OF STRESS

Health-Related Outcomes

The relationship between workplace stress and health outcomes has been well documented (Spector, Dwyer, & Jex, 1988). Excessive chronic stress has been shown to cause depression, cardiovascular disease, and problems regulating the immune system (Cohen et al., 2007). Studies have found that stressful events lead to depression, with approximately 20–25% of individuals who experienced major, social stressors developing symptoms of depression (van Praag, de Koet, & van Os, 2004). Experiments on animals, healthy adults, and cardiac patients suggest that stress can foster myocardial ischemia and other inflammatory mechanisms within the heart (Krantz & McCeney, 2002). Stress has also been linked to alterations of the immune system through the innervation of lymphatic tissue, leaving individuals susceptible to a host of other diseases (Cohen et al., 2007). Some researchers have even begun to suggest that chronic stress can result in the development and progression of cancer, although more research is needed in this area to be able to form causal conclusions (Heffner, Loving, Robles, & Kiecolt-Glaser, 2003; Reiche, Nunes, & Morimoto, 2004).

Because LGB individuals are susceptible to experiencing greater amounts of stress in the workplace, they are likely to experience more negative health outcomes compared to heterosexual individuals. Indeed, the LGB-related stressors identified above have all been shown to relate to these and other negative health outcomes. In a study comparing the effects of formal and interpersonal discrimination on an individual's wellbeing, both forms of discrimination were found to relate to negative health outcomes. Formal discrimination related to the erosion of positive affect and interpersonal discrimination was related to the development of depressive symptoms (Noh et al., 2007). Stigma consciousness has been shown to relate to psychological distress (Kelleher, 2009; Lewis, Derlega, Clark, & Kuang, 2006) and depression (Berghe et al., 2010). Studies have linked internalized heterosexism to lower levels of overall health (Lewis, Derlega, Griffin, & Krowinski, 2003), such as guilt and demoralization (Meyer, 1995), increased depressive symptoms (Berghe et al., 2010), and decreased utilization of health care resources (McGregor et al., 2001). The fear of disclosure within one's place of work has been shown to relate to anxiety and depression (Ragins, Singh, & Cornwall, 2007). And finally, studies have shown that a lack of supportive social interactions is significantly related to depressive symptoms (Berghe et al., 2010) and that social isolation is related to coronary heart disease (Grant et al., 2009; Lett et al., 2005). Thus, each of the identified LGB-workplace stressors have the potential to elicit severe health-related outcomes through their influence on workplace stress.

Work-Related Outcomes

The fact that LGB workplace stressors impact health outcomes and promote disease should be a grave concern for employers, as these outcomes can severely impact an organizations' bottom line. In a general sense, stress in the workplace has been shown to increase absenteeism (Jacobson et al., 1996) and turnover intentions, and decrease job commitment, motivation, and satisfaction (Podsakoff et al., 2007). As a result, sexual orientation minorities are at greater risk of experiencing these negative workplace outcomes. Each of the LGB workplace stressors discussed previously has been shown to influence negative workplace outcomes.

Perceived work-related discrimination has been shown to result in increased turnover intentions, and decreased organizational commitment, career commitment, organizational self-esteem, and job satisfaction (Ragins & Cornwell, 2001). Perceiving interpersonal discrimination (referred to as everyday discrimination) was strongly, negatively related to job satisfaction (Deitch et al., 2003). Having higher levels of stigma consciousness has been shown to relate to psychological disengagement from the organization as well as turnover intentions (Pinel & Paulin, 2005). Experiencing internalized heterosexism related to less satisfaction with one's work and increased absenteeism and withdrawal behaviors, even when controlling for general job stress (Waldo, 1999). Finally, concealing has been shown to relate positively to turnover intentions and negatively to job satisfaction, job commitment, career commitment, and organization-based self-esteem (Griffith & Hebl, 2002; Ragins et al., 2007). Given the evidence provided above, it seems reasonable to conclude that these LGB-related stressors produce deleterious organizational outcomes through their effect on psychological stress.

PREVENTION AND COPING STRATEGIES

Due to the aforementioned damaging health- and work-related consequences of LGB workplace stress, a critical question that follows is: what can organizations, stigmatized individuals, and their allies do to reduce such stress? Luckily, several strategies aimed at promoting inclusion and thus reducing the impact and the amount of stressors experienced by stigmatized populations have been identified in the organizational literature. Creating an inclusive environment in the workplace involves working to help sexual orientation minorities feel represented, welcome, and respected on the job (Thomas & Ely, 1996). In this section, we describe strategies that can be used by organizations, targets of prejudice, and their allies to prevent the experience of LGB-related stressors in the first place as well as remediate the negative impacts of such stressors. In so doing, we tie each strategy to the source of stress (caused by both social and individual stressors) that it is most likely to effectively ameliorate. As proposed by our model, organizational strategies are mostly useful in preventing social stressors whereas target strategies are mostly useful in preventing individual stressors. The ally supportive strategies highlighted are expected to help LGB individuals cope with the experiences of both social and individual stressors. We begin this discussion with strategies that organizations can use to prevent LGB-related workplace stressors.

Organizational Strategies

Establishing Organizationally Protective Policies

As mentioned above, one potential method for preventing social LGB-related stressors involves implementing organization-wide protective policies against discrimination of LGB individuals. This strategy is useful in that it explicitly forbids formal acts of discrimination in the workplace. Studies have shown that protective legislation is negatively related to experiencing formal discrimination. Establishing LGB-affirming organizational policies demonstrates that the organization is proactive in protecting its minority employees from minority stressors that could result in negative outcomes for the individual employees as well as the organization as a whole. Thus, establishing progressive organizational policies may ultimately reduce the prevalence of all prejudice events, whether they are formal or interpersonal in nature, by communicating to stigmatized employees that such events are not the norm and would not be tolerated.

Diversity Training

The most commonly used diversity initiative aimed at promoting inclusion and reducing stress for stigmatized individuals in the workplace is diversity training. We define diversity training as any exercise aimed at facilitating in-group and out-group interaction while also reducing stress and discrimination for marginalized groups (Pendry, Driscoll, & Field, 2007), and up to two out of three human resource managers report using such training initiatives in their organizations (Esen, 2005). Although some researchers have questioned the effectiveness of diversity training programs (see Bezrukova, Jehn, & Spell, 2012; Kulik & Roberson, 2008 for comprehensive reviews), recent research points to specific diversity training exercises that may be effective in reducing the LGB-related workplace stressor of stigma consciousness.

A recent experimental field study utilizing goal-setting theory (Locke, 1968; Locke & Latham, 1990) found that participants who developed LGB-supportive goals within a diversity training context demonstrated more positive behaviors and attitudes toward LGB individuals (Madera, King, & Hebl, 2013). In a similar study, researchers were able to demonstrate the effectiveness of perspective taking – actively considering the psychological experiences of others, with an emphasis on how those experiences may differ from our own (Todd, Bodenhausen, Richeson, & Galinsky, 2011) – in terms of improving attitudes toward a stigmatized group (Madera, Neal, & Dawson, 2011). Importantly, this work also identified empathy as a key mediator of this effect. Thus, although studies have produced mixed findings, setting goals and taking the perspective of a stigmatized individual may be effective in terms of improving attitudes and increasing supportive behaviors.

Thus, when conducted effectively, organization-wide diversity training programs have power to establish organizational norms of acceptance and positivity as well as promote more inclusive work environments for LGB minorities. These improved organizational climates will likely reduce individual levels of stigma consciousness or fears associated with being a stigmatized minority. This in turn will likely reduce overall experiences of LGB-workplace stress.

Ally Strategies

Ally Confrontation

An important shortcoming of the aforementioned strategies is that they must be enacted by organizations, which may leave LGB individuals and their allies wondering what they can do to alleviate stress and reduce discrimination in the workplace. One strategy that allies can engage in to reduce the impact of interpersonal discrimination is prejudice confrontation, defined as "verbally or nonverbally expressing one's dissatisfaction with prejudicial and discriminatory treatment to the person who is responsible for the remark or behavior" (Shelton, Richeson, & Vorauer, 2006, p. 67). Confrontation is one of the only methods that have been shown to be equally effective for targets and allies in reducing future expressions of prejudice by its perpetrators (Czopp, Monteith, & Mark, 2006). Because confrontations can sometimes be emotionally charged events, it is not surprising that the people report that they do not confront prejudiced behavior as often as they say they think they should or would (Swim & Hyers, 1999). Indeed, the Confronting Prejudiced Responses (CPR) Model describes several obstacles that get in the way of effective confrontation (Ashburn-Nardo, Morris, & Goodwin, 2008). In order to avoid these obstacles and ensure that confrontation can have its prejudice-reducing effect, the authors argue that stigmatized individuals and their allies should strive to increase discrimination detection, help people understand that prejudice is serious and needs to be dealt with immediately, and promote feelings of personal responsibility for confronting (Ashburn-Nardo et al., 2008).

Although confrontation has been primarily studied with other stigmatized groups based on racial and gender differences, we think this strategy could be particularly effective for LGB populations and their allies due to the fact that interpersonal discrimination against this group often goes undetected or unchecked in the workplace. Some individuals making prejudiced comments or engaging in interpersonally discriminatory behavior may not even be aware that they are doing anything wrong if coworkers do not confront them. For instance, people often refer to other people, things, and situations as "gay" in a derogatory manner without so much as a retort from fellow employees indicating that what they said was prejudiced and wrong. We believe that confrontation can have a beneficial impact through promoting stigma awareness and sensitivity in the workplace. Through the use of this strategy, we should be able to remove such inappropriate comments from our workplaces and move forward as a more inclusive society.

Thus, we believe that ally confrontations can be especially beneficial for LGB individuals by reducing the stress associated with interpersonal discrimination.

Ally Acknowledgment

Allies can also effectively reduce the impact of LGB stress by providing comfort, support, or other tangible resources to these individuals (Sabat, Martinez, & Wessel, 2013). Support behaviors that have been shown to be effective are those that positively acknowledge one's ally status in the workplace. This includes displaying stickers or signs signifying of one's ally identity (e.g., safe-zone stickers; Evans, 2002) or acknowledging that one supports LGB individuals and LGB-related policies.

This strategy may help LGB individuals cope with the stressor of social isolation for two reasons. First, this strategy helps signal to LGB employees that they have a potential network of supportive individuals and friends, even if those individuals do not necessarily share the same specific stigma. Second, this strategy demonstrates to LGB employees that these individuals would be supportive of disclosures of minority sexual orientation identities. The supportiveness of coworkers regarding these disclosure interactions has been shown to be the mediating factor in predicting positive workplace outcomes for these LGB employees (Griffith & Hebl, 2002).

Ally acknowledgment may also be a beneficial strategy in that it models a positive regard toward minority sexual orientation identities. Therefore, this strategy may help to reduce the impact of the LGB-workplace stressor of internalized heterosexism. Individuals suffering from this stressor may experience less stress if they witness allies outwardly demonstrating positivity and pride regarding their ally-identities. Indeed, having workplace allies that can acknowledge their ally status with confidence and positivity can greatly impact a variety of health and workplace outcomes for stigmatized LGB employees.

Individual Strategies

Identity Management

In addition to the aforementioned strategies that allies can enact to promote an inclusive workplace, there are also strategies that LGB individuals can engage in to protect themselves from experiencing individual LGB-related stress in the workplace. One strategy that sexual orientation minority members can engage in to prevent the negative outcomes associated with LGB-related workplace stress is to engage in positive identity management strategies. If organizations have positive diversity climates and few to no instances of heterosexist prejudice, then disclosing one's sexual orientation has the potential to reduce all forms of stress associated with the individual stressor of concealing one's sexual orientation identity. In general, disclosing one's minority sexual orientation significantly negatively relates to job anxiety and positively relates to job satisfaction and organizational commitment (Griffith & Hebl, 2002; Ragins & Cornwall, 2001). These positive outcomes associated with disclosure primarily occur through two main processes that help to increase social support.

First, disclosing one's LGB status allows one to gain social support and other tangible resources from organizations and organizational leaders, who may otherwise assume that no sexual orientation minorities exist within their companies. Second, disclosing allows one to develop a network of social support among supportive allies and other LGB-coworkers who may also be hiding their identities. It follows that disclosing not only protects oneself from the individual stressor of concealing but also protects other potentially vulnerable LGB employees. Importantly, disclosure exists on a continuum ranging from only signaling one's sexual identity to openly advocating on behalf of it (Clair et al., 2005). Thus, these different strategies allow LGB individuals to "feel out" a workplace environment before openly advocating on behalf of their stigmatized identity.

These identity management strategies, albeit helpful, place the burden of prejudice reduction on the stigmatized minorities themselves. Also, it is only beneficial in cases where organizations are free from high levels of social LGB-related stress. Thus, it is important to focus on the combination of organization, ally, and target strategies in order to optimally reduce the stress that LGB members face within their places of work.

CONCLUSION

This chapter highlights the antecedents and outcomes of the stress that LGB employees experience within a workplace setting. Specifically, this chapter identifies six stressors that commonly affect LGB employees (formal discrimination, interpersonal discrimination, stigma consciousness, internalizing heterosexism, concealing, and social isolation) and demonstrates how these stressors each produce workplace stress. Additionally, we discuss how this LGB-workplace stress can produce deleterious health and workplace outcomes. Finally, we discuss several strategies that may be effective in terms of reducing this stress while promoting a more inclusive work environment. Researchers and practitioners alike should continue to investigate the other causes and outcomes of LGB-related workplace stress and continue to test the effectiveness of strategies that reduce stress and promote inclusion in the workplace.

We see several potential avenues for future research in this domain. First, we would like to see more work that acknowledges that the visibility of LGB status actually exists on a continuum rather than in categorical dimensions as it has been typically studied. Indeed, most conceptualizations and studies of this stigma treat it as either completely visible or completely invisible. However, it is our belief that prior knowledge about an individual (e.g., knowledge gained from coworkers, social media, or other outlets) could render this assumption obsolete. Thus, we would like to see more work conducted that assesses the prior knowledge that individuals and organizations have about someone's LGB stigma, and how this prior knowledge may affect how they react to disclosure decisions in the workplace.

Additionally, we would like to see more work conducted on how varying levels of disclosure across life domains (i.e., work and non-work domains) can affect the stress that LGB individuals endure. Indeed, the stress associated with revealing or concealing could be exacerbated if the same disclosure decision is not made across life domains. This inconsistency could require a greater degree of monitoring and more stress associated with being "found out" among LGB individuals both inside and outside of the workplace environment. Ragins (2008) discussed this idea of "disclosure disconnects" in a theoretical piece, but to our knowledge very limited empirical research has been conducted so far on these ideas.

Finally, we would like to see more work conducted in the diversity training realm that is specific to LGB individuals and reducing the stress that they experience in the workplace. Recent reviews (Bezrukova et al., 2012; Kulik & Roberson, 2008) indicate that findings regarding diversity training programs are mixed, but we think that LGB individuals could benefit from a greater focus on target-specific training exercises that could benefit this group specifically. We have cited some of the work that has been conducted in this vein earlier in this chapter (see Madera et al., 2013), but more work remains to be done regarding which exercises are the most effective, why those exercises are most effective, and for whom those exercises are most effective. Overall, we assert that researchers should continue to identify the full set of antecedents and outcomes of LGB-related workplace stress and determine effective prevention and coping strategies to help improve working conditions for sexual orientation minorities and all stigmatized employees.

REFERENCES

Allport, G. W. (1954). *The nature of prejudice*. Reading, MA: Addison-Wesley.

Ambady, N., Hallahan, M., & Conner, B. (1999). Accuracy of judgments of sexual orientation from thin slices of behavior. *Journal of Personality and Social Psychology, 77*, 538–547.

Ashburn-Nardo, L., Morris, K. A., & Goodwin, S. A. (2008). The confronting prejudiced responses (CPR) model: Applying CPR in organizations. *Academy of Management Learning & Education, 7*, 332–342. doi:10.5465/AMLE.2008.34251671

Badgett, M. V. L., Lau, H., Sears, B., & Ho, D. (2007). *Bias in the workplace: Consistent evidence of sexual orientation and gender identity discrimination*. Retrieved from http://www.law.ucla.edu/williamsinstitue. Accessed on June 26.

Berghe, W. V., Dewaele, A., Cox, N., & Vincke, J. (2010). Minority-specific determinants of mental well-being among lesbian, gay, and bisexual youth. *Journal of Applied Social Psychology, 40*, 153–166. doi:10.1111/j.1559-1816.2009.00567.x

Bevan, S. (2010). *The business case for employee health and wellbeing*. London: The Work Foundation.

Bezrukova, K., Jehn, K. A., & Spell, C. S. (2012). Reviewing diversity training: Where we have been and where we should go. *Academy of Management Learning & Education, 11*, 207–227. doi:10.5465/amle.2008.0090

Brooks, V. R. (1981). *Minority stress and lesbian women*. Lexington, MA: D. C. Heath.

Cass, V. C. (1984). Homosexual identity formation: Testing a theoretical model. *Journal of Sex Research, 20*, 143–167. doi:10.1080/00224498409551214

Clair, J. A., Beatty, J., & MacLean, T. (2005). Out of sight but not out of mind: Managing invisible social identities in the workplace. *Academy of Management Review, 30*, 78–95. doi:10.5465/AMR.2005.15281431

Cohen, S., Janicki-Deverts, D., & Miller, G. E. (2007). Psychological stress and disease. *JAMA: The Journal of the American Medical Association, 298*, 1685–1687. doi:10.1001/jama.298.14.1685

Cohen, S., Kessler, R. C., & Gordon, L. U. (1995). Strategies for measuring stress in studies of psychiatric and physical disorders. In S. Cohen, R. Kessler, & L. U. Gordon (Eds.), *Measuring stress: A guide for health and social scientists* (pp. 3–26). New York, NY: Oxford University Press.

Coleman, E. (1982). Developmental stages of the coming out process. *Journal of Homosexuality, 7*, 31–43. doi:10.1300/J082v07n02_06

Colgan, F., Creegan, C., McKearney, A., & Wright, T. (2007). Equality and diversity policies and practices at work: Lesbian, gay and bisexual workers. *Equal Opportunities International, 26*, 590–609.

Crocker, J., Major, A., & Steele, C. (1998). Social stigma. In S. T. Fiske, G. Lindzey, & D. T. Gilbert (Eds.), *The handbook of social psychology* (Vol. 2, 4th ed., pp. 504–553). Boston, MA: McGraw-Hill.

Czopp, A. M., Monteith, M., & Mark, A. Y. (2006). Standing up for a change: Reducing bias through interpersonal confrontation. *Journal of Personality and Social Psychology*, *90*, 784–803. doi:10.1037/0022-3514.90.5.784

Deitch, E. A., Barsky, A., Butz, R. M., Chan, S., Brief, A. P., & Bradley, J. C. (2003). Subtle yet significant: The existence and impact of everyday racial discrimination in the workplace. *Human Relations*, *56*, 1299–1324. doi:10.1177/00187267035611002

Dohrenwend, B. P. (2000). The role of adversity and stress in psychopathology: Some evidence and its implications for theory and research. *Journal of Health and Social Behavior*, *41*, 1–19.

Employment Non-Discrimination Act. (2014, March 20). *Human Rights Campaign*. Retrieved from http://www.hrc.org/laws-and-legislation/federal-legislation/employment-non-discrimination-act. Accessed on April 7, 2014.

Esen, E. (2005). *Workplace diversity practices survey report*. Alexandria, VA: Society for Human Resource Management.

Evans, N. J. (2002). The impact of an LGBT Safe Zone project on campus climate. *Journal of College Student Development*, *43*, 522–539. Retrieved from http://www.eric.ed.gov/ERICWebPortal/detail?accno=EJ650166

Festinger, L. (1962). *A theory of cognitive dissonance*. Stanford, CA: Stanford University Press.

Gallup. (2006). *Americans at odds over gay rights*. Retrieved from http://www.gallup.com/poll/23140/Americans-Odds-Over-Gay-Rights.aspx. Accessed on April 8, 2013.

Gallup. (2012). *U.S. acceptance of gay/lesbian relations is the new normal*. Retrieved from http://www.gallup.com/poll/154634/acceptance-gay-lesbian-relations-new-normal.aspx. Accessed on April 8, 2013.

Goffman, E. (1963). *Stigma*. Englewood Cliffs, NJ: Prentice-Hall.

Gonsiorek, J. C. (1988). Mental health issues of gay and lesbian adolescents. *Journal of Adolescent Health Care*, *9*, 114–122. doi:10.1016/0197-0070(88)90057-5

Gonsiorek, J. C., & Weinrich, J. D. (1991). *The definition and scope of sexual orientation*. Thousand Oaks, CA: Sage Publications, Inc.

Grant, N., Hamer, M., & Steptoe, A. (2009). Social isolation and stress-related cardiovascular, lipid, and cortisol responses. *Annals of Behavioral Medicine*, *37*, 29–37. doi:10.1007/s12160-009-9081-z

Griffith, K. H., & Hebl, M. R. (2002). The disclosure dilemma for gay men and lesbians: "Coming out" at work. *Journal of Applied Psychology*, *87*, 1191–1199.

Hebl, M. R., Foster, J. B., Mannix, L. M., & Dovidio, J. F. (2002). Formal and interpersonal discrimination: A field study of bias toward homosexual applicants. *Personality and Social Psychology Bulletin*, *28*, 815–825. doi:10.1177/0146167202289010

Heffner, K. L., Loving, T. J., Robles, T. F., & Kiecolt-Glaser, J. K. (2003). Examining psychosocial factors related to cancer incidence and progression: In search of the silver lining. *Brain, Behavior, and Immunity*, *17*, 109–111.

Herek, G. M. (1992). The social context of hate crimes: Notes on cultural heterosexism. In G. M. Herek & K. T. Berrill (Eds.), *Hate crimes: Confronting violence against lesbians and gay men* (pp. 89–104). Newbury Park, CA: Sage.

Herek, G. M. (2009). Hate crimes and stigma-related experiences among sexual minority adults in the United States prevalence estimates from a national probability sample. *Journal of Interpersonal Violence*, *24*, 54–74. doi:10.1177/0886260508316477

Hicks, G. R., & Lee, T. T. (2006). Public attitudes toward gays and lesbians: Trends and predictors. *Journal of Homosexuality*, *51*, 57–77. doi:10.1300/J082v51n02_04

House, J. S., Landis, K. R., & Umberson, D. (1988). Social relationships and health. *Science*, *241*, 540–545.

Jacobson, B. H., Aldana, S. G., Goetzel, R. Z., Vardell, K. D., Adams, T. B., & Pietras, R. J. (1996). The relationship between perceived stress and self-reported illness-related absenteeism. *American Journal of Health Promotion*, *11*, 54–61. doi:10.4278/0890-1171-11.1.54

Jernigan, C., & Mistree, B. F. (2009). Gaydar: Facebook friendships expose sexual orientation. *First Monday*, *14*. Retrieved from http://firstmonday.org/ojs/index.php/fm/article/viewArticle/2611/2302

Jones, K. P., Peddie, C. I., Gilrane, V. L., King, E. B., & Gray, A. L. (2013). Not so subtle: A meta-analytic investigation of the correlates of subtle and overt discrimination. *Journal of Management*. doi:0149206313506466. Retrieved from http://jom.sagepub.com/content/early/2013/10/11/0149206313506466.abstract

Kanner, A. D., Coyne, J. C., Schaefer, C., & Lazarus, R. S. (1981). Comparison of two modes of stress measurement: Daily hassles and uplifts versus major life events. *Journal of Behavioral Medicine*, *4*, 1–39. doi:10.1007/BF00844845

Kanter, R. M. (1977). Some effects of proportions on group life: Skewed sex ratios and responses to token women. *American Journal of Sociology*, *85*, 965–990.

Kelleher, C. (2009). Minority stress and health: Implications for lesbian, gay, bisexual, transgender, and questioning (LGBTQ) young people. *Counselling Psychology Quarterly*, *22*, 373–379. doi:10.1080/09515070903334995

Krantz, D. S., & McCeney, M. K. (2002). Effects of psychological and social factors on organic disease: A critical assessment of research on coronary heart disease. *Annual Review of Psychology*, *53*, 341–369. doi:10.1146/annurev.psych.53.100901.135208

Krehely, J. (2011, June 2). *Polls show huge public support for gay and transgender workplace protections*. Retrieved from http://www.americanprogress.org/issues/lgbt/news/2011/06/02/9716/polls-show-huge-public-support-for-gay-and-transgender-workplace-protections/. Accessed on January 15, 2014.

Kulik, C. T., & Roberson, L. (2008). Common goals and golden opportunities: Evaluation of diversity education in academic and organizational settings. *Academy of Management Learning & Education*, *7*, 309–331. doi:10.5465/AMLE.2008.34251670

Lazarus, R. S. (1991). *Emotion and adaptation*. New York, NY: Oxford University Press.

Lazarus, R. S., & Folkman, S. (1984). *Stress, appraisal, and coping*. New York, NY: Springer Publishing Company.

Lett, H. S., Blumenthal, J. A., Babyak, M. A., Strauman, T. J., Robins, C., & Sherwood, A. (2005). Social support and coronary heart disease: Epidemiologic evidence and implications for treatment. *Psychosomatic Medicine*, *67*, 869–878. doi:10.1097/01.psy.0000188393.73571.0a

Lewis, R. J., Derlega, V. J., Clarke, E. G., & Kuang, J. C. (2006). Stigma consciousness, social constraints, and lesbian well-being. *Journal of Counseling Psychology*, *53*, 48–56. doi:10.1037/0022-0167.53.1.48

Lewis, R. J., Derlega, V. J., Griffin, J. L., & Krowinski, A. C. (2003). Stressors for gay men and lesbians: Life stress, gay-related stress, stigma consciousness, and depressive symptoms. *Journal of Social and Clinical Psychology*, *22*, 716–729. doi:10.1521/jscp.22.6.716.22932

Locke, E. A. (1968). Toward a theory of task motivation and incentives. *Organizational Behavior and Human Performance*, *3*, 157–189.

Locke, E. A., & Latham, G. P. (1990). *A theory of goal setting and task performance*. Englewood Cliffs, NJ: Prentice Hall.

Madera, J. M., King, E. B., & Hebl, M. R. (2013). Enhancing the effects of sexual orientation diversity training: The effects of setting goals and training mentors on attitudes and behaviors. *Journal of Business and Psychology*, *28*, 79–91. doi:10.1007/s10869-012-9264-7

Madera, J. M., Neal, J. A., & Dawson, M. (2011). A strategy for diversity training focusing on empathy in the workplace. *Journal of Hospitality & Tourism Research*, *35*, 469–487. doi:10.1177/1096348010382240

Mayfield, W. (2001). The development of an internalized homonegativity inventory for gay men. *Journal of Homosexuality*, *41*, 53–76. doi:10.1300/J082v41n02_04

Maylon, A. K. (1982). Psychotherapeutic implications of internalized homophobia in gay men. *Journal of Homosexuality*, *7*, 59–69. doi:10.1300/J082v07n02_08

Mays, V. M., Coleman, L. M., & Jackson, J. S. (1996). Perceived race-based discrimination, employment status, and job stress in a national sample of black women: Implications for health outcomes. *Journal of Occupational Health Psychology*, *1*, 319–329. doi:10.1037/1076-8998.1.3.319

McGregor, B. A., Carver, C. S., Antoni, M. H., Weiss, S., Yount, S. E., & Ironson, G. (2001). Distress and internalized homophobia among lesbian women treated for early stage breast cancer. *Psychology of Women Quarterly*, *25*, 1–9. doi:10.1111/1471-6402.00001

Meyer, I. H. (1995). Minority stress and mental health in gay men. *Journal of Health and Social Behavior*, *36*, 38–56.

Meyer, I. H. (2003). Prejudice, social stress, and mental health in lesbian, gay, and bisexual populations: Conceptual issues and research evidence. *Psychological Bulletin*, *129*, 674–697. doi:10.1037/0033-2909.129.5.674

Meyer, I. H., & Dean, L. (1998). Internalized homophobia, intimacy, and sexual behavior among gay and bisexual men. In G. M. Herek (Ed.), *Stigma and sexual orientation: Understanding prejudice against lesbians, gay men, and bisexuals. Psychological perspectives on lesbian and gay issues* (Vol. 4, pp. 160–186). Thousand Oaks, CA: Sage Publications.

Newcomb, M. E., & Mustanski, B. (2010). Internalized homophobia and internalizing mental health problems: A meta-analytic review. *Clinical Psychology Review*, *30*, 1019–1029. doi:10.1016/j.cpr.2010.07.003

Noh, S., Kaspar, V., & Wickrama, K. A. S. (2007). Overt and subtle racial discrimination and mental health: Preliminary findings for Korean immigrants. *Journal Information*, *97*, 1269–1274. doi:10.2105/AJPH.2005.085316

Oswald, D. L. (2007). "Don't Ask, Don't Tell": The influence of stigma concealing and perceived threat on perceivers' reactions to a gay target. *Journal of Applied Social Psychology*, *37*, 928–947. doi:10.1111/j.1559-1816.2007.00193.x

Pachankis, J. E. (2007). The psychological implications of concealing a stigma: A cognitive-affective-behavioral model. *Psychological Bulletin*, *133*, 328–345. doi:10.1037/0033-2909.133.2.328

Pascoe, E. A., & Richman, S. L. (2009). Perceived discrimination and health: A meta-analytic review. *Psychological Bulletin*, *135*, 531–554. doi:10.1037/a0016059

Pendry, L. F., Driscoll, D. M., & Field, C. T. (2007). Diversity training: Putting theory into practice. *Journal of Occupational and Organizational Psychology*, *80*, 227–250. doi:10.1348/096317906X118397

Pinel, E. C. (1999). Stigma consciousness: The psychological legacy of social stereotypes. *Journal of Personality and Social Psychology*, *76*, 114–128. doi:10.1037/0022-3514.76.1.114

Pinel, E. C. (2004). You're just saying that because I'm a woman: Stigma consciousness and attributions to discrimination. *Self and Identity*, *3*, 39–51. doi:10.1080/13576500342000031

Pinel, E. C., & Paulin, N. (2005). Stigma consciousness at work. *Basic and Applied Social Psychology*, *27*, 345–352. doi:10.1207/s15324834basp2704_7

Pizer, J. C., Sears, B., Mallory, C., & Hunter, N. D. (2012). Evidence of persistent and pervasive workplace discrimination against LGBT people: The need for federal legislation prohibiting discrimination and providing for equal employment benefits. *Loyola of Los Angeles Law Review*, *45*, 715–779.

Podsakoff, N. P., LePine, J. A., & LePine, M. A. (2007). Differential challenge stressor-hindrance stressor relationships with job attitudes, turnover intentions, turnover, and withdrawal behavior: A meta-analysis. *Journal of Applied Psychology*, *92*, 438–454. doi:10.1037/0021-9010.92.2.438

Powers, B. (1996). The impact of gay, lesbian, and bisexual workplace issues on productivity. *Journal of Gay & Lesbian Social Services*, *4*, 79–90. doi:10.1300/J041v04n04_05

Ragins, B. R. (2008). Disclosure disconnects: Antecedents and consequences of disclosing invisible stigmas across life domains. *Academy of Management Review*, *33*, 194–215. doi:10.5465/AMR.2008.27752724

Ragins, B. R., & Cornwell, J. M. (2001). Pink triangles: Antecedents and consequences of perceived workplace discrimination against gay and lesbian employees. *Journal of Applied Psychology*, *86*, 1244–1261. doi:10.1037/0021-9010.86.6.1244

Ragins, B. R., Singh, R., & Cornwell, J. M. (2007). Making the invisible visible: Fear and disclosure of sexual orientation at work. *Journal of Applied Psychology*, *92*, 1103–1118. doi:10.1037/0021-9010.92.4.1103

Reiche, E. M. V., Nunes, S. O. V., & Morimoto, H. K. (2004). Stress, depression, the immune system, and cancer. *The Lancet Oncology*, *5*, 617–625. doi:10.1016/S1470-2045(04)01597-9

Ruggs, E. N., Martinez, L. R., & Hebl, M. R. (2011). How individuals and organizations can reduce interpersonal discrimination. *Social and Personality Psychology Compass*, *5*, 29–42. doi:10.1111/j.1751-9004.2010.00332.x

Sabat, I. E., Martinez, L. R., & Wessel, J. L. (2013). Neo-activism: Engaging allies in modern workplace discrimination reduction. *Industrial and Organizational Psychology*, *6*, 480–485. doi:10.1111/iops.12089

Schein, E. H. (1985). *Organizational culture and leadership*. San Francisco, CA: Jossey-Bass.

Shelton, J. N., Richeson, J. A., & Vorauer, J. D. (2006). Threatened identities and interethnic interactions. In W. Stroebe, & M. Hewstone (Eds.), *European review of social psychology* (Vol. 17, pp. 312–358). New York, NY: Psychology Press.

Smart, L., & Wegner, D. M. (2000). The hidden costs of hidden stigma. In T. Heatherton, R. Kleck, & J. Hull (Eds.), *The social psychology of stigma* (pp. 220–242). New York, NY: Guilford Press.

Spector, P. E., Dwyer, D. J., & Jex, S. M. (1988). Relation of job stressors to affective, health, and performance outcomes: A comparison of multiple data sources. *Journal of Applied Psychology*, *73*, 11–19. doi:10.1037/0021-9010.73.1.11

Sue, D. W., Capodilupo, C. M., Torino, G. C., Bucceri, J. M., Holder, A., Nadal, K. L., & Esquilin, M. (2007). Racial microaggressions in everyday life: Implications for clinical practice. *American Psychologist*, *62*, 271–286. doi:10.1037/0003-066X.62.4.271

Swann, W. B. (1983). Self-verification: Bringing social reality into harmony with the self. *Psychological Perspectives on the Self*, *2*, 33–66.

Swim, J. K., & Hyers, L. L. (1999). Excuse me – What did you just say?!: Women's public and private responses to sexist remarks. *Journal of Experimental Social Psychology*, *35*, 68–88.

Thomas, D. A., & Ely, R. J. (1996). Making differences matter: A new paradigm for managing diversity. *Harvard Business Review*, *74*, 79–90.

Todd, A. R., Bodenhausen, G. V., Richeson, J. A., & Galinsky, A. D. (2011). Perspective taking combats automatic expressions of racial bias. *Journal of Personality and Social Psychology*, *100*, 1027–1042. doi:10.1037/a0022308

van Praag, H. M., de Koet, E. R., & Van Os, J. (2004). *Stress, the brain and depression*. Cambridge, England: Cambridge University Press.

Waldo, C. R. (1999). Working in a majority context: A structural model of heterosexism as minority stress in the workplace. *Journal of Counseling Psychology*, *46*, 218–232. doi:10.1037/0022-0167.46.2.218

Ward, A., & Brenner, L. (2006). Accentuate the negative: The positive effects of negative acknowledgment. *Psychological Science*, *17*, 959–962.

Wegner, D. M., & Lane, J. D. (1995). From secrecy to psychopathology. In J. W. Pennebaker (Ed.), *Emotion, disclosure, and health* (pp. 25–46). Washington, DC: American Psychological Association.

Williamson, I. R. (2000). Internalized homophobia and health issues affecting lesbians and gay men. *Health Education Research*, *15*, 97–107. doi:10.1093/her/15.1.97

OCCUPATIONAL STRESS: CONSIDERING THE COMPLEX INTERPLAY OF SEX, GENDER, AND JOB ROLES

Shannon L. Rawski, Emilija Djurdjevic and Leah D. Sheppard

ABSTRACT

Findings regarding the relationship between biological sex and job stress remain inconsistent. In the present chapter, we suggest that this is due to the overly simplistic and synonymous treatment of biological sex and gender. Specifically, researchers have operationalized gender as sex, neglecting the inherent complexity of the gender construct. To address this, we take a more nuanced approach and develop a theory around the effects of biological sex and gender on job stress, considering how sex, gender, sex-based prescribed gender roles and work roles interact to create role conflict. We predict that a lack of congruence between any of the aforementioned variables results in various types of role conflict, leading to stress, and requiring coping. Drawing on the literature on role conflict, emotional labor, and facades of conformity, we introduce the

The Role of Demographics in Occupational Stress and Well Being
Research in Occupational Stress and Well Being, Volume 12, 199–233

ISSN: 1479-3555/doi:10.1108/S1479-355520140000012006

concept of gender façades as a coping mechanism. Theoretical and practical implications are discussed.

Keywords: Gender; façades; biological sex differences; occupational stress

It's becoming a hard HRM environment, and sometimes I feel that I'm exposing myself to criticism from other managers about being too soft, especially if I come across as being a bit effeminate. (Tom, homosexual man, Rumens & Kerfoot, 2009, p. 778)

I felt like they only employed me because I was a girl and yet they didn't want me to act feminine. (Debra, quantity surveying engineering student, Powell, Bagilhole, & Dainty, 2009, p. 422)

Occupational stress researchers have long been interested in how men and women differ in terms of experiencing stress in the workplace. These scholars have focused on determining whether men and women are exposed to different workplace stressors and whether the stress-related outcomes they experience are different. Though this has been a topic of interest for some time, the findings have been inconsistent (Vagg, Speilberger, & Wasala, 2002), with some meta-analytic studies finding no sex differences in occupational stress (Davis, Matthews, & Twamley, 1999; Martocchino & O'Leary, 1989). Yet, there seem to be good theoretical reasons to believe that workplace stressors and stress-related outcomes differ for men and women. For example, large status differences between men and women at work remain a reality (Catalyst, 2012), which may result in different types of stressors, and potentially different stress-related outcomes.

The seeming lack of gender differences in the experience of occupational stress may be due, in part, to the overly simplistic treatment of gender. That is, researchers have generally operationalized gender simply as biological sex. Investigating relationships between biological sex (male vs. female) and occupational stress cannot, however, reveal how the construct of *gender* is related to occupational stress. Although often used synonymously, gender is distinct from biological sex and refers to the femininity or masculinity of an individual's traits and behaviors. Gender also captures whether an individual identifies more with masculinity or femininity. Therefore, gender should play an important role in explaining the effects of biological sex on the experience of occupational stress.

In the present chapter, we suggest that gender interacts with biological sex and the requirements of a particular work role to predict varying levels of occupational stress, via role conflict. We posit that understanding the relationship between biological sex and occupational stress lies in the social construction of gender and the gendered requirements of the work role. Throughout this chapter, we take this more nuanced approach to develop a theory of role conflicts that specifically relate to an individual's sex, gender, and gendered work role. We suggest that these role conflicts may be the source of sex-related differences in occupational stress, although we maintain that these differences are more complex than mere differences between men and women.

Further, we propose that individuals cope with these role conflicts by creating gender façades. Gender façades constitute false representations of gender (masculine or feminine), constructed by an employee to meet social expectations and/or work role requirements. Gender façades are similar to emotional labor (i.e., the regulation of emotions in workplace settings; see Ashforth & Humphrey, 1993) in that they require individuals to suppress their normal displays of masculinity or femininity and, instead, present false displays of masculinity or femininity at work in order to meet societal and/or occupational role demands. Façades, however, are also distinct from emotional labor, since constructing a false gender requires altering behaviors, attitudes, and identity symbols (e.g., clothing style) *in addition to* emotional displays (Hewlin, 2003). Gender façades may help alleviate occupational stress in some circumstances – to the extent that they allow employees to "fit in" and obtain the benefits that come from social inclusion at work – but we assert that they may also exacerbate occupational stress and lead to forms of strain, such as burnout.

Our theoretical model contributes to the literature on occupational stress by considering biological sex differences in a complex way that also accounts for gender and the requirements of social roles. We assert that this complexity may help clarify exactly how biological sex relates to occupational stress. Today, more than ever, work roles are becoming more sex-integrated, especially with campaigns urging women to pursue STEM (science, technology, engineering, and math) careers (Lichtman, 2013) and economic hardships motivating men to take traditionally feminine occupations such as nursing (Census Bureau, 2013). This sex-integration may have an impact on the nature of work, expectations, and the experience of job stress. Thus, our nuanced theory of sex, gender, and role requirements is timely and may shed light on new sources of occupational stress as demographic factors in the workplace change.

In the remainder of this chapter, we begin by explicating the difference between biological sex and gender, followed by a detailed description of social role theory, which has been used by past researchers to explain sex differences in occupational stress. Next, we review the empirical results of past research on biological sex and occupational stress. By integrating social role theory with role conflict theory, we consider how the gendered requirements of a person's work role interact with his or her dispositional masculinity and femininity and his or her sex-based gender roles, to produce different types of role conflict, coping mechanisms, and stress-related outcomes. Our goal for this chapter is two-fold. First, we attempt to develop a comprehensive theory of sex and gender-related role conflict, taking into consideration the inherent complexities of biological sex, gender, and gendered work demands. Second, drawing from the social identity, façades of conformity, and emotional labor literatures, we propose a mechanism (i.e., gender façades) that individuals employ to cope with sex and gender-related role conflict. Fig. A1 depicts our conceptual model. We first consider how sex, gender, and gendered role requirements may combine to represent a stressor – in the form of role conflicts. Next, we suggest that gender façades can be used as a way of coping with the stress resulting from role conflict. Finally, the potential negative and positive outcomes of this complex interaction and the gender façade coping mechanism are discussed.

REVIEW OF BIOLOGICAL SEX, GENDER, AND OCCUPATIONAL STRESS

Defining and Disentangling Biological Sex and Gender

Biological sex represents the anatomical characteristics (e.g., primary and secondary sex characteristics) that distinguish men and women from each other (Borna & White, 2003). Although biological sex technically only refers to physical characteristics, it is one of the primary factors used to place individuals into socially constructed categories (Tajfel & Turner, 1985). This grouping, based on sex, results in two main categories or gender types: masculine and feminine. Gender, then, represents a category individuals are assigned to on the basis of their biological sex. Men are assigned a masculine gender while women are assigned a feminine gender by society.

Research suggests that in western cultures, masculinity is synonymous with an instrumental or agentic orientation and encompasses traits such as dominance, assertiveness, and aggressiveness (Bem, 1974; Eagly, 1987; Williams & Best, 1982). Femininity, on the other hand, is associated with an expressive, communion, or other-orientation, and comprises traits such as understanding, compassion, and friendliness (Bem, 1974; Eagly, 1987). Unlike biological sex, wherein individuals most typically fall into one category or the other, people can vary in the degree to which they conform to *both* of these socially constructed gender categories, masculine and feminine (Bem, 1974). As such, masculinity and femininity represent two distinct dimensions rather than a continuum, such that individuals can be high, low, or moderate on both dispositional traits (Bem, 1974). Throughout this chapter, we distinguish between biological sex and gender, and contend that both biological sex and gender should be considered in order to fully understand sex- and gender-based differences in occupational stress. We begin this discussion by reviewing social role theory (Eagly, 1987), which explains why biological sex and gender differences may exist with respect to job stress, and has been used by various researchers to account for these differences (e.g., Barnett & Baruch, 1985; Davis et al., 1999; Purvanova & Muros, 2010).

Social Role Theory

The main tenet of social role theory is that men and women differ in their behaviors and characteristics – not because they are inherently different, but because they are expected to adapt to, and fulfill different social roles (Eagly, 1987). The theory suggests that the current assignment of men and women to different social roles is a result of the historically sex-based division of labor (Eagly, 1987; Eagly & Wood, 1999). For example, the physical nature of plowing and other agricultural work during preindustrial times and the physicality of early factory work during the industrial revolution, combined with sex differences in physical strength positioned, men to occupy roles outside of the home (e.g., construction) during those time periods. Men adapted to these roles by developing dominant, assertive, and agentic characteristics and skills (Eagly & Wood, 1999). Meanwhile, women have the ability to bear children and lactate, and these physical abilities combined with the highly dependent nature of human infants, made women more physiologically suited for social care roles (e.g., child care). Additionally, because women needed to stay in the home to care for dependent infants, they were also efficiently located to perform other domestic roles that could be completed simultaneously with child care (e.g., cooking and cleaning within the home). In order to successfully fulfill these roles, women adapted by developing nurturing, compassionate, and communal characteristics and skills (Eagly & Wood, 1999).

Overtime, this sex-based division of social roles developed into what is now referred to as gender roles. Gender roles are defined as society's shared expectations for men and women regarding the preferred, desirable, or appropriate characteristics, skills, and behaviors based on biological sex (Eagly, 1987, p. 12). Gender role expectations may be beneficial in helping individuals hone skills that are advantageous for certain social roles (e.g., mother). However, when applied indiscriminately to all men and women, prescribed gender roles may hinder performance in other important roles (e.g., one's role as a manager). Gender stereotypes influence human interactions by prescribing gender roles to men and women based on assumptions that men are, and should be masculine, and that women are, and should be, feminine (Eagly, 1987; Skrypnek & Snyder, 1982; Wood & Karten, 1986). Eagly and Carli (2007) have suggested that these stereotypes are also a product of the division of labor between men and women, similar to gender roles.

There were advantages to sex-based prescriptions and the division of labor before modern conveniences was introduced. Today, however, the opportunities for men and women to serve in a wide range of social roles have significantly increased (Eagly & Wood, 1999). For example, men can care for children with the use of baby formula and bottles, while women can move large objects at a construction site with the use of fork lifts and cranes. The social construction of men's and women's social roles, however, has been slower to evolve (Eagly & Wood, 1999). Behavioral, attitudinal, and emotional prescriptions for men and women are still based on socially constructed gender roles and beliefs rooted in an antiquated division of labor between the sexes, rather than the modern capabilities of men and women (Eagly, 1987). Therefore, gender roles continue to have an effect on behavior (Ridgeway, 1997), even though the sex-segregation of societal roles has begun to erode (e.g., female CEOs; stay-at-home dads) in modern times.

Biological Sex Differences and Occupational Stress

Past research that has investigated whether and why biological sex differences exist with respect to job stress has drawn from social role theory as a basis for these explanations (e.g., Barnett & Baruch, 1985; Davis et al., 1999; Purvanova & Muros, 2010). Social role theory, as previously summarized, suggests that sex differences are a direct result of the differential distributions of men and women into different social roles (Eagly, 1987). Davis and colleagues (1999) have noted that social role theory has been used to support conflicting arguments. For example, scholars have used the theory to predict that men will experience more work-related stress than women because masculine gender roles encourage instrumentality, achievement, competition, and agency (e.g., Eisler & Skidmore, 1987; Eisler, Skidmore, & Ward, 1988; Goldberg, 1987). These prescriptions set the bar high for men and may cause significant stress as men try to meet increasingly high standards for achievement (Vandello & Bosson, 2013).

However, social role theory has also been used by researchers to suggest that women experience more stress than men (Barnett & Baruch, 1985; Netterstrom, Kristensen, Damsgaard, Olsen, & Sjol, 1991). The logic in these cases has generally been that the feminine gender role requires the prioritization of others' needs ahead of one's own and structurally supports discrimination by relegating women to less powerful positions (Eagly, 1987; Nelson & Quick, 1985). Women, then, are prescribed roles within which they have less control, fewer resources, and a requirement to use those limited resources to help others ahead of themselves (Eagly, 1987). Together, these factors are theorized to result in women experiencing more work-related stress than men, taxing and exceeding their coping capacities (Barnett & Baruch, 1985; Netterstrom et al., 1991).

Interestingly, both assertions have been empirically supported (see Davis et al., 1999 for a review of social role explanations of biological sex differences in stress). Meanwhile, other studies suggest that there are no differences in the amount of occupational stress that men and women experience (Beehr & Schuler, 1980; Guppy & Rick, 1996). In fact, meta-analytic studies focusing on biological sex and job stress suggest that men and women experience similar amounts of stress in the workplace, and that the experience of stress tends to manifest similarly in terms of the psychological and physiological outcomes (Davis et al., 1999; Martocchino & O'Leary, 1989).

Some scholars have argued that social role theory is consistent with these non-significant findings because gender differences should occur in the *types* of stressors experienced, not in the *amount* of stress or strain (Aneshensel & Pearlin, 1987; Davis et al., 1999; Wethington, McLeod, & Kessler, 1987). Specifically, men will tend to experience more stress related to the organizational hierarchy (e.g., Hendrix, Spencer, & Gibson, 1994;

McDonald & Korabik, 1991), whereas women will experience more stress related to work-family conflict and discrimination (e.g., Hendrix et al., 1994; Loosemore & Waters, 2004; McDonald & Korabik, 1991). These findings, however, are overshadowed by results suggesting men and women experience many of the same stressors at work (e.g., Hendrix et al., 1994; Loosemore & Waters, 2004; McDonald & Korabik, 1991). Taken together, the findings are inconclusive regarding the effects of sex-based differences in the experience of stressors and job stress.

Though occupational stress researchers have found inconsistent and often non-significant relationships between sex and occupational stress, gender researchers have had more success identifying consistent gender-based variations in stress-related (though, not necessarily job stress-related) outcomes (Eisler & Skidmore, 1987; O'Neil, 2008; Pleck, 1981, 1995). Research in this domain has identified a construct called gender role conflict, whereby gender role prescriptions result in negative outcomes for the individual (O'Neil, 2008). In other words, gender role conflict occurs when a person is unable to fulfill his or her gender role without failing to fulfill another social role. For instance, a man who desires to fulfill a traditional masculine gender role by succeeding at work may neglect his familial roles as a spouse and/or as a father (O'Neil, 2013). Another form of gender role conflict could occur when men abuse drugs or alcohol in an attempt to reduce the expression of emotions in accordance with the stoic masculine gender role (O'Neil, 2013). Such substance abuse may also hinder work role or family role performance. A final example may include women who act submissively at work in accordance with a feminine gender role, only to be passed up for promotion because they are not "leadership material" (Eagly & Carli, 2007). Gender role conflict then represents a specific type of role conflict and has been linked to stress-related outcomes such as anxiety and increases in the stress hormone, cortisol (Caswell, Bosson, Vandello, & Sellers, 2014; O'Neil, 2008, 2013; Vandello, Bosson, Cohen, Burnaford, & Weaver, 2008).

Gender role conflict has also been connected to occupational stress (Luhaorg & Zivian, 1995). For example, Luhaorg and Zivian (1995) discovered that men in traditionally feminine occupations and women in traditionally masculine occupations experience more stress due to perceived gender role conflict than individuals in traditional sex-typed occupations. Although much of the work on gender role conflict (with the exception of Luhaorg & Zivian, 1995) has concentrated on men and largely neglected to study women (see O'Neil, 2008 for a review), the findings suggest that sex-based differences in occupational stress are more complex than mere differences between men and women or even differences in gender roles. The scant research that exists suggests a complex relationship among an individual's biological sex, his or her gender, and the context and requirements of his or her gendered work role. The limited body of work on this topic corresponds with a more familiar theory from the occupational stress domain: role conflict theory.

ROLE CONFLICT THEORY

Role conflict theory (Kahn, Wolfe, Quinn, Snoek, & Rosenthal, 1964) is commonly used in management and occupational stress research (Jackson & Schuler, 1985; Travis & Collins, 2000) to understand potential sources of stress for employees. The theory suggests that, ceteris paribus, individuals encounter more stressors and experience increased stress and strain when they endure some form of role conflict. Role conflict can be a result of a mismatch between the demands of an individual's environment (e.g., assigned roles) and the individual's ability to fulfill the role requirements (Kahn et al., 1964). Role conflict may also result from the competing requirements of different roles (Kahn et al., 1964). This theory emphasizes the complex relationships that occur between an individual's characteristics and those of the individual's social and organizational environment. Therefore, to further inform our understanding of the potential effects of biological sex and gender on the experience of job stress, it is important to consider not only the individuals' biological sex, but also his or her (1) gender, (2) socially prescribed gender roles directly resulting from the his or her biological sex, and (3) gender-related work-role demands.

This approach is not entirely novel as some work has investigated how gender roles interact with work roles to produce conflict and subsequent negative outcomes for individuals (see O'Neil, 2008 for a review). The gender role conflict construct, however, was developed to understand what happens when men experience conflict because of their prescribed gender role, and how this affects them and others (O'Neil, 2008). Following the lead of gender researchers, we develop comprehensive theory that considers both men's and women's sex, gender, gendered work-role expectations, the potential conflicts (e.g., gender role conflict) that may arise and represent stressors, and how these stressors may result in stress-related outcomes (e.g., burnout).

TYPES OF GENDER ROLE CONFLICT

Table B1 presents a chart predicting specific types of role conflict, based on the interaction of an individual's sex, gender, sex-based gender roles, and gendered work-role requirements. Table B1 also illustrates whether and how the individual will create and enact a gender façade in order to cope with the role conflict(s). In the following section, we describe these specific types of role conflict, and subsequently, delineate how gender façades can help an individual cope with these conflicts in the workplace. As previously noted, an individual's biological sex determines whether the person is labeled as a man or a woman and the associated societal gender role expectations (masculine for men and feminine for women). At the same time, the work role an individual occupies may have a masculine or feminine gender-orientation, requiring gendered behaviors for successful job performance. For example, a kindergarten teacher would need to display many characteristics that are also required by a feminine gender role, such as nurturance. Likewise, a police officer would need to display many of the same characteristics required by the masculine gender role, such as assertiveness. Considering these factors in combination provides a more nuanced understanding of both the types of stressors and amount of stress male and female employees are likely to encounter in different jobs.

We propose that employees can experience two types of role conflict discussed by Kahn and colleagues (1964) as a result of potential misalignments between sex, gender, and gendered work-role requirements. These include inter-role conflict and person-role conflict. Inter-role conflict occurs when role prescriptions associated with membership in the organization are mismatched with the role prescriptions from another social group (Kahn et al., 1964). We suggest that the expectations stemming from the employee's work role may conflict with those arising from the gender role assigned to the employee based on his or her biological sex, thereby creating inter-role conflict. For example, female attorneys may need to enact masculinity by demonstrating dominance to be successful in the courtroom. At the same time, this masculine requirement is counter to their proscribed feminine gender role, which calls for submissive behavior.

Moreover, person-role conflict can also occur when the prescriptions of a work role are at odds with an individual's needs, values, and personal abilities (Kahn et al., 1964). We suggest that both the employee's gender role and work role may conflict with the employee's gender (i.e., his or her personal need or value for and/or identification with masculinity or femininity) resulting in person-role conflict. For example, a masculine person may desire to be aggressive and confrontational, but if this individual is working in a customer service role, or if this individual is female and therefore expected to be feminine, her need to enact masculinity will be at odds with both of her roles. Below, we theorize about the effects of the various combinations of sex, gender, and gendered work-role expectations on the experience of role conflict and subsequent stress-related outcomes.

Person-Role Matches

Masculine men who find themselves in masculine-oriented jobs (e.g., firefighting) will experience alignment between their sex, gender, and work role. Similarly, feminine women working in feminine-oriented jobs (e.g., nursing) should experience relative synergy between their sex, gender, and work role. As a result, these individuals will not face many challenges meeting the expectations of their assigned gender roles and work roles because their actual and authentic gender is aligned with societal and job expectations. In essence, these individuals represent a good fit with both their gender role and their work role. As such, they will not be likely to experience any form of role conflict at work related to sex or gender. Although these employees may experience other types of role conflict and stressors (e.g., role overload, politics), consideration of this is beyond the scope of the present chapter. It is also worth noting that the fit between a person and the social roles he or she fills may change as the specific role changes. Therefore, a masculine male street cop may experience a great fit with his masculine job role in his early career, but this degree of fit my subside if he is promoted to a desk job where the expression of masculine aggression is no longer necessary to fulfill his job role. Below, we elaborate more on potential mismatches between individuals and the work and social roles they occupy.

Person-Role Mismatches

Person-Work Role Conflict

Masculine and feminine employees may experience a type of person-role conflict that is directly related to the work role being occupied.

When a work role includes gender-related behaviors and characteristics (e.g., professional football players, day care workers), individuals whose self-identified genders do not match the gendered-orientation of their work role will experience what we refer to as person-work role conflict. Similar to the person-role conflict discussed by Kahn et al. (1964), person-work role conflict occurs when an individual's gender (i.e., his or her need to enact masculinity or femininity) does not meet the requirements of his or her work role. Although general forms of person-work role conflict have been discussed by others (e.g., Kahn et al., 1964; Latack, 1981), our treatment of this construct is unique in that it focuses on the interplay between gender and the gendered-orientation of work roles.

A masculine-oriented work role requires agentic behaviors from both masculine and feminine employees, regardless of whether they are men or women. For example, in the case of police officers, both masculine and feminine officers, no matter their biological sex, must be assertive and authoritative to successfully execute the role. At the same time, a feminine-oriented work role requires communal behaviors from both masculine and feminine employees. A personal assistant represents an example of a feminine-oriented work role that requires the individual occupying the role to be caring and considerate of another's needs. Both men and women employed as personal assistants, regardless of their actual authentic gender, must meet the communal requirements of the personal assistant role if they are to be successful. Masculine employees in feminine-oriented roles and feminine employees in masculine-oriented roles are, therefore, likely to experience role interference, or challenges in negotiating these roles (Settles, Sellers, & Damas, 2002) for which they are mismatched.

This conceptualization of person-work role conflict is also similar to the need-supplies view and the demands-abilities view of person-organization fit theory (Kristof, 1996). Essentially, when an individual has their needs satisfied by the organization (e.g., their need to enact an authentic gender) and when an individual satisfies the organization's demands (e.g., the individual's enacted gender contributes to job performance), then there will be a good fit between the person and his or her organization (Kristof, 1996). When there is a lack of fit between the individual's needs and the organization's demands, person-work role conflict occurs (Kahn et al., 1964). Person-organization fit, for example, has been shown to have a negative relationship with occupational stress such that those who are poor fits with their organization experience more stress (Chesney & Rosenman, 1980; Ivancevich & Matteson, 1980; Matteson & Ivancevich, 1982). We propose that when individuals have a poor fit with their organizational role, based on a mismatch between their own masculinity or femininity and that required by their job role, similar stress outcomes will ensue. Therefore, we propose that person-work role conflict will result in the increased experience of stress.

Person-Gender Role Conflict

Employees may also experience another type of role conflict that is not directly affected by the work role occupied in the organization. Due to individual variations in masculinity and femininity, not all men and women meet the requirements of their socially prescribed gender roles. When this is the case, we suggest that these individuals experience a form of role conflict that we label person-gender role conflict. Although the workplace is not the only salient source of this type of role conflict – indeed, society is the primary dictator of gender roles – employees are nevertheless likely to experience person-gender role conflict at work. This is because organizations generally espouse societal norms. Furthermore, individuals spend a large portion of their time and experience considerable social interactions within their work organizations. In fact, an employee's supervisor, coworkers, subordinates, or customers may function as societal role senders of gender norms (Deaux & Major, 1987; Gherardi & Poggio, 2001).

As such, feminine men and masculine women may receive signals, in the form of verbal comments, body language, or social exclusion, that their enacted genders (i.e., behavioral, attitudinal, and emotional tendencies) violate societal gender expectations for their biological sex group (Eagly, 1987). In fact, research has found a variety of negative outcomes (e.g., sex-based harassment and prejudice: Berdahl, 2001; Lehavot & Lambert, 2007) associated with violations of gender norms at work. As such, we propose that regardless of the gendered-orientation of the work role, feminine men and masculine women will experience person-gender role conflict in the workplace, resulting in subsequent stress, and potential stress-related outcomes.

Person-Gender Role Conflict and Person-Work Role Conflict

The role conflict that feminine men and masculine women experience could be further complicated by the work roles these individuals occupy. For instance, feminine men in masculine-oriented work roles and masculine women in feminine-oriented work roles will also experience person-work role conflict. The person-work role conflict will stem from the discrepancy of the employee's gender and the gender expectations of the work role that the employee occupies. Unfortunately, these individuals are faced with both negative social and work outcomes because their genders do not fit the requirements of their gender roles or their work roles. Therefore, these individuals are likely to perceive a threat to their legitimacy as employees as well as prototypical members of their biological sex groups.

Legitimacy threats are those that dispute whether an individual is a member of a valued social identity group (Breakwell, 1986; Ellemers, Spears, & Doosje, 2002). This perceived threat represents another potential stressor, resulting in additional stress (Petriglieri, 2011), as the individual perceives that his or her status as a member in two groups (e.g., employees and men or women) is at risk. The negative effects resulting from the lack of fit with the gender and work roles are greater for these individuals experiencing both types of person-role conflict. Interestingly, though, the demands of both roles are aligned, which has implications for the coping strategies discussed in the next section.

Inter-Role Conflict

When individuals are employed in sex-typed jobs that are inconsistent with their sex, they will experience conflicting demands from their gender role and their work role. For example, a male nurse will have to meet requirements for femininity to fulfill his communion-oriented work role. At the same time, he will continue to face social demands to fulfill his masculine gender role. As another example, women employed as police officers will be required to display masculinity to fulfill their agentic-oriented work roles. These women will also be expected to simultaneously fulfill their gender role by being feminine. Thus, under these conditions, gender roles and work roles are at odds, requiring employees to demonstrate both genders. This poses a conflict for individuals as the fulfillment one gender role is typically characterized in part by the absence of the other gender (e.g., fulfillment of a masculine gender role requires the absence of femininity; Vandello & Bosson, 2013). In this way, inter-role conflicts can occur when employees' biological sexes (and subsequent assigned gender roles) are mismatched with the gender orientations of their work roles. The extant stress research suggests that inter-role conflict is related to increased job stress (Kahn & Langlieb, 2003; Kahn et al., 1964). We expect a similar relationship with the experience of occupational stress when employees experience inter-role conflict between gender roles and work roles.

Inter-Role Conflict and Person-Gender Role Conflict

Inter-role conflict may also occur *simultaneously* with person-role conflict. Feminine men in feminine-oriented work roles and masculine women in masculine-oriented work roles are predicted to experience both inter-role conflict and person-gender role conflict. These employees will likely experience inter-role conflict stemming from the discrepancy between their prescribed gender and work roles. At the same time, these employees will experience person-gender role conflict stemming from the discrepancy between their sex and gender. As previously discussed, an employee experiencing person-gender role conflict will face legitimacy threats to his or her status as a man or woman in society. While these individuals face challenges meeting their gender roles, however, they are well suited for their work roles. Their ability to be good performers for the organization may, to some extent, alleviate some of the negative social outcomes that occur in response to gender role violations. We theorize about this issue in more detail in the section on coping.

Inter-Role Conflict and Person-Work Role Conflict

Masculine men in feminine-oriented work roles and feminine women in masculine-oriented work roles will also face both inter-role conflict and person-work role conflict. These individuals easily conform to the expectations of their gender roles, but will likely struggle to be effective at their job, as their gender is inconsistent with the gendered requirements of the job. In addition, attempting to fulfill their work roles may result in violating their gender roles. Although individuals facing multiple forms of gender role conflict may seem to be in an impossible situation, strategically employed gender façades will help address these role stressors and may alleviate the stress they experience, thereby helping them navigate the complexity of fulfilling gender requirements at work.

GENDER FAÇADES AS A COPING MECHANISM

To cope with the stress caused by the various types of role conflict, individuals may engage in problem-focused or emotion-focused coping (Lazarus & Folkman, 1984). Emotion-focused coping, intended to regulate the emotional response to the stressor, is most likely to occur in situations where the stressor is appraised to be outside the individual's control (Folkman & Lazarus, 1980; Lazarus & Folkman, 1984). Problem-focused coping, on the other hand, is intended to deal with the stressor, by managing or altering it, and should occur when a stressor is appraised as amenable to change (Folkman & Lazarus, 1980; Lazarus & Folkman, 1984).

Employees are likely to perceive little to no control over prescribed gender and organizational roles for a number of reasons. First, gender roles represent societal norms and are largely outside of any one employee's control. Second, the gendered traits needed to perform the work role may be legitimately needed for in-role performance. For instance, nurturing children while in the role of a kindergarten teacher is a feminine gendered behavior that is legitimately needed for successful performance in the work role. The specific gender-related behaviors demanded by work roles are a product of the specific tasks that need to be completed. Organizations determine how tasks are assigned to work roles. Therefore, employees typically have little to no control over their work role and the gender-related behaviors required to fulfill that the work role.

Although employees have little to no control over their gender role and work role (aside from self-selection into a particular work role), they have control over their own behaviors, attitudes, and emotional displays. Research on impression management tactics (Roberts, 2005) and emotional labor (Hochschild, 1983) suggests that individuals alter their behavioral and emotional responses to work situations in order to accomplish goals or meet role requirements. These same tactics can be used to enact gender role and work-role appropriate behaviors and emotional expressions. Therefore, when experiencing the types of role conflict discussed in this chapter, individuals are likely to appraise the enactment of gender-related behaviors and emotions as controllable, and thereby engage in problem-focused coping.

Gender role and work-role conflicts can be managed to the extent that individuals are able and willing to alter their in-role behaviors and displayed emotions. Behavioral alterations have been referred to as façades of conformity, defined as "false representations created by employees to appear as if they embrace organizational values" (Hewlin, 2003, p. 634). Hewlin (2003) theorized that façades are conscious choices to mask one's true self by hiding the values of one's identity and purposefully enacting (either verbally or non-verbally) the values desired by the organization. Facades of conformity have been theoretically distinguished from emotional labor (Hewlin, 2003), or the regulation of emotions in workplace settings (e.g., Ashforth & Humphrey, 1993). Although creating a façade may indeed involve altering ones emotional display as in emotional labor, façades also involve other forms of identity work, including altering behaviors, attitudes, and identity symbols (e.g., style of dress or office décor). Both theoretical and empirical research indicates that employees can create façades of conformity to fit in organizational settings that are inconsistent with their values and beliefs (Hewlin, 2003, 2009; Stormer & Devine, 2008). At the same time, theory on emotional labor, a component of façade creation, suggests that employees alter their emotions to meet organizational display rules and goals (e.g., Ashforth & Humphrey, 1993; Grandey, 2000; Hochschild, 1983). Emotional labor can be a component of a holistic façade created in order to fit into a specific prescribed role. Below, we elaborate on how individuals may use such techniques to manage the gender-related role conflicts they face in the workplace.

Gender Façade Creation Strategies

Creating a gender façade, in part by engaging in emotional labor, is a potential strategy for directly managing gender-related role conflicts, by changing one's enacted gender to better fit role prescriptions. As such, gender façade creation and enactment represents a problem-focused coping mechanism in response to role-conflict(s). It also constitutes a dynamic and iterative identity negotiation process. Individuals are constantly involved in identity work, the forming, repairing, maintaining, and revising of identities (Alvesson & Willmott, 2002; Ashforth, Harrison, & Corley, 2008). The construction of a façade involves just as much identity work, but this identity work may be limited to only contexts where the façade is needed (i.e., work tasks, social situations, or both). In essence, gender façade creation and enactment requires engaging in behaviors and emotional displays affiliated with a gender that the employee does not actually identify with.

Individuals have a core motive to maintain positive distinctiveness with regards to their valued identities (Tajfel & Turner, 1985). It may, therefore, appear counterintuitive that anyone would choose to violate their own valued gender identity by enacting a gender that they do not identify with. According to social interactionism, however, individuals form identities by reproducing roles across social interactions (Goffman, 1959, 1974). Therefore, the ability to successfully execute roles is highly identity-relevant. When role conflicts occur, not only will successful role performance be jeopardized, but also any associated identities will be threatened due to the possibility that the individual will not be able to enact that role (and corresponding identity) in the future (Petriglieri, 2011).

We have already argued that sex and gender-related role conflicts at work can be a source of identity threats for individuals, by threatening their legitimacy as members of a valued social identity group. When a valued identity is threatened, concealment of that identity, and attempts to enact a non-threatened identity, can be a protective response to threats (Petriglieri, 2011; Tajfel, 1978). Additionally, identity threats have been suggested to be a source of stress-motivating coping processes (Lazarus & Folkman, 1984; Petriglieri, 2011). If an employee is faced with a legitimacy threat, then the employee will have a confirmation goal and will seek to confirm that he or she is a valid member of a valued social identity group (Roberts, 2005). Individuals can accomplish this confirmation by capitalizing on the social identity group's stereotypes (Roberts, 2005). In other words, the employee may try to portray himself or herself as a more prototypical member of the valued social identity group in order to cope with role conflicts. Therefore, individuals facing sex and gender-related role conflicts at work will be motivated to create and enact gender façades in order to cope with the stress of the role conflicts and protect their threatened identities.

Once an employee is motivated to create a gender façade, he or she will begin to enact the façade in work contexts when it is perceived as beneficial. This enactment may take on two forms: (1) fabrication or (2) concealment (Herek, 1996).

Fabrication

"Fabrication occurs when a person deliberately provides false information about himself or herself to others" (Clair, Beatty, & Maclean, 2005, p. 82; Herek, 1996). This false information could come in several forms of observable characteristics, including behaviors and identity markers such as clothing style and office decor (Ashforth, 2001). By behavior, we mean any work-related behaviors the focal employee may use to convey a false gender.

The work behaviors displayed could be gendered in how the work is done. For example, a masculine individual may be trying to appear more feminine at work. As a result, this individual may consult coworkers for their opinions on a project, without any intention of considering those opinions, to create the appearance of someone who is communion-oriented. Indeed, research on impression management suggests that individuals may intentionally engage in certain behaviors (e.g., opinion conformity) to portray a desired image to others (e.g., Turnley & Bolino, 2001). Here, behavior may also refer to actions that have little to do with the employee's job, but nonetheless occur at work. For instance, an employee trying to meet male gender role expectations that men should like sports may fake his way through sports talk during breaks with his coworkers even though he has very little interest in sports.

Finally, behaviors may also include emotional displays. Gender norms dictate how men and women should emotionally react to different stimuli. Typically, these norms suggest that women should be more emotionally expressive than men (Bem, 1974; Eagly, 1987). According to emotional labor theory (e.g., Hochschild, 1983), employees engage in emotional labor through surface acting (i.e., projecting an emotion that is not actually experienced) and deep acting (i.e., changing feelings to actually experience the needed emotions). Expressing organizationally sanctioned emotions (i.e., engaging in emotional labor) requires effort, planning, and control (Morris & Feldman, 1996), and represents an important component of successful gender façade creation.

Beyond behaviors, individuals can use identity markers, such as a particular style of dress, hairstyle, or office décor to enact their gender façade. For instance, a feminine woman may try to symbolize masculinity by dressing more masculine at work (e.g., wearing pantsuits instead of dresses). Employees who find it difficult to fake the behaviors and emotions that are associated with a gender other than their own may be more likely to use symbols of that gender to create a gender façade. However, identity markers will be most effectively used in conjunction with behaviors and emotional displays. This is because identity markers and behaviors lead to a more credible identity when used together (Roberts, 2005).

Concealment

Concealment may be used as another gender façade strategy and involves keeping others from obtaining information about oneself (Clair et al., 2005; Herek, 1996). In the case of gender façades, individuals will conceal and suppress characteristics that do not conform to the gendered requirements of prescribed roles. When a masculine employee creates a feminine gender façade, he or she must simultaneously feign femininity while suppressing masculinity. Indeed, the emotional labor literature suggests that employees may meet organizational demands by suppressing undesirable emotions (Grandey, 2000). Concealment, like fabrication, can manifest in the concealment of behaviors, emotions, and/or identity markers that would give away one's authentic gender.

Just as emotion regulation involves continuous emotion expression and suppression (Grandey, 2000), we suggest that fabrication and concealment can be used in isolation or simultaneously in order to create and maintain gender façades. Depending on the specific types of role conflict experienced, individuals may create a gender façade when engaging in organizationally sanctioned behaviors. These behaviors can include work tasks, social interactions, or both. We suggest that the task-relevant gender demands of a work role will require employees to conform to a specific gender in order to successfully perform tasks. Likewise, gender roles will demand certain gendered behaviors from employees for social interactions. Past research suggests that when it comes to expectations for social helping behaviors (i.e., citizenship behaviors), men and women are held to different gender role prescriptions (Hart et al., 2009). As such, gender façades can be useful for employees during both work tasks and day-today social interactions that occur in the workplace. Table B1 depicts patterns of gender façade creation and enactment across the different types of role conflicts. It also categorizes these specific responses according to the gender being concealed or fabricated and the type of situation (i.e., work tasks or social interactions) for which the gender façade is enacted. These specific gender façade creation and enactment strategies are explicated below.

Types of Role-Conflict and Gender Façade Strategies

Individuals who do not experience any type of role conflict related to their sex or gender will not have any need or motivation to create a gender façade. These individuals' genders match their prescribed gender and work roles, and they will, therefore, not experience any pressures to, or benefits from, enacting an inauthentic gender. However, as previously suggested, individuals who experience role conflict related to gender will be motivated to create and enact a gender façade. This will be done through the fabrication and concealment of gendered behaviors and emotional displays. We will now discuss the specific coping strategies outlined in our typology for the three categories of co-occurring role conflicts: (i) person-gender role conflict and person-work role conflict, (ii) person-gender role conflict and inter-role conflict, and (iii) person-work role conflict and inter-role conflict.

Coping with Person-Gender Role Conflict and Person-Work Role Conflict

Individuals who experience both person-gender role conflict (i.e., mismatch between sex and gender) and person-work role conflict (i.e., mismatch between gender and gendered work-role) can create an effective gender façade by concealing their authentic gender and fabricating their prescribed gender. This may be done for both work tasks and social interactions. For example, feminine men in masculine roles can fabricate masculine behaviors and emotional displays while concealing feminine behaviors and emotional displays. The creation of the gender façade fulfills the man's prescribed masculine gender role and the masculine requirements of his work role. Likewise, a masculine woman employed in a feminine work role could conceal her masculine tendencies and fabricate feminine behaviors and emotional displays to fulfill both her feminine gender role and work role. As individuals in these situations are responding to coinciding demands for gendered behaviors and emotions from the gender and work roles, one consistent gender façade will be used. Thus, across both work tasks and social situations, individuals experiencing person-gender role conflict along with person-work role conflict will conceal their real genders and fabricate false genders in order to meet both role demands.

Coping with Person-Gender Role Conflict and Inter-Role Conflict

Individuals may also experience both person-gender role (i.e., mismatch between sex and gender) conflict and inter-role conflict (i.e., mismatch between requirements of gender role and work-role). These individuals should be able to easily conform to their work roles, but not their gender roles. As such, these individuals will typically be able to successfully perform gendered requirements during work tasks. Despite their likely high task performance, however, others (e.g., supervisors, coworkers) in their work environment may still hold expectations that the focal employee also fulfill his or her gender role. In response to simultaneous person-gender role conflict and inter-role conflict, an individual will need to create a gender façade only for non-task-related social situations in the workplace (e.g., break time, lunch time, happy hours, or office parties). For example, a feminine man in a feminine work role, such as kindergarten teacher, may be very successful enacting feminine behaviors and emotional displays when caring for his young students. This individual may, however, feel the need to conceal these tendencies and simultaneously fabricate masculine behaviors and emotional displays when interacting with other teachers and the principal during faculty meetings. Others in this man's work context may expect him to be assertive and take charge in accordance with a masculine gender role in these faculty meetings, which may present a struggle for him.

Coping with Person-Work Role Conflict and Inter-Role Conflict
Alternatively, individuals who experience person-work role conflict (i.e., mismatch between gender and gendered work-role) and inter-role conflict (i.e., mismatch between requirements of gender role and work-role) easily fulfill their assigned gender role, but struggle to authentically fulfill the gender requirements of their work role. In order to cope with this situation, these individuals will need to enact a gender façade when engaging in task-related behaviors. For instance, a feminine female construction worker may need to act masculine and tough when working on a job site, perhaps by concealing emotional displays of pain, discomfort, or difficulty when lifting heavy objects. Her supervisor and coworkers will likely expect her to be both emotionally stoic and physically strong at the work site. These expectations, however, may be lifted for the construction company's holiday party, where the woman should have more freedom from her work tasks to enact her femininity. This example also illustrates how the reactions and expectations of role senders (e.g., supervisors and coworkers) dictate whether an employee will create a gender façade in any given situation.

Social Feedback and Façade Enactment

An important component to the success of a gender façade relies on the reactions of others who observe it. Gender façade creation does not occur in a vacuum. Rather, "people learn their identities by projecting them into an environment and observing the consequences" (Weick, 1995, p. 23). As with a real identity, a façade must be tested out on others. The focal employee will engage in fabrication and concealment to meet the requirements of his or her prescribed roles. The success or failure of the gender façade created lies in the social feedback the focal employee receives while enacting the façade. Social feedback and façade creation and enactment are a reoccurring, iterative process, whereby the focal employee enacts his or her façade, interprets feedback from others, and then edits his or her façade accordingly.

Ashforth et al. (2008) suggested that sensemaking, by observing the reactions of others to one's enacted identity, is an established component of identity creation. The same will be true for gender façades because a façade represents a faked identity. In order for the façade to be successful, others must buy into it. In other words, an employee's gender façade must be credible. The enactment of a person's personal or social identity is considered to be credible when others believe that the enactment is an accurate portrayal of that person's attributes (Roberts, 2005; Schlenker, 1985). If an employee's coworkers or supervisor sense that his or her gender façade is not credible, they will be more likely to give the employee negative social feedback about the gender façade, in the form of body language, verbal comments, or other non-verbal behaviors. Negative social feedback will in turn motivate the focal employee to readjust his or her gender façade until it is perceived as credible.

Authenticity and Outcomes of Façade Enactment

In addition to the credibility of a gender façade, as perceived by others, the authenticity of the gender façade, as perceived by the individual enacting it, is also an important component of the identity negotiation process. Although the definition of gender façades suggests that individuals are choosing to enact gender-related behaviors and emotions that they do not identify with and are, therefore, inherently inauthentic, identification with the work role may actually increase the degree of authenticity perceived by the gender façade creator. Ashforth and Humphrey (1993) have suggested that the degree to which an individual identifies with a social identity group or work role will affect the authenticity of feigned emotions at work. Specifically, the authors argue that when an employee strongly identifies with the work role, he or she will affirm this valued identity by conforming to emotional display rules (Ashforth & Humphrey, 1993). Therefore, somewhat counterintuitively, for high identifiers, enacting prescribed emotions, actually feels authentic to the individuals, as they strive to emulate the requirements of a valued work role. However, when employees do not strongly identify with work roles, engaging in emotional labor will feel inauthentic to the individuals (Ashforth & Humphrey, 1993).

Drawing on this logic, we argue that a similar relationship will exist for those who create and enact gender façades. Although employees who create gender façades, by definition, do not identify with the gender they enact, they may still identify with their work role. Identification with the work role can increase the authenticity of the gender façade if that façade helps the individual successfully fulfill his or her work role. The degree of authenticity perceived by the façade creator will have important implications for stress-related outcomes of gender façade creation. Past research on emotional labor, impression management, and façades of conformity has identified both positive and negative consequences of creating false representations of the self at work. For instance, Roberts (2005) has suggested that impression management will lead to increased psychological well-being, while Clair and colleagues (2005) suggest that hiding one's true identity results in strain. According to Ashforth and Humphrey (1993), those who identify with the work role they are conforming to will actually experience increased psychological well-being, while those who do not identify with the work role they are conforming to will experience negative outcomes.

In general, we predict a similar effect of work role identification on the relationship between gender façade enactment and stress-related consequences. For instance, individuals who experience both types of person-role conflict, and subsequently enact a gender façade for both work tasks and social interactions, are likely to feel overwhelmed by the inauthenticity of their gender façade. The inauthenticity of enacting a false gender for a work role that is not important to the individual's sense of self will be a cause of these negative outcomes. As such, increased job stress and subsequent burnout, especially emotional exhaustion and negative self-evaluations (Maslach & Jackson, 1981), are most likely to occur when the individual does not identify with his or her work role. However, when the individual identifies with his or her work role, enacting a false gender to be successful in that role should increase the authenticity of the gender façade, neutralizing the person-role conflict and leading to increased psychological well-being, as the individual emulates a valued work role identity. Overtime, it is likely that the individual's façade will become a real identity in the same way the deep-level acting during emotional labor often leads to authentic emotional responses that align with organizational display rules (Ashforth & Humphrey, 1993).

When more than one identity is salient in a given context, role conflicts become more likely (Wiesenfeld & Hewlin, 2003). In our case, we have already detailed how demands from gender roles and work roles may lead to sex- and gender-related role conflicts at work and how these conflicts can threaten the legitimacy of an employee's gender and work role identities. When an individual's gender role and work role directly oppose each other and inter-role conflict is experienced, the consideration of that individual's work role identification is insufficient to predict stress-related outcomes. We must also consider whether that individual has integrated his or her gender identity with his or her work role identity. Individuals who can separate, segment, or compartmentalize their conflicting identities may be able to reduce inter-role conflicts (Ashforth, 2001). Hewlin (2003, p. 638) suggests that "individuals who are better able to segment their personal and work identities will be less likely to experience negative outcomes when they create facades of conformity." Likewise, we suggest that individuals who are able to compartmentalize their actual gender identity from their work role identity will be better able to switch their gender façade on and off, as it is needed for work tasks or social interactions. The ability to switch between valued identities thereby reduces role-conflict and the potential experience of job stress by allowing the individual to concentrate on enacting one valued identity at a time without the risk of perceiving threats to other valued identities.

Those individuals who integrate their identities, however, will be especially stressed by inter-role conflicts between their work and gender roles. When two identities are merged or integrated within a person's sense of self, the individual perceives enactment of one identity as relevant to the other and vice versa (Roccas & Brewer, 2002). As such, inter-role conflicts will be especially overwhelming to those who integrate their gender and work role identities because satisfying one role identity will threaten the other. Therefore, we suggest that individuals will experience positive outcomes such as increased psychological well-being *if* they identify with their work role *and* if they compartmentalize their work role identity from their gender identity. If one or both of these conditions are not met, then the individual will experience negative outcomes, including increased job stress, burnout, and decreased well-being.

Burnout, Well-Being, and Job-Related Outcomes

We suggest that among individuals who fail to identify with their work role and/or to compartmentalize their work role identity from their gender identity, stress-related outcomes, such as burnout and decreased well-being, will be exacerbated. Burnout is conceptualized as a product of amassed work-related stress, comprising three distinct components: emotional exhaustion, depersonalization, and reduced personal accomplishment (Maslach, 1982). We would expect that individuals who fail to identify with their work role and/or to compartmentalize their work role identity from their gender identity are particularly likely to experience emotional exhaustion and reduced personal accomplishment. Specifically, these individuals would need to utilize substantial cognitive and emotional resources while "faking" certain components of their work roles and/or gender roles, leaving them depleted, and resulting in emotional exhaustion. These individuals may also consistently feel that they fail to fulfill requirements of their work role and/or gender role, which is consistent with a sense of reduced personal accomplishment. The experience of burnout, in turn, will lead to decreased well-being, including sleep problems and illness that can result in time away from work (Kristensen, Borritz, Villadsen, & Christensen, 2004), as well as decreased job satisfaction and commitment (Singh, Goolsby, & Rhoads, 1994) and increased turnover intentions (Geurts, Schaufeli, & De Jonge, 1998; Kristensen et al., 2004).

DISCUSSION

Biological sex differences are often the subject of organizational research. Biological sex, however, is closely intertwined with socially constructed gender and socially prescribed gender roles. Thus, any scholarly inquiry into biological sex differences would benefit from also taking into account individuals' genders and conformity to gender roles. It is equally important for organizational researchers to take into consideration the roles prescribed by the organization itself, namely, work roles. In an attempt to consider all of these relevant factors, the current chapter has developed a theory of sex- and gender-related role conflict, occupational stress, and gender façade coping strategies. Our theory accounts for the complexity of the interactions among sex, gender, sex-based prescribed gender roles, and gendered work expectations. As such, it holds a number of implications for future stress research.

First, this chapter presents theory that may aid in explaining the inconsistent results of past research on biological sex differences in occupational stress. Our theory suggests that sex-related differences in occupational stress cannot be fully understood without considering the possible differences in masculinity and femininity. Additionally, these individual characteristics interact with prescribed gender roles and work roles to create role conflicts. Mismatches among these variables act as stressors and induce work stress. Taken together, our theory suggests that researchers interested in biological sex differences in occupational stress would benefit from also considering these other variables. We encourage others to empirically test the assertions of this chapter, so that we can begin to better understand these complex relationships between sex, gender, and job stress.

Second, our chapter helps bridge the gap between gender research and occupational stress research. There are many topics, typically considered by gender researchers that can be investigated from an occupational stress perspective. First, the increasing number of women in "men's" jobs is a generational phenomenon that warrants research from occupational stress researchers. Not only will the women in these masculine roles experience role conflict, as our theory suggests, but the men inhabiting these roles may face other stressors such as fears of job insecurity. Third, our theory provides some insight into the topic of glass ceilings, often considered a stressor unique to women. Management positions, which are typically associated with masculinity (Eagly & Carli, 2007), may seem impossible to reach for individuals who must work their way up from more feminine-oriented work roles. For these individuals, in order to be successful at their current job (e.g., kindergarten teacher), they must refrain from enacting the masculine behaviors that are typically associated with managing positions (e.g., principals; superintendents). By the very act of performing a feminine job well, employees may be creating their own glass ceiling as others observing their feminine actions may judge them to be "not management material." Fourth, our theory holds insights for understanding the unique stressors encountered by LGBT employees. These individuals are sometimes stereotyped as having an opposite sex-typed gender, for example, gay men may be assigned feminine gender roles (Kite & Deaux, 1987). Our theoretical framework could be applied to LGBT employees to help understand how gender roles applied on the basis of sexuality can affect stress, coping, and stress-related outcomes.

Although our chapter contributes to a theoretical understanding of sex- and gender-based variations in occupational stress, our theory is also limited. These limitations, however, provide additional avenues for future research. First, our theory is limited temporally. As times change, so do social constructions of gender and the acceptance of individuals who identify with a wide range of genders. The acceptance of a wide set of nuanced genders may, in time, eliminate gender-related role conflicts. Therefore, we not only encourage researchers of today to empirically test our theory, but we also encourage future generations of researchers to revisit our assertions and inquire as to whether they stand the test of time. Furthermore, we mainly focus on work roles with a clear gendered-orientation. There are many jobs that are gender-neutral, however. Future researchers may benefit from investigating how the theory presented here may change when applied to jobs that do not require gendered behaviors or that require androgynous behaviors. Additionally, our chapter represents an initial theoretical basis for future research on biological sex, gender, and occupational stress. As such, there are many questions that our theory does not specifically address. For instance, it is possible that, due to a gender hierarchy that ranks masculinity above femininity, it is more socially acceptable for a woman to be masculine than for a man to be feminine (Berdahl, 2007). Considering this insight from gender research, we may expect that for those individuals experiencing person-gender role conflict, men will experience more negative outcomes than women. Future research would benefit from building on our initial theory by considering this possibility a as well others. Finally, although our chapter makes a contribution by considering the complexity of sex, gender, and social roles, and the introduction of the gender façades construct as an individual-level response to gender role conflicts, we do not address organizational-level factors or organizational-level actions that can be taken to reduce the types of role conflict identified. We see benefit in future research that considers factors such as organizational culture, political climate, and diversity training and their effects on sex- and gender-related role conflicts and subsequent occupational stress. Additionally, attempting to identify how sex- and gender-related occupational stress can be alleviated could be an additional, promising avenue for future research.

CONCLUSION

In the present chapter, we provide a nuanced theoretical examination of the interplay between sex, gender, and gendered job requirements on the experience of job stress. To inform our theorizing, we drew on identity, façades, and emotional labor theories, as well as the extant research on stress. Our theory suggests that to fully understand the role of sex in occupational stress, we must consider sex, gender, proscribed gender roles, and gendered work role requirements in combination. The theory presented here also posits that individuals may cope with sex- and gender-related role conflicts at work by creating and enacting a gender façade, or a false representation of masculinity and/or femininity. The result of this coping mechanism could lead to either reduced or exacerbated occupational stress, depending on the employee's level of identification with relevant work and/or gender roles and the integration of those identities. It is our hope that this chapter will stimulate more nuanced empirical investigations of the relationships among biological sex, gender, role demands, and occupational stress.

ACKNOWLEDGMENTS

The authors would like to thank Anne O'Leary-Kelly, the editors of this volume, especially Chris Rosen, and our anonymous reviewer for their comments on earlier drafts of this chapter. Additionally, we thank Samantha Conroy and Joshua Foster for their support and encouragement throughout the development of this chapter.

REFERENCES

Alvesson, M., & Willmott, H. (2002). Identity regulation as organizational control: Producing the appropriate individual. *Journal of Management Studies*, *39*, 619–644.

Aneshensel, C. S., & Pearlin, L. I. (1987). Structural contexts of sex differences in stress. In R. C. Barnett, L. Biener, & G. K. Baruch (Eds.), *Gender and stress* (pp. 75–95). New York, NY: Free Press.

Ashforth, B. E. (2001). *Role transitions in organizational life: An identity based perspective.* Mahwah, NJ: Erlbaum.

Ashforth, B. E., Harrison, S. H., & Corley, K. G. (2008). Identification in organizations: An examination of four fundamental questions. *Journal of Management*, *34*(3), 325–374.

Ashforth, B. E., & Humphrey, R. H. (1993). Emotional labor in service roles: The influence of identity. *Academy of Management Review*, *18*(1), 88–115.

Barnett, R. C., & Baruch, G. K. (1985). Women's involvement in multiple roles and psychological distress. *Journal of Personality and Social Psychology*, *49*(1), 135–145.

Beehr, T., & Schuler, R. (1980). Stress in organizations. In K. Rowland & G. Ferris (Eds.), *Personnel management* (pp. 390–419). Boston, MA: Allyn and Bacon.

Bem, S. L. (1974). The measurement of psychological androgyny. *Journal of Counseling Psychology*, *42*(2), 155–162.

Berdahl, J. L. (2007). Harassment based on sex: Protecting social status in the context of gender hierarchy. *Academy of Management Review*, *32*(2), 641–658.

Borna, S., & White, G. (2003). "Sex" and "gender": Two confused and confusing concepts in the "women in corporate management" literature. *Journal of Business Ethics*, *47*(2), 89–99.

Breakwell, G. (1986). *Coping with threatened identities.* New York, NY: Methuen.

Caswell, T., Bosson, J. K., Vandello, J. A., & Sellers, J. (2014). Testosterone and men's stress responses to gender threats. *Psychology o f Men & Masculinity*, *15*(1), 4–11.

Catalyst. (2012). *2012 Catalyst Census: Fortune 500 women executive officers and top earners.* Retrieved from http://www.catalyst.org/knowledge/2012-catalyst-census-fortune-500-women-executive-officers-and-top-earners. Accessed on April 6, 2013.

Census Bureau. (2013). *Male nurses becoming more commonplace.* Census Bureau reports. Retrieved from http://www.census.gov/newsroom/releases/archives/employment_occupations/cb13-32.html. Accessed on January 12, 2014.

Chesney, M. A., & Rosenman, R. H. (1980). Type A behavior in the work setting. In C. L. Cooper & R. Payne (Eds.), *Current concerns in occupational stress* (pp. 187–212). New York, NY: Wiley.

Clair, J. A., Beatty, J. E., & Maclean, T. L. (2005). Out of sight but not out of mind: Managing invisible social identities in the workplace. *Academy of Management Review*, *30*(1), 78–95.

Davis, M. C., Matthews, K. A., & Twamley, E. W. (1999). Is life more difficult on Mars or Venus? A meta-analytic review of sex differences in major and minor life events. *Annals of Behavioral Medicine*, *21*(1), 83–97.

Deaux, K., & Major, B. (1987). Putting gender into context: An interactive model of gender-related behavior. *Psychological Review*, *94*(3), 369–389.

Eagly, A. H. (1987). *Sex differences in social behavior: A social-role interpretation*. Hillsdale, NJ: Erlbaum.

Eagly, A. H., & Carli, L. L. (2007). *Through the labyrinth: The truth about how women become leaders*. Boston, MA: Harvard Business School Press.

Eagly, A. H., & Wood, W. (1999). The origins of sex differences in human behavior. *American Psychologist*, *54*(6), 408.

Eisler, R. M., Skidmore, J. R., & Ward, C. H. (1988). Masculine gender-role stress: Predictor of anger, anxiety, and health-risk behaviors. *Journal of Personality Assessment*, *52*(1), 133.

Eisler, R., & Skidmore, J. (1987). Masculine gender role stress. Scale development and component factors in the appraisal of stressful situations. *Behavior Modification*, *11*(2), 123–136.

Ellemers, N., Spears, R., & Doosje, B. (2002). Self and social identity. *Annual Review of Psychology*, *53*, 161–186.

Folkman, S., & Lazarus, R. S. (1980). An analysis of coping in a middle-aged community sample. *Journal of Health and Social Behavior*, *21*, 219–239.

Geurts, S., Schaufeli, W., & De Jonge, J. (1998). Burnout and intention to leave among mental health-care professionals: A social psychological approach. *Journal of Social and Clinical Psychology*, *17*, 341–362.

Gherardi, S., & Poggio, B. (2001). Creating and recreating gender order in organizations. *Journal of World Business*, *36*(3), 245.

Goffman, E. (1959). *The presentation of self in everyday life*. New York, NY: Doubleday.

Goffman, E. (1974). *Frame analysis: An essay on the organization of experience*. Boston, MA: Northeastern University Press.

Goldberg, H. (1987). *The hazards of being male: Surviving the myth of masculine privilege* (2nd ed.). New York, NY: Signet.

Grandey, A. A. (2000). Emotion regulation in the workplace: A new way to conceptualize emotional labor. *Journal of Occupational Health Psychology*, *5*(1), 95–110.

Guppy, A., & Rick, J. (1996). The influences of gender and grade on perceived work stress and job satisfaction in white collar employees. *Work & Stress*, *10*(2), 154–164.

Hart, W., Albarracín, D., Eagly, A. H., Brechan, I., Lindberg, M. J., & Merrill, L. (2009). Feeling validated versus being correct: A meta-analysis of selective exposure to information. *Psychological Bulletin*, *135*(4), 555–588.

Hendrix, W. H., Spencer, B. A., & Gibson, G. S. (1994). Organizational and extraorganizational factors affecting stress, employee well-being, and absenteeism for males and females. *Journal of Business and Psychology*, *9*(2), 103–128.

Herek, G. M. (1996). Why tell if you are not asked? Self-disclosure, intergroup contact, and heterosexuals' attitudes toward lesbians and gay men. In G. M. Herek, J. B. Jobe, & R. M. Carney (Eds.), *Out in force: Sexual orientation and the military* (pp. 197–225). Chicago, IL: University of Chicago Press.

Hewlin, P. (2009). Wearing the cloak: Antecedents and consequences of creating facades of conformity. *Journal of Applied Psychology*, *94*(3), 727–741.

Hewlin, P. F. (2003). An the award for best actor goes to …: Façades of conformity in organizational settings. *Academy of Management Review*, *28*(4), 633–642.

Hochschild, A. R. (1983). *The managed heart: Commercialization of human feeling*. Berkeley, CA: University of California Press.

Ivancevich, J. M., & Matteson, M. T. (1980). Nurses and stress: Time to examine the potential problem. *Supervisor Nurse*, *11*, 17–22.

Jackson, S. E., & Schuler, R. S. (1985). A meta-analysis and conceptual critique of research on role ambiguity and role conflict in work. *Organizational Behavior & Human Decision Processes*, *36*(1), 16.

Kahn, J. P., & Langlieb, A. M. (2003). *Mental health and productivity in the workplace: A handbook for organizations and clinicians*. San Francisco, CA: Jossey-Bass.

Kahn, J. P., Wolfe, D. M., Quinn, R. P., Snoek, J. D., & Rosenthal, R. A. (1964). *Organizational stress: Studies in role conflict and ambiguity*. New York, NY: Wiley.

Kite, M. E., & Deaux, K. (1987). Gender belief systems: Homosexuality and the implicit inversion theory. *Psychology of Women Quarterly*, *11*, 83–96.

Kristensen, T. S., Borritz, M., Villadsen, E., & Christensen, K. B. (2004). The Copenhagen burnout inventory: A new tool for the assessment of burnout. *Work and Stress*, *19*(3), 192–207.

Kristof, A. L. (1996). Person-organization fit: An integrative review of its conceptualizations, measurement, and implications. *Personnel Psychology*, *49*(1), 1–49.

Latack, J. C. (1981). Person/role conflict: Holland's model extended to role-stress research, stress management, and career development. *Academy of Management Review*, *6*(1), 89–103.

Lazarus, R. S., & Folkman, S. (1984) *Stress, appraisal, and coping*. New York, NY: Springer.

Lehavot, K., & Lambert, A. J. (2007). Toward a greater understanding of antigay prejudice: On the role of sexual orientation and gender role violation. *Basic & Applied Social Psychology*, *29*(3), 279–292.

Lichtman, F. (NPR Host). (2013, August 16). *The STEM gender gap*. National Public Radio. Retrieved from http://www.npr.org/2013/08/16/212613885/the-stem-gender gap. Accessed on January 12, 2014.

Loosemore, M., & Waters, T. (2004). Gender differences in occupational stress among professionals in the construction industry. *Journal of Management in Engineering*, *20*(3), 126–132.

Luhaorg, H., & Zivian, M. T. (1995). Gender role conflict: The interaction of gender, gender role, and occupation. *Sex Roles*, *33*(9–10), 607–620.

Martocchino, J. J., & O'Leary, A. M. (1989). Sex differences in occupational stress: A meta-analytic review. *Journal of Applies Psychology*, *74*(3), 495–501.

Maslach, C. (1982). *Burnout: The cost of caring*. Englewood Cliffs, NJ: Prentice Hall.

Maslach, C., & Jackson, S. E. (1981). The measurement of experienced burnout. *Journal of Occupational Behavior*, *2*(2), 99–113.

Matteson, M. T., & Ivancevich, J. M. (1982). Type A and B behavior patterns and health symptoms: Examining individual and organizational fit. *Journal of Occupational Medicine*, *24*, 585–589.

McDonald, L. M., & Korabik, K. (1991). Sources of stress and ways of coping among male and female managers. *Journal of Social Behavior & Personality*, *6*(7), 185–198.

Morris, J., & Feldman, D. C. (1996). The dimensions, antecedents, and consequences of emotional labor. *Academy Of Management Review*, *21*(4), 986–1010.

Nelson, D. L., & Quick, J. C. (1985). Professional women: Are distress and disease inevitable? *Academy of Management Review*, *10*, 206–213.

Netterstrom, B., Kristensen, T. S., Damsgaard, M. T., Olsen, O., & Sjol, A. (1991). Job strain and cardiovascular risk factors: A cross-sectional study of employed Danish men and women. *British Journal of Industrial Medicine*, *48*, 684–689.

O'Neil, J. M. (2008). Complexity, contextualism, and multiculturalism: Responses to the critiques and future directions for the gender role conflict research program. *Counseling Psychologist*, *36*(3), 469–476.

O'Neil, J. M. (2013). Gender role conflict research 30 years later: An evidence-based diagnostic schema to assess boys and men in counseling. *Journal of Counseling & Development*, *91*, 490–498.

Petriglieri, J. (2011). Under threat: Responses to the consequences of threats to individuals' identities. *Academy of Management Review*, *36*(4), 641–662.

Pleck, J. H. (1981). *The myth of masculinity*. Cambridge, MA: MIT Press.

Pleck, J. H. (1995). The gender role strain paradigm: An update. In R. F. Levant & W. S. Pollack (Eds.), *A new psychology of men* (pp. 11–32). New York, NY: Basic Books.

Powell, A., Bagilhole, B., & Dainty, A. (2009). How women engineers do and undo gender: Consequences for gender equality. *Gender, Work & Organization*, *16*(4), 411–428.

Purvanova, R. K., & Muros, J. P. (2010). Gender differences in burnout: A meta-analysis. *Journal of Vocational Behavior*, *77*(2), 168–185.

Ridgeway, C. L. (1997). Interaction and the conservation of gender inequality: Considering employment. *American Sociological Review*, *62*, 218–235.

Roberts, L. M. (2005). Changing faces: Professional image construction in diverse organizational settings. *Academy of Management Review*, *30*(4), 685–711.

Roccas, S., & Brewer, M. (2002). Social identity complexity. *Personality and Social Psychology Review*, *6*(2), 88–106.

Rumens, N., & Kerfoot, D. (2009). Gay men at work: (Re)constructing the self as professional. *Human Relations*, *62*(5), 763–786.

Schlenker, B. (1985). Introduction: Foundations of the self in social life. In B. R. Schlenker (Ed.), *The self and social life* (pp. 1–28). New York, NY: McGraw-Hill.

Settles, I. H., Sellers, R. M., & Damas, A., Jr. (2002). One role of two? The function of psychological separation in role conflict. *Journal of Applied Psychology*, *87*(3), 574–582.

Singh, J., Goolsby, J. R., & Rhoads, G. K. (1994). Behavioral and psychological consequences of boundary spanning burnout for customer service representatives. *Journal of Marketing Research*, *31*, 558–569.

Skrypnek, B. J., & Snyder, M. (1982). On the self-perpetuating nature of stereotypes about women and men. *Journal f Experimental Social Psychology*, *18*(3), 277–291.

Stormer, F., & Devine, K. (2008). Acting at work. *Journal of Management Inquiry*, *17*(2), 112–134.

Tajfel, H. (1978). *Differentiation between social groups: Studies in the social psychology of intergroup relations*. New York, NY: Academic Press.

Tajfel, H., & Turner, J. C. (1985). The social identity theory of intergroup behavior. In S. Worchel & W. G. Austin (Eds.), *Psychology of intergroup relations* (2nd ed., pp. 7–24). Chicago, IL: Nelson Hall.

Tubre, T. C., & Collins, J. M. (2000). Jackson and Schuler (1985) revisited: A meta-analysis of the relationships between role ambiguity, role conflict, and job performance. *Journal of Management*, *26*(1), 155–169.

Turnley, W. H., & Bolino, M. C. (2001). Achieving desired images while avoiding undesired images: Exploring the role of self-monitoring in impression management. *Journal of Applied Psychology*, *86*(2), 351–360.

Vagg, P. R., Speilberger, C. D., & Wasala, C. F. (2002). Effects of organizational level and gender on stress in the workplace. *International Journal of Stress Management*, *9*(4), 243–261.

Vandello, J. A., & Bosson, J. K. (2013). Hard won and easily lost: A review and synthesis of theory and research on precarious manhood. *Psychology of Men & Masculinity*, *14*(2), 101–113.

Vandello, J. A., Bosson, J. K., Cohen, D., Burnaford, R., & Weaver, J. (2008). Precarious manhood. *Journal of Personality and Social Psychology*, *95*, 1325–1339.

Weick, K. E. (1995). *Sensemaking in organizations*. Thousand Oaks, CA: Sage.

Wethington, E., McLeod, J. D., & Kessler, R. C. (1987). The importance of life events for explaining sex differences in psychological distress. In R. C. Barnett, L. Biemer, & G. K. Baruch (Eds.), *Gender and stress* (pp. 144–156). New York, NY: Free Press.

Wiesenfeld, B. M., & Hewlin, P. (2003). Splintered identities and organizational change. In B. Mannix, M. Neale, & J. Polzer (Eds.), *Research on managing groups and teams* (Vol. 5, pp. 27–52). New York, NY: Elsevier Science.

Williams, J. E., & Best, D. L. (1982). *Measuring sex stereotypes: A thirty nation study*. Beverly Hills, CA: Sage.

Wood, W., & Karten, S. J. (1986). Sex differences in interaction style as a product of perceived sex differences in competence. *Journal of Personality and Social Psychology*, *5*, 341–347.

APPENDIX A

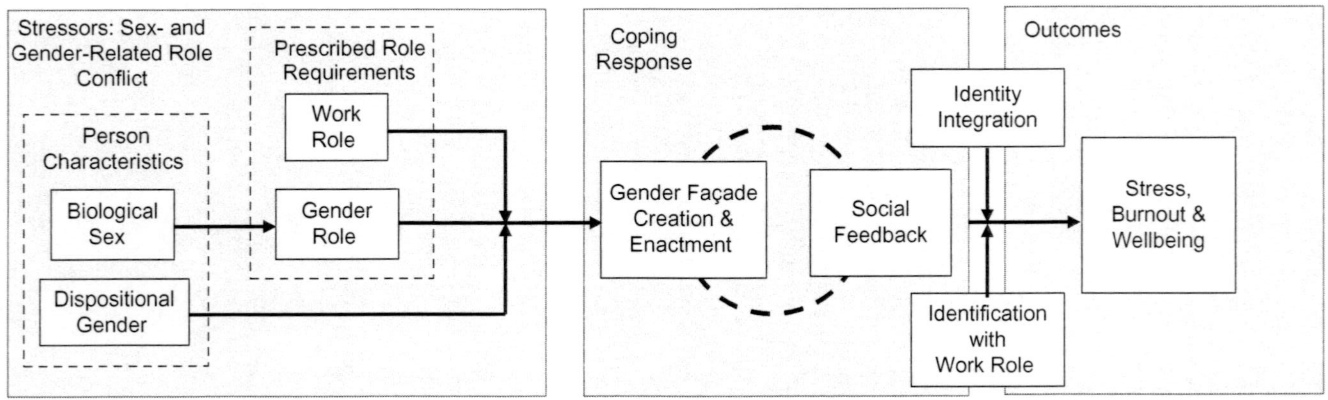

Fig. A1. Theoretical Model of Sex- and Gender-Based Role Conflict and Gender Façades.

APPENDIX B

Table B1. Sex, Gender, and Role-Based typology of Role Conflict and Gender Façade Creation.

Person Characteristics		Prescribed Role Requirements		Person-Role Conflict		Inter-Role Conflict	Façade Creation							
							During work tasks				During social interactions			
							Fabricate		Conceal		Fabricate		Conceal	
Biological sex	Dispositional gender	Gender role	Work role	Gender role	Work role		Mas	Fem	Mas	Fem	Mas	Fem	Mas	Fem
Male	Mas	Mas	Mas											
			Fem		✓	✓		✓	✓					
	Fem	Mas	Mas	✓	✓		✓			✓	✓			✓
			Fem	✓		✓					✓			✓
Female	Mas	Fem	Mas	✓		✓						✓	✓	
			Fem	✓	✓			✓	✓			✓	✓	
	Fem	Fem	Mas		✓	✓	✓			✓				
			Fem											

Mas = Masculine; Fem = Feminine.

DEMOGRAPHIC FACTORS AND WORKER WELL-BEING: AN EMPIRICAL REVIEW USING REPRESENTATIVE DATA FROM THE UNITED STATES AND ACROSS THE WORLD

Louis Tay, Vincent Ng, Lauren Kuykendall and Ed Diener

ABSTRACT

The relationship between demographic factors and worker well-being has garnered increased attention, but empirical studies have shown to inconsistent results. This chapter addresses this issue by examining how age, gender, and race/ethnicity relate to worker well-being using large, representative samples. Data from the Gallup Healthways Index and Gallup World Poll provided information on both job and life satisfaction outcomes for full-time workers in the United States and 156 countries, respectively. In general, results indicated that increasing age was associated with more workers reporting job satisfaction and fewer people

The Role of Demographics in Occupational Stress and Well Being
Research in Occupational Stress and Well Being, Volume 12, 235–283

ISSN: 1479-3555/doi:10.1108/S1479-355520140000012007

reporting stress and negative affect. Women were comparable to men in reported job satisfaction and well-being, but more women reported experiencing negative affect and stress. Less consistent well-being differences in ethnic/racial groups were found. Finally, we found strong evidence for direct and indirect national demographic effects on worker well-being showing need for considering workforce demography in future theory building. Theoretical and practical implications are discussed.

Keywords: Well-being; stress; emotions; age; gender; race/ethnicity

There is growing interest in the role of demographic factors and the well-being of workers. While meta-analyses (e.g., Brush, Moch, & Pooyan, 1987; Ng & Feldman, 2010) have summarized how age, gender, and race/ethnicity are linked to worker well-being, there continue to be concerns about the consistency of demography effects (Joshi, Liao, & Roh, 2011). As such, recent representative sampling of workers by the Gallup Organization within the United States and across the world can offer new insights into the role of demographic factors play in worker well-being. With representative polling of more than 450,000 full-time workers within the United States, we seek to provide an empirical review of the relation between demographic factors and well-being. Further, we heed the call for a greater cross-national emphasis on worker well-being (Judge, Parker, Colbert, Heller, & Ilies, 2001) by using demographic information of more than 150,000 full-time workers across 156 nations. The data can provide a reliable empirical yardstick to evaluate the generalizability of individual level demographic theories and also serve to address the call for a multilevel perspective on workplace demography research (Joshi et al., 2011) by considering for the demographic makeup of the societal workforce.

We take a cross-domain perspective on worker well-being with an emphasis on psychological well-being. This includes evaluative components such as job satisfaction and affective components such as positive or negative feelings within the domain of work (e.g., Judge & Klinger, 2007; McKee-Ryan, Song, Wanberg, & Kinicki, 2005; Tay & Harter, 2013; Wright & Cropanzano, 2000). Additionally, it encompasses the general life domain, which includes life satisfaction and daily affective experiences (Erdogan, Bauer, Truxillo, & Mansfield, 2012; Judge & Watanabe, 1993). We advocate for this integrative view as work and non-work domains are closely intertwined and have spillover effects on work and non-work well-being (Judge & Iles, 2004; Judge, Iles, & Scott, 2006). This is also in line with the recent emphasis in research on the holistic study of the worker and their occupational well-being (Danna & Griffin, 1999; Weiss & Rupp, 2011) and public health strategies such as the NIOSH Total Worker Health (TWH) Initiative.

The chapter is structured as follows: (a) we review key theoretical perspectives and extant empirical findings[1] on age, gender, race/ethnicity, and their relations to worker well-being; (b) we describe the Gallup data and the relevant demographic and well-being variables; (c) we present the analyses of worker well-being by demographic categories within the United States and across the world; (d) we propose new empirical and theoretical directions for future exploration.

THEORETICAL PERSPECTIVES

Age

Table 1 displays large-scale studies assessing the relationship between age and job satisfaction.[2] As can be seen, several studies have indicated a significant positive relationship between age and job satisfaction (e.g., Herzog & Rodgers, 1981; Wunder & Wiencierz, 2013). Nevertheless, uncertainty remains about the exact form of this relationship. Some researchers have proposed that job satisfaction rises linearly as age increases because older individuals are more proactive in pursuing satisfying work (Ng & Feldman, 2010). A life-span perspective, namely, the socioemotional selectivity theory (SES; Carstensen, 1992) provides a similar explanation. The SES theory states that as time-horizons (i.e., perceptions of time available left) reduce with age, individuals choose to engage in more emotionally meaningful activities. By implication, older workers are more likely to invest more in emotionally meaningful work; this can lead to choosing a more intrinsically satisfying job or lowered expectations for extrinsic rewards at work. Advocates of this perspective expect an upward linear trend between age and worker well-being. Broadly, SES theory also suggests that workers' overall life satisfaction should also increase as workers age. While not focusing exclusively on workers, some large-scale studies have shown increases in life satisfaction during ages typically associated with the late career life stage (e.g., Baird, Lucas, & Donnellan, 2010; Blanchflower & Oswald, 2008, 2009; Wunder &Wiencierz, 2013). Table 2 displays large-scale studies assessing the relationships between life satisfaction and age.

Table 1. Studies Assessing the Relationship between Age and Job Satisfaction.

Author (Date)	Data Source	*N*	Age	Instrument	Shape (Shape with controls)	Controls	Notes
Birdi, Warr, and Oswald (1995)	International Social Survey Program	4,356	18–64	One item	U-shaped (Null)	Gender, marital status, country, length of education, supervisory, working hours, income, job rewards, poor work conditions, work relations, employment commitment, and work values	Non-significant relationship between age and job satisfaction after control variables taken into account
Herzog and Rodgers (1981)	Quality of Life 1971, Quality of Life 1978, General Social Surveys 1972–1978, Social Indicator Study 1972, Omnibus 1973–1975		20–90		Linear-positive		
	Quality of Life 1971 and Quality of Life 1978		20–90		(Linear-positive)	Religion; length in residence; social desirability; last three (simultaneously); life evaluations;	

						income, education and health; last two (simultaneously); and all variables except income, education, and health (simultaneously)	
Wunder and Wiencierz (2013)	German Socio-Economic Panel Study 1986–2007				Curvilinear-positive		Relatively flat until rising at 10–15 years prior to retirement
	British Household Panel Study 1996–2006				Curvilinear-positive		Slight decline and then rising 10–15 years prior to retirement
Easterlin (2006)	General Social Survey 1973–1994	29,651	18–89	One item (happiness)	(Inverted U-shape)	Gender, race, education, and birth cohort	Rise from 18 to 60 and then decline
Lange (2009)	European Values Study (Central and Eastern Countries)	2,026 (M) 1,827 (F)		One item	(U-shape)	Age, marital status, education, occupational skills level, chief earner in household status, size of town, job characteristics, values/beliefs,	

Table 1. *(Continued)*

Author (Date)	Data Source	*N*	Age	Instrument	Shape (Shape with controls)	Controls	Notes
						institutional confidence, and country	
Clark et al. (1996)	British Household Panel Study 1991	5,140		One item	(U-shape)	Gender, health, race, education, income, work hours, manager status, union member status, establishment size, region, industry, occupation, tenure, work values, marital status, number of own children, and number in household	
Kalleberg and Loscocco (1983)	Quality of Employment Survey 1973	1,455		Five item scale		Education, gender, race, work structures, family life cycles, job rewards, work-related work values	Can be modeled by a cubic function

Table 2. Studies Assessing the Relationship between Age and Life Satisfaction.

Author (Date)	Data Source	*N*	Age	Instrument	Shape (Shape with Controls)	Controls	Notes
Baird, Lucas, and Donnellan (2010)	German Socio-Economic Panel Study	20,696	16–91	One item	Curvilinear		Flat and then declining
	British Household Panel Study	21,448	16–91	One item	Wave		Starts high at age 16, low at 40, high at 70, and drops; U-shaped and then declining
Blanchflower and Oswald (2004)	US General Social Surveys 1972–1998	37,711		One item (happiness)	Convex (U-shape)	Marital status, demographics, and education	Minimum at ~40 years all with controls held constant
	Eurobarometer Surveys	56,863		One item	U-shape (U-shape)	Marital status, demographics, and education	Minimum at ~40 years all with controls held constant
Blanchflower and Oswald (2008)	US General Social Surveys 1972–2006	20,316 (M) 25,837 (F)		One item (happiness)	U-shape (U-shape)	Race, education, workforce status, marital status, no living with both parents at age 16, cohort effects, and income	For both sexes

Table 2. (*Continued*)

Author (Date)	Data Source	*N*	Age	Instrument	Shape (Shape with Controls)	Controls	Notes
	Eurobarometers 1976–1980, 1982–2002 (17 countries)	293,612 (M) 314,431 (F)		One item	U-shape (U-shape)	Race, education, workforce status, marital status, no living with both parents at age 16, cohort effects, and income	Analysis with control variables excluded years 1979, 1981, 1995, and 1996 from data due to missing income variables
	World Values Survey 1981–2004 (Western Europe)	33,470 (M) 35,448 (F)		One item	(U-shape)	Workforce status, marital status, education, country, year, and income	For both sexes
	World Values Survey 1981–2004 (Eastern Europe)	12,806 (M) 14,419 (F)		One item	(U-shape)	Workforce status, marital status, education, country, year, and income	For both sexes
	World Values Survey 1981–2004 (Developing countries)	33,631 (M) 33,072 (F)		One item	(U-shape)	Workforce status, marital status, and country	For both sexes
	Latinobarometers 1997, 2000, 2001, and 2003–2005	45,177 (M) 54,128 (F)		One item	(U-shape)	Workforce status, marital status, education, country, year, and income	For both sexes

	Asianbarometers 1997–2005 (15 countries)	8,592 (M) 5,025 (F)		One item	(U-shape)	Workforce status, marital-status, year, and education	For both sexes
Blanchflower and Oswald (2009)	Eurobarometers 1976–2006	546,083		One item	(U-shape)	Country and gender	
Frijters and Beatton (2012)	German Socio-Economic Panel Study 1984–2002	176,770	44.26	One item	(Late wave)	Selectivity and time-in-panel effects	Flat to ~55 years, peaks at ~65 years, and drops sharply at ~75 years
	Household, Income and Labor Dynamics in Australia Survey (waves 2–8)	72,108	45.50	One item	(Late wave)	Selectivity and time-in-panel effects	Flat to ~55 years, peaks at ~65 years, and drops sharply at ~75 years
	British Household Panel Study (waves 6–10, 12–18)	153,886	46.65	One item	(Late wave)	Selectivity and time-in-panel effects	Flat to ~55 years, peaks at ~65 years, and drops sharply at ~75 years
Herzog and Rodgers (1981)	Quality of Life 1978		20–90		Linear-positive [(Linear-positive)] [(Null)]	[Religious activity; length in residence; both (simultaneously); life events; income, education, and health] [Life evaluation; education, income, health, life events,	

Table 2. (*Continued*)

Author (Date)	Data Source	*N*	Age	Instrument	Shape (Shape with Controls)	Controls	Notes
						and life evaluation (simultaneously); and all variables except income, education, and health (simultaneously)]	
	Omnibus 1973–1975		20–90		Linear-negative		
	Quality of Life 1971, General Social Surveys 1972–1978, Social Indicator Study 1972		20–90		Null		
	Quality of Life 1971		20–90		[(Linear-positive)] [Null]	[Income, education, and health, all variables exception income, education and health (simultaneously)] [Religious activity; length in residence; social desirability; last three (simultaneously);	

						life evaluation; and income, education, health, and life evaluation (simultaneously)]	
Wunder and Wiencierz (2013)	German Socio-Economic Panel Study 1986–2007				Wave		Falls from 18 to 52, rises from 53 to 65, and falls after 66
	British Household Panel Study 1996–2006				Wave		Falls from 18 to 48, rises from 49 to 70, and falls after 71
Clemente and Sauer (1976)	General Social Survey 1973	1,347	18 and older	Four items (residence, friends, family, activities)	(Linear-positive)	Race, education, income, marital status, perceived health, vote, church attendance, and sex	
Easterlin (2006)	General Social Survey 1973–1994	29,651	18–89	One item (happiness)	(Inverted U-shape)	Gender, race, education, and birth cohort	Rise from 18 to 51 and then decline

These studies include working-age populations and are not restricted to only workers.

In contrast, others have contested the argument that the relationship between age and job satisfaction is linear, pointing to evidence that the relationship between age and job satisfaction is primarily U-shaped with higher levels of satisfaction occurring for younger and older workers (Clark, Oswald, & Warr, 1996). Higher levels of job satisfaction in younger workers may stem from initial novelty and overly positive beliefs (Clark et al., 1996; Wanous, 1973). As the novelty of working wears off, job satisfaction may then decline through early to mid-thirties and then ascend as efforts are redirected toward finding more emotionally fulfilling work as implied by SES theory. As can be seen in Table 2, several large-scale studies have also shown support for this perspective (Clark et al., 1996; Lange, 2009).

Alternatively, differences in the observed relationship between age and job satisfaction may stem from the types of job satisfaction constructs measured. For example, Kacmar and Ferris (1989) found that the relationship between age and job satisfaction followed a U-shaped relationship for more extrinsic aspects of work (e.g., coworkers), but a linear relationship for intrinsic aspects (i.e., the work itself). This finding stands in contrast to Clark et al.'s (1996) finding that the U-shaped relationship was found between age and both extrinsic and intrinsic job satisfaction.

In the current chapter, we examine the relationship between age and job satisfaction using a representative sample from the United States and across the world to more fully clarify the nature of their association. Beyond job satisfaction, we also seek to capture how age and other broader measures of worker well-being are associated.

Gender and Race/Ethnicity

Apart from age, other important demographic factors include gender and race/ethnicity. In this literature, some research has shown links between minority status and lower levels of worker well-being (Greenhaus, Parasuraman, & Wormley, 1990; Lyness & Thompson, 1997, 2000). Such findings may be due to the perception on the part of minority members that they experience less favorable job outcomes compared to their majority counterparts. As such, one would expect minority membership to be associated with lower levels of job satisfaction. An extension of this idea in sociological research, known as "double jeopardy," suggests that the negative outcomes of being a member of more than one historically disadvantaged group would interact multiplicatively to create worse outcomes than the additive direct effects of each group (Lincoln & Allen, 2004). We label this intuitive phenomenon of having lowered well-being due to receiving objectively less favorable work outcomes as "direct disadvantage." Further, because job dissatisfaction can have bottom-up influences on general life satisfaction (Lance, Lautenschlager, Sloan, & Varca, 1989; Tay & Harter, 2013), the effects of minority membership may result not only in reduced job satisfaction but also in diminished levels of overall life satisfaction and other general indicators of worker well-being.

Our review of the large-scale studies assessing the relationship between gender and job satisfaction and life satisfaction (see Tables 3 and 4) reveals that, despite theoretical arguments implying that female workers should have lower job satisfaction than male workers, females appear to have equal or even greater job satisfaction and life satisfaction as men (Blanchflower & Oswald, 2004; Lange, 2009; Mukerjee, 2013), despite negative conditions such as lower pay. Such findings are consistent with an emerging perspective within sociology, which states that although objective conditions such as pay may be worse for members of a group, they may experience proportionately greater psychological rewards from gains in relevant contexts such as work due to an activation of group member schema and the recognition of being in a disadvantageous position (Schieman, 2002). For individuals in a group that has historically experienced obstacles in a particular context, gains in that context will be particularly rewarding because they will be aware of their status advantage relative to their historical counterparts. Thus, when traditional role gender schemas are activated for working women, they will likely gain greater satisfaction from successes in the work domain. This idea is also congruent with findings from the social comparison literature that *downward social comparison* is preferred when under threat because it serves to buffer self-esteem (Taylor & Lobel, 1989). Yet, this does not fully explain why men who might engage in similar self-protecting interests would not yield similar levels of job satisfaction unless the objective referent point is lower for women than men. Indeed, Clark (1997) noted that the gender differential in job satisfaction may ultimately be a transitory effect that will disappear as women continue to gain equality in the work context. In contrast to "direct disadvantage," we label these processes as "disadvantage adjustment."

These contrasting theories may also be applied to racial/ethnic minority groups. Tables 5 and 6 display large-scale studies assessing the relationship between race/ethnicity and job satisfaction. Most of these studies have

Table 3. Studies Assessing the Relationship between Gender and Job Satisfaction.

Author (Date)	Data Source	*N*	Age	Instrument	Relative to Males	Controls	Notes
Weaver (1980)	General Social Survey 1972–1978	4,709	18 and older	One item	Equal		Mean values not significantly different for each of the seven years
Mukerjee (2013)	General Social Survey 1972–2008	20,501		One item	Greater	Income, benefits, and education	
	National Longitudinal Surveys of Youth 1997				Greater	Income, benefits, and education	
Weaver (1977)	General Social Survey 1974	633	18 and older	One item	Equal	Pay, sex, occupational prestige, supervisory position, and work autonomy	Equal job satisfaction before and after accounting for effect of control variables
Lange (2009)	European Values Study (Central and Eastern Countries)	2,026 (M) 1,827 (F)		One item	Greater	Age, marital status, education, occupational skills level, chief earner in household status, size of town, job characteristics, values/beliefs, institutional confidence, and country	

Table 4. Studies Assessing the Relationship between Gender and Life Satisfaction.

Author (Date)	Data Source	*N*	Age	Instrument	Females Compared to Males	Controls	Notes
Blanchflower and Oswald (2004)	General Social Surveys of the United States 1972–1998	15,548 (M) 21,163 (F)		One item	Greater		Small difference
	Eurobarometer Surveys	27,082 (M) 29,781 (F)		One item	Greater		
Clemente and Sauer (1976)	General Social Survey 1973	1,347	18 and older	Four items (residence, friends, family, activities)	Equal		

Table 5. Studies Assessing the Relationship between Race/Ethnicity and Job Satisfaction.

Author (Date)	Data Source	*N*	Age	Instrument	Ranking (Ranking with Control)	Controls	Notes
Weaver (2003)	General Social Survey 1972–2000	40,933		One item	Euro-Americans Asian-Americans African-Americans		Ranking is for males. Same ranking was found for females, but differences in mean job satisfaction not significantly different between Euro-Americans and Asian-Americans
Barger, Donoho, and Wayment (2009)	National Health Interview Survey Behavioral Risk Factor Surveillance System	29,243 329,004		One item	Whites African-Americans and Whites Hispanics		Difference lessens after controlling for socio-economic status, health, and relationships
Weaver (1980)	General Social Survey 1972–1978	4,709	18 and older	One item	Whites African-Americans		
Mukerjee (2013)	General Social Survey 1972–2008 National Longitudinal Surveys of Mature Men 1997	20,501			(Whites African-Americans) (Whites African-Americans)	Income, benefits, and education Income, benefits, and education	
Bartel (1981)	National Longitudinal Surveys of Mature Men 1966, 1969, and 1971	3,222 2,728 2,515		Two item composite	(Blacks Whites)	Education, experience, health status, union membership, job characteristics and location characteristics	Blacks did not have significantly less job satisfaction compared to Whites even when not controlling for pay and occupation type. Blacks had increasingly greater job satisfaction even after controlling for sampling selection bias
Weaver (1977)	General Social Survey 1974	633		One item	Whites Blacks (Equal)	Pay, sex, occupational prestige, supervisory position, and work autonomy	Differences in job satisfaction between races disappears after accounting for control variables
Tuch (1991)	General Social Survey 1985, 1987, 1988, and 1989	2,517		One item	Whites Blacks		
Weaver (1998)	General Social Survey 1972–1996 (except 1979, 1981, 1992, and 1995)			One item	White Black		Based on percentage that were very satisfied with their job

Table 6. Studies Assessing the Relationship between Race/Ethnicity and Life Satisfaction.

Author (Date)	Data Source	*N*	Age	Instrument	Ranking	Controls	Notes
Blanchflower and Oswald (2004)	General Social Surveys of the United States 1972–1998	5,078		One item	Whites African-Americans		African-Americans exhibit an upward trend in happiness over time despite being lower in happiness relative to Whites
Clemente and Sauer (1976)	General Social Survey 1973	1,347	18 and older	Four item composite (residence, friends, family, activities)	Whites African-Americans		
Mookherjee (1992)	General Social Survey 1978 and 1988	1,532	18–89	Seven item composite (satisfaction with residence, family, hobbies, friendship, health, income, and life)	Whites Non-whites		
Thomas and Hughes (1986)	General Social Survey 1972–1985			Five item composite (satisfaction with family life, health, friendship, non-work activities, and residence) One item (happiness)	White Blacks	Income, education, employment status, age, and marital status	
Weaver and Hinson (2000)	General Social Surveys 1972–1996 (except 1979, 1981, 1992, and 1995)	12,139		One item	Whites African-Americans Asian-Americans		Difference between Whites and both Asian-Americans and African-Americans; Asian-American and African-American are similar

shown lower job satisfaction and life satisfaction for minorities compared to non-minorities, lending support for direct disadvantage. However, not all findings have supported the direct disadvantage hypothesis (e.g., Bartel, 1981) and some have even shown minority workers to be more satisfied with their jobs. For example, in a study comparing white Canadian workers to Chinese, South Asian, and Black minorities, Chinese workers were the most satisfied with their jobs followed by Whites, South Asians, and Blacks (Yap, Cukier, Holmes, & Hannan, 2010). Such findings suggest that it may not be minority status itself that determines higher or lower levels of worker well-being relative to the majority.

Our goal is to explore the contrasting perspectives of direct disadvantage and disadvantage adjustment in gender and race/ethnic groupings using the Gallup data. We seek to provide a representative picture of the recent trends of these possible effects within the United States and across the world. In doing so, it may reveal a more nuanced understanding of the ways in which subjective well-being (SWB) outcomes vary by different demographic groups.

Bridging Multiple Levels Via Workforce Demography

Organizational research has evolved to capture the complexities of the world of work through the development of multilevel theories and methods (Kozlowski & Klein, 2000; Tay, Woo, & Vermunt, 2014). A recent review has pointed out that demography research has been primarily conducted at single levels of analysis (*viz.* individual, work group, and organization), but most of the variation occurs through the interplay between multiple levels (Joshi et al., 2011). This has now led to some research exploring interactive effects of individuals with workgroups (van Knippenberg & Schippers, 2007) and organizations/communities (Sacco & Schmitt, 2005). And yet, to our knowledge, despite inherent national and policy-related interests in diversity and demography, no work has explicitly examined national workforce demography and its interaction with individual demography on worker well-being.

We propose that workforce demography represents an important socioecological factor that can influence worker well-being outcomes. There is currently a re-emphasis on social habitats at the community and national level (Oishi & Graham, 2010) that serves to influence psychological processes. One channel of influence is via cultural processes, where in this instance, workforce demography affects the perceptions, assumptions, and motivations of workers. The cultural stereotype of a typical worker can potentially contrast or complement the self-identity of a worker leading to lower or higher well-being, respectively. Another channel of influence stems from ecological environments, where in this case workforce demography represents the likelihood of conditions and interactions directly experienced by the worker. While the cultural and ecological channels are conceptually distinct, their effects are mutually codetermined from workforce demography: demographic culture is a reaction to the ecology of workforce demography and the ecology of workforce demography is shaped by the demographic culture. This integrated channel can vitally influence the well-being of the worker over and above individual demography.

Workforce demography may further act as a contextual moderator between individual demography and well-being. One pattern of interaction observed in cross-national contexts is a matching trend: individuals who share characteristics with the dominant societal characteristic tend to be happier (Fulmer et al., 2010; Tay, Morrison, & Diener, 2014). When one shares more similarities with the dominant societal characteristics, uncertainty is decreased and one's self-concept is validated, resulting in higher self-esteem and happiness. By extension, the matching of workforce demography and individual demography can potentially enhance worker well-being. Research has shown that individuals who match the dominant gender composition within the workplace have higher job satisfaction, providing direct support for the matching proposition (Peccei & Lee, 2005). The matching proposition has also garnered indirect support from research showing that perceived age similarity in the workplace was related to higher levels of work engagement among older workers who were satisfied with their coworkers (Avery, McKay, & Wilson, 2007). As such, we seek to determine whether this matching hypothesis holds for workforce demography and individual demography.

Summary

Questions about the effects of individual demography have generated contrasting perspectives. With regard to age, researchers have reached different conclusions about whether the form of the upward function through which job satisfaction rises is primarily linear or U-shaped. With regard to gender and race/ethnicity, it is unclear whether minorities are negatively affected in their well-being from direct disadvantage or show resilience through a reframing process which we term as disadvantage adjustment. These contrasting views are difficult to adjudicate at present, but the recent large-scale representation of worker data from The Gallup Organization can provide a robust empirical base to evaluate these perspectives. Further, we are able to expand the boundaries of demographic research by incorporating national workforce demography and its effects on worker well-being. We examine the extent to which national workforce demography can exert direct effects on well-being beyond individual demography and demonstrate moderating effects as well.

THE GALLUP WORKER DATA

The Gallup Healthways Index (GHI) surveys about 1,000 US residents on non-holidays with the goal of representing the health and well-being of 98% of the adult US population. Surveys are conducted over the phone with about 850 landline respondents and 150 cellphone respondents. Interviews are conducted primarily in English and with interviews conducted in Spanish for Spanish speaking respondents. The initial data consisted of 1,415,515 respondents with a subset of 468,367 full-time workers (i.e., ≥30 hours worked per week) that was analyzed.

The Gallup World Poll (GWP) seeks to provide representative information of the opinions and attitudes of 95% of all adults aged 15 and older across the world. The GWP employed representative sampling of 162 nations where surveys were conducted over the telephone for countries where there was telephone coverage for at least 80% of the population; otherwise, face-to-face interviews were undertaken. Surveys were translated from English into the major language of each nation using a two-stage process whereby an initial translation is undertaken by one translator and reviewed and refined by a second translator. Survey data were collected over the years of 2005–2013 providing information for 1,101,692 individuals across the world of which 510,737 were workers. Because we were only interested in full-time workers, and at the point of data analysis, information on full-time work status was only made available for 2010, our sample consisted of the subset of full-time workers ($n = 172{,}949$) in 2010 from 156 nations.

Table 7 shows the well-being dimensions, item content, response format, and reliabilities of the measures used in our analysis for both the GHI and the GWP. Notably, the reliabilities were low for positive and negative feelings due to the dichotomous response format. In economics, each indicator is analyzed as perfectly reliable (e.g., Kahneman & Deaton, 2010).

Table 7. Well-being Variables of Interest in the Gallup Healthways Index (GHI) and the Gallup World Poll (GWP).

	Item Content	Response	GHI	GWP
Work-related well-being				
Job satisfaction	Are you satisfied or dissatisfied with your job or the work you do?	Yes/No	X	X
Sense of mastery	In your work, do you have an opportunity to do what you do best every day, or not?	Yes/No	X	
General well-being				
Current life evaluations	Life satisfaction today	0–10	X	X
Positive feelings	Experience a lot of the following emotions yesterday: enjoyment, smile/laugh ($\alpha_{GHI}=0.57$; $\alpha_{GWP}=0.60$)	0–1	X	X
Negative feelings	Experience a lot of the following emotions yesterday: worry, anger, sadness ($\alpha_{GHI}=0.61$; $\alpha_{GWP}=0.63$)	0–1	X	X
Stress	Experience a lot of the following emotion yesterday: stress	Yes/No	X	X

However, we felt it was preferable to use a composite where possible rather than individual indicators in which scale reliability cannot be assessed.

In our GHI analysis, we also included control variables health (1 = "poor" to 5 = "excellent"), monthly income (1 = <$60, 2 = $60–$499, 3 = $500–$999, 4 = $1,000–$1,999, 5 = $2,000–$2,999, 6 = $3,000–$3,999, 7 = $4,000–$4,999, 8 = $5,000–$7,499, 9 = $7,500–$9,999, 10 = $10,000–$14,999, 11 = $15,000–$19,000, 12 = >$20,000), education levels (1 = "less than high school diploma"; 2 = "High school degree or diploma"; 3 = "Technical/Vocational school"; 4 = "Some college"; 5 = "College graduate"; 6 = "Post-graduate work or degree"), and dummy coded job type categories (1 = "Professional"; 2 = "Manager, Executive or Official"; 3 = "Business Owner or Self-Employed"; 4 = "Clerical or Office Worker"; 5 = "Sales"; 6 = "Service"; 7 = "Construction or Mining"; 8 = "Manufacturing or Production"; 9 = "Transportation"; 10 = "Installation or Repair"; 11 = "Farming, Fishing or Forestry"; 12 = "Other"). The GWP analysis made use of the control variables with some differences in response categories for health (0 = "dissatisfied"; 1 = "satisfied"), household income (absolute annual income converted to international dollars), and education levels (1 = "elementary education (<= 8 years)"; 2 = "tertiary/secondary education (9–15 years)"; 3 = "4 years beyond high school or College Degree").

WORKER WELL-BEING WITHIN THE UNITED STATES

We seek to present a descriptive picture of age, gender, and race/ethnicity while applying statistical procedures, specifically linear regression or logistic regression, to obtain predicted levels of worker well-being. In the following, we present both descriptive information as well as regression-based predicted levels – with the white Caucasian group weighted by the observed gender proportions as the referent – in the figures. We also narratively report the estimated coefficients of worker well-being by demographic variables while controlling for health, income, education level, and job type. For intuitive reporting of logistic regression, we use "odds" in place of "log-odds".

Age

As shown in Fig. 1, the descriptive information presented show that with regard to well-being at work, the relationship is more complex than a simple linear or U-shaped function as previously anticipated. A cubic function of age ($p < 0.05$) was significantly related to work-related well-being outcomes even after controlling for other demographics, health, income, and education levels. From the descriptive information and the predicted levels of well-being, the proportion of respondents reporting job satisfaction appears to increase initially in the early years, followed by a plateau before slight increases closer to the retirement years. It is also helpful to note that there are fewer workers in the younger age category of 15–20, resulting in more variability as shown from the wide 95% confidence intervals, and the regression line may weigh this age group less in the overall model.

For job satisfaction, we observe a general increase in those reporting job satisfaction from about 88% to about 92% from age category 21–25 to 65–70, although there is some stability across ages 31–55. With regard to mastery-related experiences at work, we observe a similar upward trend as well with similar levels of stability in middle-aged workers from 31 to 60.

How is age related to the overall pattern of general well-being? In Fig. 2, we find that unlike work-specific well-being, there is less evidence of a plateau effect during the middle age. Interestingly, general SWB (Diener, 1984) which includes life satisfaction, positive feelings, and negative feelings exhibited U-shaped patterns, where middle-aged workers experienced lower levels of SWB. Importantly, the trends continue to provide support for the

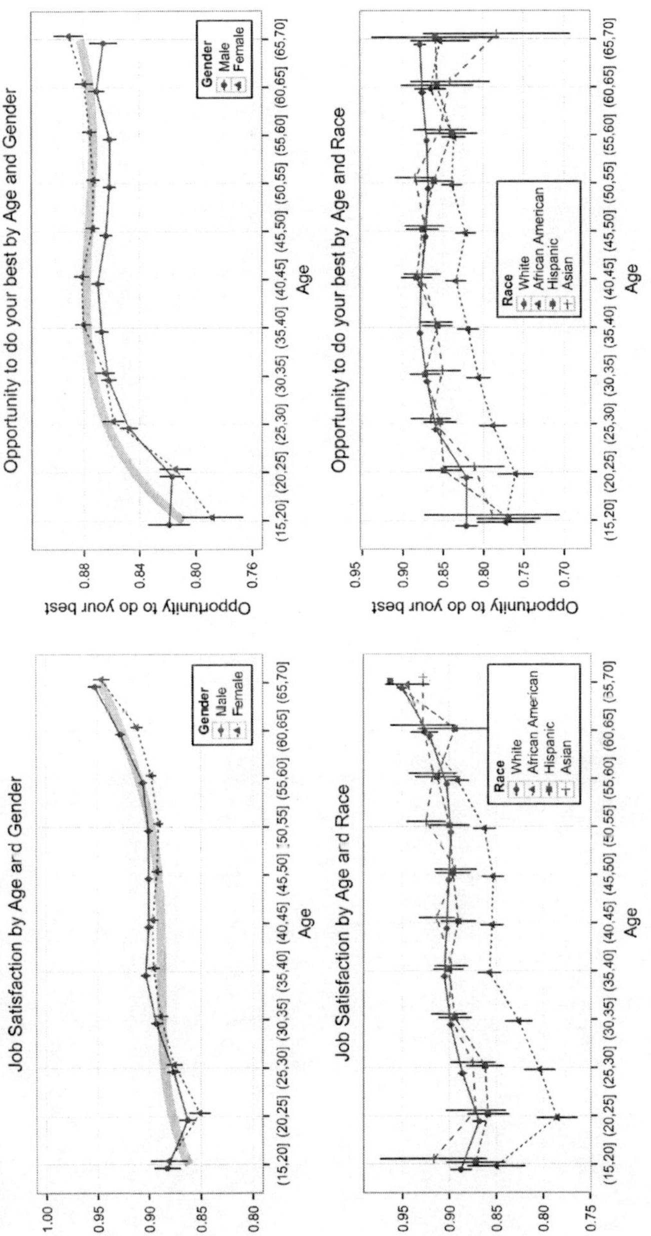

Fig. 1. Well-being of Workers within the United States in the Work Domain. *Note*: Light gray line represents overall predicted regression line for well-being outcome of interest controlling for health, income, education levels, and job type. 95% confidence intervals are represented using the error bars around the mean values.

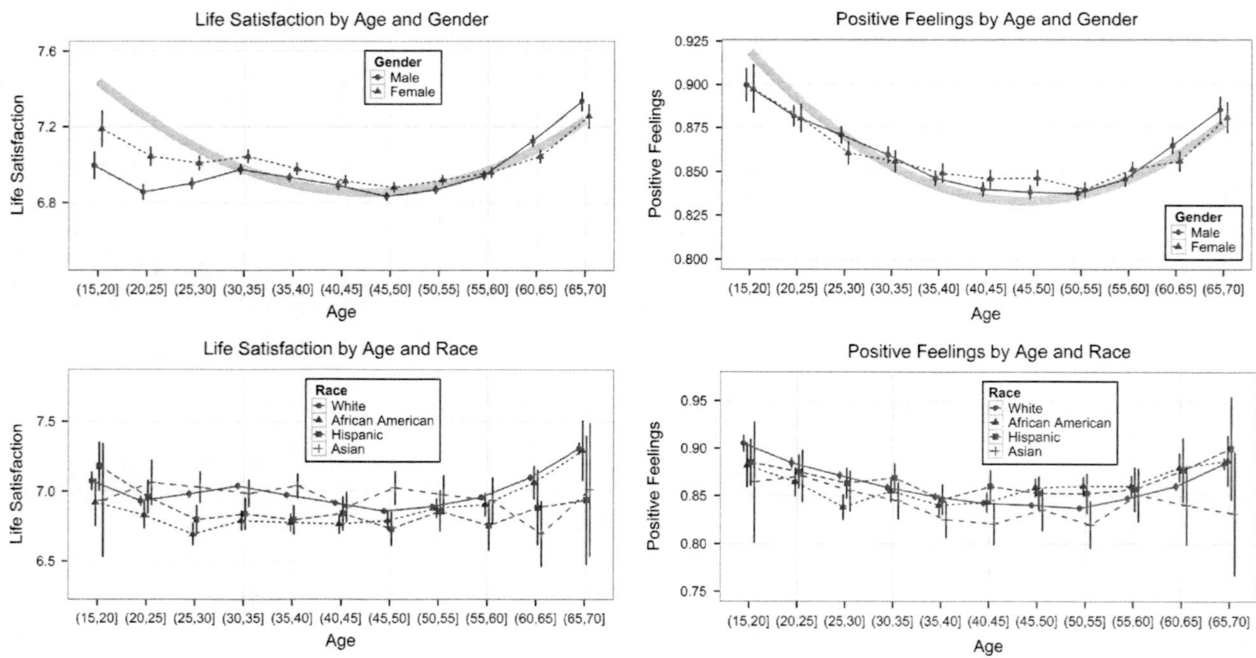

Fig. 2. Well-being of Workers within the United States in General Life. *Note*: Light gray line represents overall predicted regression line for well-being outcome of interest controlling for health, income, education level, and job type. 95% confidence intervals are represented using the error bars around the mean values.

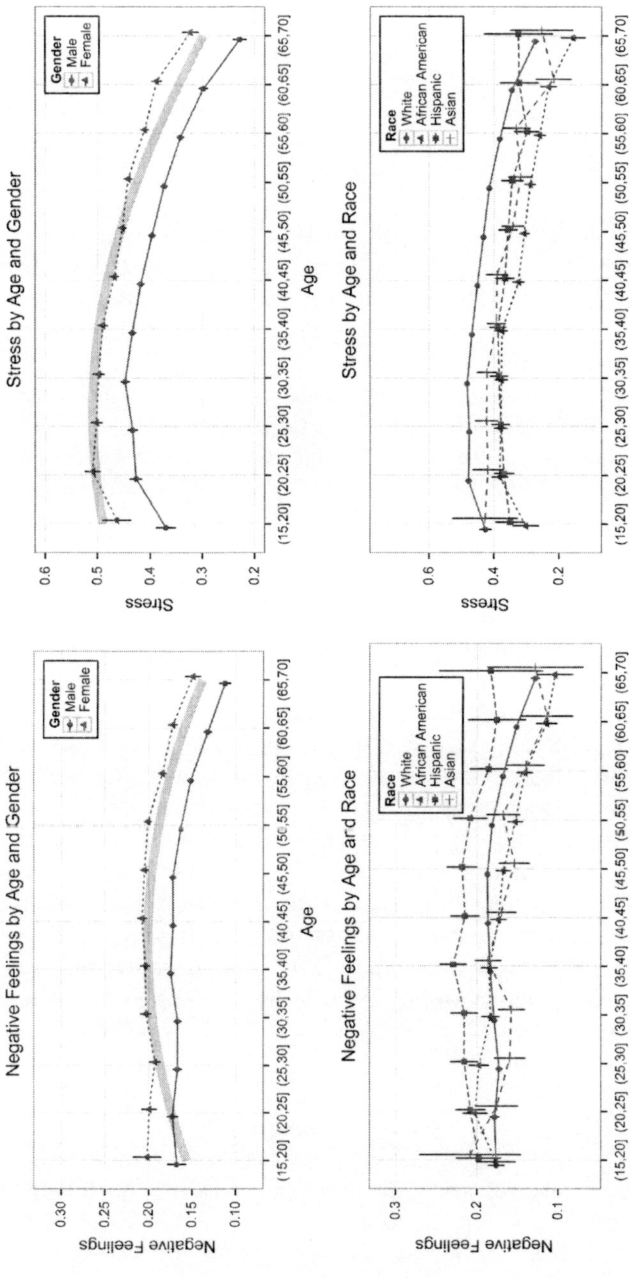

Fig. 2. *(Continued)*

SES theory, with increases in SWB occurring particularly during later stages in life. With regard to the experience of stress on a daily basis, fewer people report experiencing stress as age increases.

Gender

Fig. 1 shows similar levels in job satisfaction across the age groups for job satisfaction but it appears that female full-time workers tended to feel that the work context provided them more opportunity to do their best. In our initial logistic regression models, controlling for health, income, education, we found that there was no significant difference between males and females in reporting job satisfaction ($b_{\text{female}}=0.03$, $p>0.05$), but there were greater odds of females reporting opportunity to do their best at work ($b_{\text{female}}=0.17$, $p<0.05$). Nevertheless, when job types were further controlled for, we found that females did not have greater odds compared to males to report opportunities to do their best at work ($b_{\text{female}}=0.01$, $p>0.05$).

With regard to general SWB, women workers had similar levels of life satisfaction and similar proportion reporting positive feelings compared to male workers. Although females had significantly higher levels of life satisfaction and greater odds of reporting positive feelings (LS [0–10 scale] $b_{\text{female}}=0.12$, $p<0.05$; PA [0–1 scale] $b_{\text{female}}=0.00$, $p<0.05$), the predicted mean scale differences were very small. Indeed Fig. 2 reflects this minor difference. While there were no differences between males and females on the positive dimensions of SWB, we found that female workers experienced more negative emotions ($b_{\text{female}}=0.03$, $p<0.05$) and more stress ($b_{\text{female}}=0.07$, $p<0.05$) than men. As shown in Fig. 2, negative emotion and stress were greater for women compared to men, respectively, and consistently reflected across all the age categories. Overall, this finding is consistent with SWB research indicating that women tend to have similar levels of positive feelings but higher levels of negative feelings compared to men (Fujita, Diener, & Sandvik, 1991).

Race/Ethnicity

Consistent with past research, the findings of worker well-being by race/ethnicity were more complicated than can be easily explained by direct disadvantage or disadvantage adjustment. Table 8 presents the estimated

Table 8. Estimated Unstandardized Coefficients for Race/Ethnic differences by Worker Well-being Outcomes.

	Black vs. White	Hispanic vs. White	Asian vs. White
Workplace well-being			
Job satisfaction	−0.23***	0.15**	0.05
Do your best	−0.26***	0.10*	−0.09
General well-being			
Life satisfaction	0.05***	0.36***	−0.11***
Positive feelings	0.01***	0.03***	0.00
Negative feelings	−0.03	0.00	−0.02***
Stress	−0.14***	−0.10***	−0.10***

Note: $^{*}p<0.05$, $^{**}p<0.01$, $^{***}p<0.001$. Estimated coefficients are based on logistic (job satisfaction, do your best, and stress) and linear (life satisfaction, positive feelings, negative feelings) regressions that include age, gender, income, health, education, and job type as controls.

unstandardized coefficients for race/ethnic differences by different well-being outcomes. Two findings appear to be relatively large and consistent. First, African American workers have lower odds of reporting workplace well-being as compared to white workers and even compared to other race/ethnic groups as depicted in Fig. 1. This suggests that direct disadvantage may primarily affect African American workers, but not Hispanic and Asians. Second, more Caucasian workers report daily stress compared to all the other race/ethnic groups as seen in Table 8 and in Fig. 2. This is somewhat surprising given that job characteristics such as job type cannot account for this difference as this was controlled for in the regression analysis. Further, when examining other aspects of general well-being among full-time workers, other race/ethnic groups had comparable or higher reported well-being. These results cannot be straightforwardly interpreted with either direct disadvantage or disadvantage adjustment.

WORKER WELL-BEING ACROSS THE WORLD

Parallel to the GHI analysis, we seek to present a descriptive picture of worker well-being by age and gender. We integrate this with the predicted levels of worker well-being using hierarchical linear modeling (HLM; Raudenbush & Bryk, 2002) controlling for other variables such as health, income, education levels, and job type. Using the nation as a grouping variable, moderate levels of intra-class correlations for job satisfaction (0.09), life satisfaction (0.20), positive emotions (0.07), negative emotions (0.06), and stress (0.07) were obtained, indicating that the use of HLM was appropriate. Random coefficients modeling was used to account for the nested outcomes; specifically, all individual level predictors were nation-centered (Enders & Tofighi, 2007) and were specified as random with the exception of dummy coded job type. In all our analyses, the random effects were significant at $p < 0.05$. In addition, nation level variables were entered as grand-mean centered. Again, for intuitive reporting of logistic regression, we use "odds" in place of "log-odds".

Age

With regard to job satisfaction, there was a general incline between job satisfaction and age over time. Unlike that of the US worker job satisfaction data, this was a linear incline ($b_{\text{centered age}} = 0.108$, $p < 0.001$) and not a quadratic effect ($b^2_{\text{centered age}} = 0.000$, $p > 0.05$). We also found that the average worker age of the nation predicts odds of reporting job satisfaction ($b_{\text{nation age}} = 0.691$, $p < 0.001$) and this effect was significantly larger than the individual level age effect, implying that the average level of worker age in a nation positively predicts job satisfaction over and above individual level worker age. This provides evidence for the impact of workforce demography – specifically age – on worker well-being.

We performed additional analyses and found that the effects of individual level age were moderated by the average age in the nation workforce, but not by national income levels. Even when using HLM for analyses, we continued to find that average worker age in a nation was associated with higher levels of job satisfaction ($b_{\text{nation age}} = 0.651$, $p < 0.001$). However, we also found a significant cross-level interaction between average worker age and individual level age-squared ($b = 0.043$, $p < 0.001$). This finding is shown in Fig. 3 in which societies that have on average older workers also tended to have greater odds of reported job satisfaction for older workers. Interestingly, the job satisfaction trend is very similar to the United States, which has workers with an average age of 41. We see a general plateau from ages 20–55 but a steep incline in the later years. Although we see increasing odds of reported job satisfaction in societies with on average younger workers, the increase is not as pronounced. This strongly alludes to the matching hypothesis between workforce demography and individual

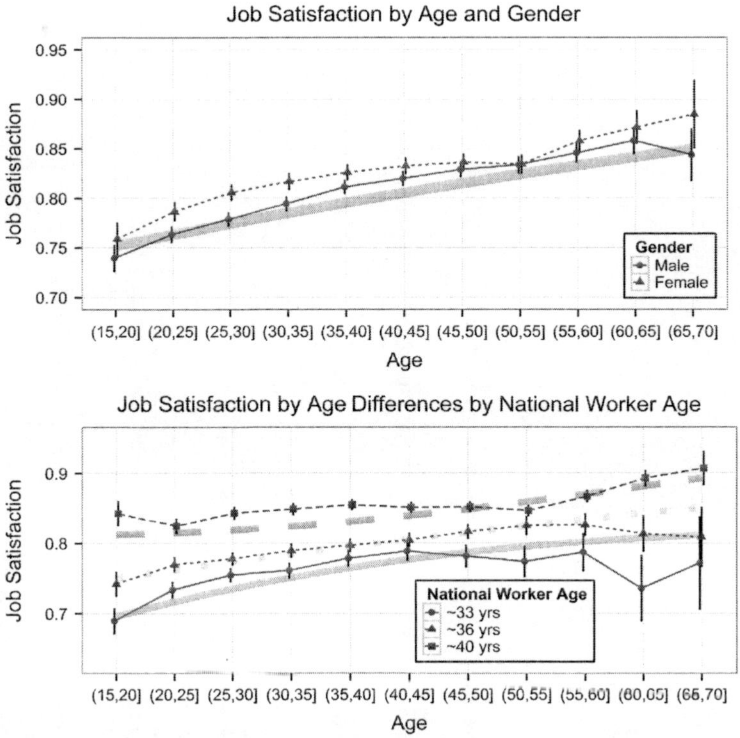

Fig. 3. Well-being of Workers across the World in the Work Domain. *Note*: Translucent lines represent predicted regression line for well-being outcome of interest controlling for health, income, education level, and job type. 95% confidence intervals are represented using the error bars around the mean values.

demography: there are older workers satisfied with their jobs in nations that have a greater proportion of older workers.

In Fig. 4, we present the descriptive and predicted levels of SWB for full-time workers across the world. Notably, the predicted levels of general well-being control for other characteristics and so may appear to differ from the actual levels of SWB. We find that the predicted levels of life satisfaction and negative feelings appear to be fairly consistent over different age groups. Positive feelings decline slightly as age increases and stress levels decline more with older workers. Overall, this presents a picture of fairly stable levels of SWB for full-time workers with slightly lower levels of positive feelings, but even lower levels of daily stress.

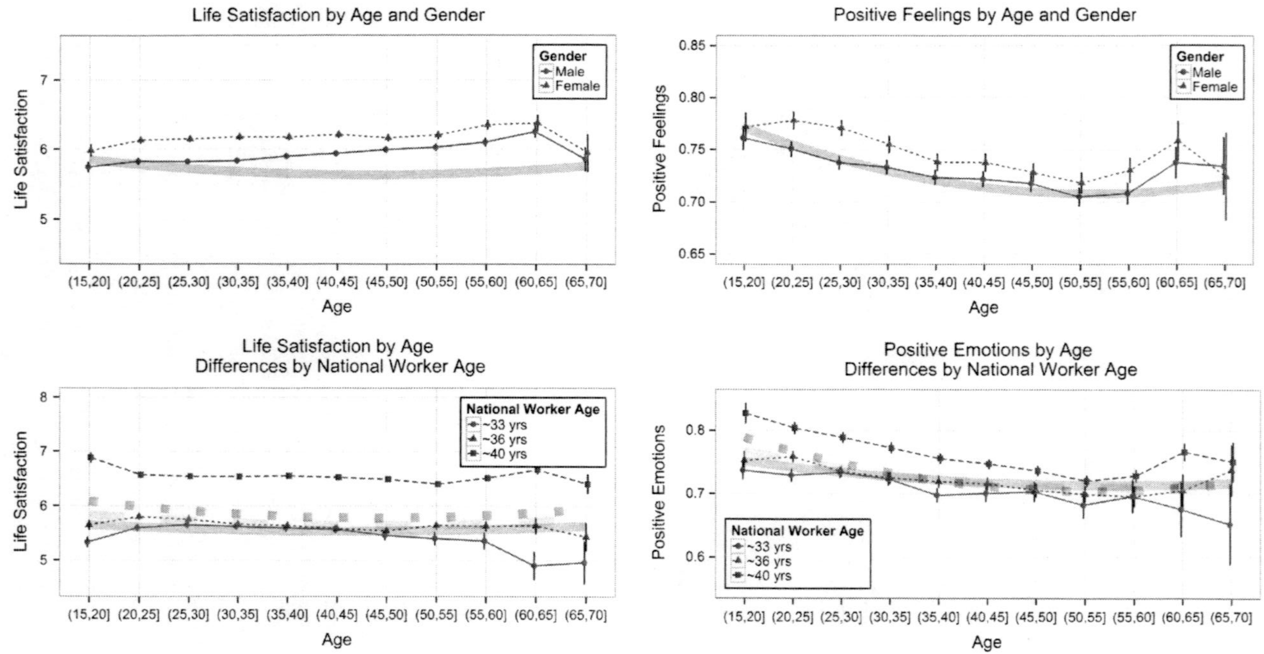

Fig. 4. Well-being of Workers across the World in General Life. *Note*: Translucent lines represent predicted regression line for well-being outcome of interest controlling for health, income, education level, and job type. 95% confidence intervals are represented using the error bars around the mean values.

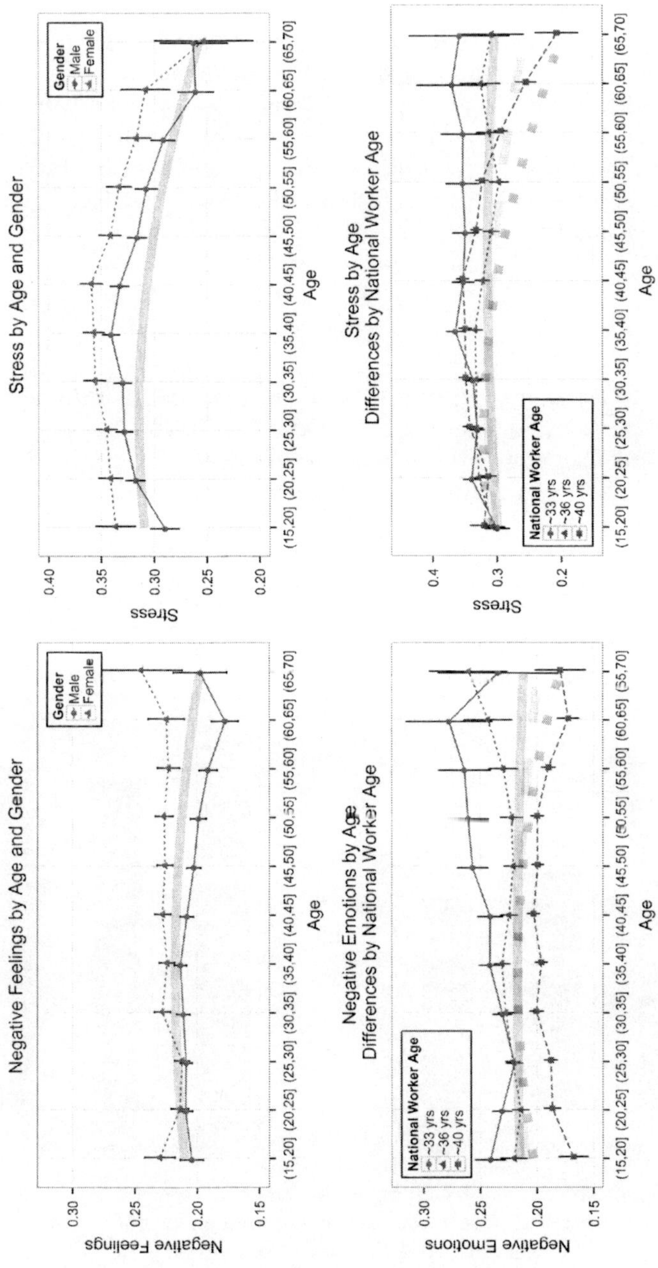

Fig. 4. (*Continued*)

When examining the potential contextual moderating effects of national worker age, we find that the strongest exhibited effects can be seen for negative feelings and stress. Consistent with the matching hypothesis, older workers had lower levels of negative feelings and lower odds of stress in a national workforce that consists on average of older workers. On the other hand, while we found statistically significant matching interaction effects for life evaluations and positive feelings, the observed effects appear to be substantially smaller as seen in Fig. 4.

Gender

For job satisfaction, gender effects were not significantly different between males and females at both the individual level ($b_{\text{centered female}} = -0.004$, $p > 0.05$) and the nation level (i.e., proportion of females; $b_{\text{nation female}}$ -0.197, $p > 0.05$). An examination of the matching hypothesis showed opposite effects than expected. A clear disordinal interaction ($b = -0.395$, $p < 0.05$) in Fig. 5 shows that as the proportion of females within a nation increases, the proportion of females being satisfied with their job decreases;

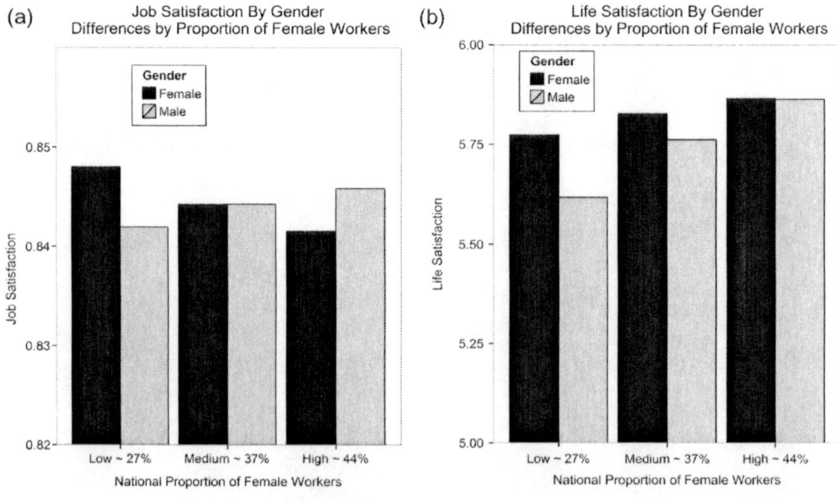

Fig. 5. Predicted Levels of Well-being of Male and Female Workers across the World. *Note*: Predicted levels for well-being outcomes controlling for health, income, education level, and job type.

by contrast, the proportion of males reporting job satisfaction increased as the proportion of females increase. These findings are consistent with a uniqueness effect of non-majority status. That is, higher job satisfaction among female workers may be due to their unique status as workers within society compared to other women. Importantly, because our analyses controlled for variables such as health, education, income, and job type, concerns about potential confounds for the uniqueness effect were reduced.

Unlike the US data, we found that across the world, life evaluations were significantly higher for females at both the individual level ($b_{\text{centered female}} = 0.062$, $p < 0.001$) and nation level ($b_{\text{nation female}} = 1.358$, $p < 0.05$). This difference appears to hold across most of the age groups shown in Fig. 4. Unlike the matching or uniqueness effects, we found that being female ($b_{\text{centered female}} = 0.057$, $p < 0.001$) and having more women in the workforce ($b_{\text{nation female}} = 1.103$, $p < 0.05$) has positive effects on life satisfaction; the life satisfaction gap between males and females becomes smaller as the proportion of females working becomes larger ($b = -0.774$, $p < 0.001$). The plot for this interaction is displayed in Fig. 5.

While the world data for job and life satisfaction revealed different trends between males and females than the US data, we found similarities in both datasets for the daily experience of emotions. Consistent with the US worker data, positive feelings was not significantly different between males and females for the individual level ($b_{\text{centered female}} = 0.003$, $p > 0.05$) or the nation level ($b_{\text{nation female}} = 0.128$, $p > 0.05$). Further, we found that women reported more negative feelings compared to men ($b_{\text{centered female}} = 0.031$, $p < 0.001$), but not positive feelings ($b_{\text{nation female}} = -0.120$, $p > 0.05$). Being female was associated with greater odds of experiencing stress ($b_{\text{centered female}} = 0.165$, $p < 0.001$). Interestingly, a higher level of female workers within a society was associated with lower odds of daily stress ($b_{\text{nation female}} = -1.024$, $p < 0.05$). Unlike life evaluations, experienced emotions were not influenced by an interactive effect of gender composition in the workforce and gender effects.

DISCUSSION

In one of the first representative US and global analyses of the relationship between demographics and worker well-being, we found support for prior perspectives, but also new trends that require further development of theoretical and empirical work. In the following, we provide an integrative summary of the findings and discuss the implications and future directions on worker demography and well-being research.

Key Findings

Age

We found strong support that job satisfaction increases with age. Nevertheless, the form of this increase is moderated by the context in which we study job satisfaction. Within the United States (average worker age = 41) and in societies that have a workforce with older workers (average worker age = 40) such as Sweden, Japan, Denmark, and the Netherlands, the proportion of individuals satisfied with their jobs plateaus among young- and middle-aged workers, but increases when workers are over 50. These findings are consistent with the SES theory as applied to workers, which posits that age-associated changes in time perspectives orient and motivate older workers toward more satisfying work (Carstensen, 1992). Yet the salience of the limited time perspective may occur in the later part of one's life prompting increased selectivity and optimization for higher job satisfaction. Within the context of work, individuals may also face greater constraints during the middle-aged years due in part to non-work domain commitments (e.g., family), which may limit flexibility to switch jobs or job craft. Supporting this idea, we also found that the proportion of workers reporting opportunities to do their best at work remained relatively unchanged among middle-aged workers, but increased for older workers.

Importantly, the rising gradient in percentage of those reporting job satisfaction toward later years is tempered when the average worker age of the nation decreases, suggesting that the workforce demographic norm of older workers could enhance the job satisfaction of older workers as implied by the matching hypothesis. Workers who share age similarity with the workforce demographic may share more similar cohort experiences and work attitudes that enhance job satisfaction (Avery et al., 2007). Aside from psychological connection, societies with an older workforce may have better workplace policies to better accommodate the desires and needs of older workers compared to societies with a smaller prevalence of older workers; such policies can promote job satisfaction as well.

Apart from job satisfaction, negative feelings and daily stress also exhibited consistent trends across the United States and the world. Older workers reported more negative feelings than younger workers. Also, a smaller proportion of older workers reported daily stress whereas a substantial proportion of younger workers reported experiences of daily stress. These findings support the SES theory with older workers optimizing their experiences for fewer stressful encounters. Moreover, we found support for the matching hypothesis, with older individuals reporting less daily negative feelings (or less older individuals reporting stress) in societies that have a prevalence of older workers. As such, results for job satisfaction, daily negative feelings, and daily stress were very consistent with the SES theory and provided strongest evidence for the matching hypothesis.

By contrast, for full-time workers, the other general indicators of SWB, life satisfaction and positive feelings, were not as consistent with SES theory and did not display strong trends for the matching hypothesis. One explanation for these findings may be that life satisfaction among workers captures uncontrollable circumstances such as losses in relationships or health that can diminish life satisfaction more than satisfaction in a specific domain like job satisfaction. Further, older age is generally associated with less unregulated emotional reactivity (Kunzmann, Kupperbusch, & Levenson, 2005) implying that older workers may experience less intense emotions on a daily basis compared to younger workers. Gains in positivity may be counterbalanced with less emotional reactivity, whereas gains in lowered negativity may be accentuated with the decline in reactivity.

Gender

Within the United States and in the worldwide sample of workers, women and men have very similar levels of job satisfaction and a sense of doing their best at work. Results showed little to no differences in job satisfaction between male and female workers. As such, the direct disadvantage with regard to issues such as discrimination or wage gap (e.g., Ostroff & Atwater, 2003) does not surface in the form of job dissatisfaction or a sense of lowered competence among women. Within the United States, our results suggest that the types of jobs women engage in may play a mediating role, influencing their sense of doing their best at work. That is, women may choose jobs in which they derive a greater sense of workplace mastery. In accordance with previous research showing that women do not necessarily have lower workplace wellness (Clark, 1997), our results show that within the United States, both men and women are equally happy in their jobs – although the types of jobs chosen may be different. Our data is therefore suggestive of the notion that females tend to choose work in which they can achieve comparable levels of workplace well-being to men. However, our results are also consistent with disadvantage adjustment: females workers derive greater satisfaction from overcoming more obstacles; or in-group social comparisons with other working or non-working women may have contributed to the higher than expected levels of worker wellness.

For other indicators of well-being, females also have similar levels of well-being with the exception that more female workers tended to experience negative emotions and stress, which is consistent with known gender difference in the experience of negative emotions (Fujita et al., 1991). Overall, the main effect of gender displays a disadvantage adjustment where women, despite known disadvantages, have equally high levels of well-being.

The effects of gender composition in the workforce showed a different trend than the matching hypothesis found with age. The matching hypothesis suggests that an individual demographic matching with the dominant trait in the workforce benefits well-being, but we found an opposite effect occurring with gender. A uniqueness effect occurred where more females (compared to males) were satisfied with their jobs when the proportion of female workers in the nation was small. In nations with more female workers, the rates of job satisfaction among females were substantially lower as shown in Fig. 4. One possible explanation for the contrasting workforce demographic contextual effects between age and gender is that gender has been shown to be more salient for self-categorization than age (Thatcher & Patel, 2011). Worker demographic variables like age can be distributed across gender groups but gender is fairly static. Strong self-categorization effects in gender could lead to discrepant effects from age. According to the disadvantage adjustment hypothesis, women who work in a workforce with fewer female workers would encounter a substantially strong gender stereotype resulting in greater job satisfaction from successes in the work domain. Another related possibility is that women as workers stand in a unique space in society and they derive greater satisfaction from the ability to work in spite of the inherent difficulties in the national context. This uniqueness effect can also account in part for the trend in male workers as the proportion of men satisfied with their jobs increased as the proportion of male workers in the workforce decreases. The effect could also be a function of motivations for working. As an anonymous reviewer pointed out, a smaller proportion of women in the workplace may indicate that women in that nation do not need or are not expected to work. Consequently, those women who do work are more likely to be working out of choice and a desire to engage in a career, which would yield a larger proportion of those women workers reporting job satisfaction.

However, these gender composition effects do not necessarily generalize to life satisfaction: the greater levels of equality in workforce demography enhance the general life satisfaction of both female and male workers. Moreover, greater equality reduced the discrepancy between male and female life satisfaction as well. As such, for female workers, although there may be higher levels of job satisfaction in the presence of fewer female workers, their life evaluations are not as high as that of female workers in a society that has a larger proportion of female workers. Declines in job satisfaction are compensated with higher levels of life satisfaction as there are more women in the workforce. This is suggestive of a positive spillover effect where the presence of more women in the workforce is associated with gains in the life satisfaction of the workforce.

Race/Ethnicity

We found that the direct disadvantage for minorities could not fully account for all the trends in the data. African American workers within the United States were less satisfied with their work as compared to White Caucasian workers. Nevertheless, this trend was not found in Hispanic workers. One possible explanation for these results relates to the effect supervisors have on their direct reports. Simons, Friedman, Liu, and McLean Parks (2007) have argued that, compared to other minorities, Blacks are more likely to be hyper-vigilant to instances of hypocrisy in those higher in the hierarchy due to their unique history of being subject to discrimination and deceit by authority figures and institutions. They found that Blacks perceived greater levels of word-deed misalignment in managers than non-Blacks and this effect fully mediated the negative relationship between being Black and global satisfaction with various job aspects. This heightened sensitivity to transgressions of behavioral integrity of managers (Simons, 2002) may be one mechanism that explains fewer African-Americans experiencing job satisfaction compared to other racial/ethnic minorities. Yet this effect may not generalize across all domains as African American as well as Hispanic workers tended to have slightly higher life satisfaction as compared to White Caucasian workers. Further, more White Caucasians tended to report a high level of daily stress as compared to all the other race/ethnic groups. The lack of consistency for direct disadvantage or disadvantage adjustment may point to general changes in diversity perceptions as there have been a strong emphasis and promotion of workplace diversity within the United States.

National Demography

Advancing the multilevel perspective to demography research, we found evidence aforementioned on the moderating effects of national demography on the relation between individual demography and well-being. Further, it is important to point out that there was evidence of national demographic effects that were significantly associated with worker well-being above and beyond individual level effects for some evaluative indicators. Average worker age predicted job satisfaction beyond individual age, demonstrating that as national worker age increases, overall job satisfaction increases as well. Moreover, a higher proportion of females in the workforce was associated with greater life satisfaction over and above being female. There were smaller and less consistent contextual effects for daily affective well-being indicators as daily affect has been shown to be less dependent on national contexts (Tay, Chan, & Diener, 2014).

Theoretical and Practical Implications

The patterns of demographic factors and worker well-being reveal clear-cut instances of theoretical correspondence but also deviations that raise questions about the generalizability across all contexts or departures that necessitate theoretical development and empirical research.

First, a clear instance of theoretical correspondence is the application of SES (Carstensen, 1992) to job satisfaction, doing one's best at work, and the experiences of daily negative feelings and stress. In general, well-being improved over time particularly for older workers. Nevertheless, in the context of the workplace, the SES theory may be most applicable to societies with workers with an older average age as the gains in well-being are more pronounced in this type of workforce demographic. In other societies, these psychological gains may be attenuated by the absence of workplace policies that foster the well-being of older workers.

Second, the simple application of direct disadvantage or disadvantage adjustment to gender and race/ethnicity on all aspects of well-being does not appear to be sufficient to explain the complexity of the data at hand. With respect to gender, female and male workers show small differences on well-being measures generally. With respect to race/ethnicity, although African-Americans have lower job satisfaction that White Caucasians, they do not have lower well-being across all indicators. Moreover, another traditionally marginalized group, Hispanics, did not show clear signs of lowered well-being. By contrast, White Caucasian workers reported more daily stress than all the other minority race/ethnic groups. This could point to the importance of considering issues beyond simple race/ethnic demography to understand sources of disparity. Indeed, Lawrence (1997) proposed that intervening psychological variables will need to be considered in demography research. Additionally, as we discussed, our findings could also be indicative of a change in the current work climate for minority groups within the United States.

Third, while gender differences in worker well-being were small at the aggregate, we did find well-being differences dependent on the workforce gender distribution. Supporting the uniqueness perspective, job satisfaction of female (male) workers was greater compared to male (female) workers in societies that have a relatively smaller proportion of female (male) workers. In addition, we found greater life satisfaction with a more equal gender distributed workforce. While we have suggested fundamentally socio-psychological effects accounting for these differences, there could also be larger labor market forces that could also help account for such effects. For example, there may be a distribution of inherently (dis)satisfying jobs of a relatively fixed quantity for a certain national labor force. Women who initially enter the workforce may be more selective about jobs because reversion to the traditional gender role of say, being a homemaker, is culturally acceptable; as more women enter the workforce, less selectivity may, resulting in fewer inherently satisfying jobs being available. Clearly, future research needs to disentangle the relative socio-psychological and labor market effects. Such research questions illuminate opportunities for cross-disciplinary work between labor economists and organizational researchers.

Fourth, we found strong evidence for the need to consider workforce demography as impinging on worker well-being directly and indirectly. Within workforce demography, past research has focused on demography at the individual level (e.g., Greenhaus et al., 1990; Ng & Feldman, 2010), or demography at a meso level such as work groups (van Knippenberg & Schippers, 2007), or organizational units (McCain, O'Reilly, & Pfeffer, 1983). While some have alluded to the possibility of industry level of demographic composition (Lawrence, 1997), to our knowledge no work has been done at the national level of workforce demography, which is a key contribution of our chapter.

The aspect of workforce demography broadens the socio-psychological processes in demography research. Relational demography research, which emphasizes the interaction between worker demography and workplace demography (Tsui, Egan, & O'Reilly, 1992), has posited three main forms of social processes that occur for minority employees – social creativity, social competition, and social mobility (Chattopadhyay, Tluchowska, & George, 2004). Social creativity occurs when individuals use an alternate dimension or reframe negative attributes as positive. Social competition is a process by which minority employees strive for equal opportunities within the organization. Social mobility is engaged when minority members disassociate themselves from the low status group to adopt a majority higher status identity. However, additional socio-psychological processes may be important for understanding how workers are embedded in social relationships outside of work. One possibility is the use of downward social comparison within the in-group such that an emphasis is placed not on the objective difference between minority and majority members, but on the difference between minority members. Another possibility is the effort-justification perspective whereby individuals experience greater satisfaction with the knowledge that they overcame broader disadvantaged circumstances. Theoretical work needs to be further developed in light of evidence that is suggestive of such processes.

One policy implication derived from this study is that governments and policy makers focusing on improving equality in the workplace or protecting the rights of minority groups cannot focus solely on SWB indicators to measure whether conditions are improving. Indeed, these indicators, while important in their own right, are not sufficient for revealing potential objective disadvantages that specific demographic groups might face. Conversely, improving equality, as in the case of having a greater proportion of women workers, may not invariably lead to higher job satisfaction among female workers. Successful attempts to improve equality would require a careful consideration of a range of cultural and social factors. As such, the goal of enhancing diversity will require the tracking of both objective and subjective indicators to gain an integrative picture of the impact of labor and workplace policies.

SUMMARY AND CONCLUSION

Our empirical review using the expansive Gallup datasets has provided a detailed picture of the relation between demographic factors and different aspects of worker well-being. With respect to age, increases in job satisfaction, and decreases in negative feelings and stress, for older workers provided strong support for the SES theory. Nevertheless, the extent of the rise in worker well-being with age depends on the type of workforce demographic context. Findings on gender revealed an important trend that, compared to men, women were similarly satisfied with their jobs within the United States and across the world. While some race/ethnic difference in well-being were identified, the patterns were not easily interpretable through a single theoretical framework. Lastly, workforce demography was emphasized as an important factor to consider and was shown to influence work well-being both directly and indirectly. We encourage researchers to further develop theoretical frameworks and research seeking to understand demographic influences on worker well-being that can enable better policy decisions surrounding diversity and well-being in the workforce and workplace.

NOTES

1. A literature review was conducted to ensure adequate coverage of research relating demographics variables to various aspects of worker well-being. Articles were searched for in the *PsycInfo* and *Business Source Premiere* databases. The terms that were used to represent worker well-being included *life satisfaction, job satisfaction, well-being, occupational well-being,* and *subjective well-being*. These worker well-being terms were crossed with the terms *age, gender, race, ethnicity, racial differences, ethnic differences,* and *demographic characteristics* as subject terms for the literature search.

Many different criteria were used to decide on what articles would be included in the review. First, empirical articles published in peer-reviewed journals were the main focus of the search; book chapters, dissertations, and conference papers were not included. Second, only those articles that focused on the direct relationships between overall job or life satisfaction and demographic variables of interest were included. Those articles that looked at facets of job or life satisfaction were not included. Articles that equated well-being with mental health or constructs that did not directly relate to daily affective experiences or evaluations of job or life satisfaction were also not included. Articles that involved summing up scores from items to arrive at a job or life satisfaction score were not included if the items seemed to tap into information other than the constructs of interest. Third, the articles had to use nationally representative or cross-national samples. Fourth, the sample used in the articles had to encompass a relatively wide age range that included the ages were during which people are likely to be working.

The search yielded a total of 5,209 articles of which 33 articles met the criteria. Some articles came up across several of the searches. After these duplicates were removed, a final total of 24 unique articles were reviewed. Each article was reviewed and the relationships between demographic and well-being variables of interest were included. Results were tabulated (see Tables 1–6).

2. Our literature review (Tables 1–6) includes articles that were: (1) published in a peer-reviewed journal; (2) focused on the relationship between job and/or life satisfaction and gender, age, or race/ethnicity; and (3) large national samples.

REFERENCES

Avery, D. R., McKay, P. F., & Wilson, D. C. (2007). Engaging the aging workforce: The relationship between perceived age similarity, satisfaction with coworkers, and employee engagement. *Journal of Applied Psychology*, *92*, 1542–1556.

Barger, S., Donoho, C., & Wayment, H. (2009). The relative contributions of race/ethnicity, socioeconomic status, and social relationships to life satisfaction in the United States. *Quality of Life Research*, *18*(2), 179–189. doi:10.1007/s11136-008-9426-2

Bartel, A. (1981). Race differences in job satisfaction: A reappraisal. *Journal of Human Resources*, *16*, 294–303.

Birdi, K., Warr, P., & Oswald, A. (1995). Age differences in three components of employee well-being. *Applied Psychology*, *44*(4), 345–373. doi:10.1111/j.1464-0597.1995.tb01085.x

Blanchflower, D. G., & Oswald, A. J. (2004). Well-being over time in Britain and the USA. *Journal of Public Economics*, *88*(7–8), 1359–1386. doi:10.1016/S0047-2727(02)00168-8

Blanchflower, D. G., & Oswald, A. J. (2008). Is well-being U-shaped over the life cycle? *Social Science & Medicine*, *66*(8), 1733–1749. doi:10.1016/j.socscimed.2008.01.030

Blanchflower, D. G., & Oswald, A. J. (2009). The U-shape without controls: A response to Glenn. *Social Science & Medicine*, *69*(4), 486–488. doi:10.1016/j.socscimed.2009.05.022

Brush, D. H., Moch, M. K., & Pooyan, A. (1987). Individual demographic differences and job satisfaction. *Journal of Occupational Behaviour*, *8*, 139–156.

Carstensen, L. L. (1992). Social and emotional patterns in adulthood: Support for socioemotional selectivity theory. *Psychology and Aging*, *7*, 331–338.

Chattopadhyay, P., Tluchowska, M., & George, E. (2004). Identifying the ingroup: A closer look at the influence of demographic dissimilarity on employee social identity. *Academy of Management Review*, *29*, 180–202.

Clark, A. E. (1997). Job satisfaction and gender: Why are women so happy at work? *Labour Economics*, *4*, 341–372.

Clark, A. E., Oswald, A. J., & Warr, P. (1996). Is job satisfaction U-shaped in age? *Journal of Occupational and Organizational Psychology*, *69*, 57–81.

Clemente, F., & Sauer, W. (1976). Life satisfaction in the United States. *Social Forces*, *54*(3), 621–631. Retrieved from http://sf.oxfordjournals.org/content/54/3/621.short

Danna, K., & Griffin, R. W. (1999). Health and well-being in the workplace: A review and synthesis of the literature. *Journal of Management*, *25*, 357–384.

Diener, E. (1984). Subjective well-being. *Psychological Bulletin*, *95*, 542–575.

Easterlin, R. A. (2006). Life cycle happiness and its sources. *Journal of Economic Psychology*, *27*(4), 463–482. doi:10.1016/j.joep.2006.05.002

Enders, C. K., & Tofighi, D. (2007). Centering predictor variables in cross-sectional multilevel models: A new look at an old issue. *Psychological Methods*, *12*, 121–138.

Erdogan, B., Bauer, T. N., Truxillo, D. M., & Mansfield, L. R. (2012). Whistle while you work: A review of the life satisfaction literature. *Journal of Management*, *38*, 1038–1083.

Frijters, P., & Beatton, T. (2012). The mystery of the U-shaped relationship between happiness and age. *Journal of Economic Behavior & Organization*, *82*(2–3), 525–542. doi:10.1016/j.jebo.2012.03.008

Fujita, F., Diener, E., & Sandvik, E. (1991). Gender differences in negative affect and well-being: The case for emotional intensity. *Journal of Personality and Social Psychology*, *61*, 427–434.

Fulmer, C. A., Gelfand, M. J., Kruglanski, A. W., Kim-Prieto, C., Diener, E., Pierro, A., & Higgins, E. T. (2010). On "feeling right" in cultural contexts: How person-culture match affects self-esteem and subjective well-being. *Psychological Science*, *21*, 1563–1569.

Greenhaus, J. H., Parasuraman, S., & Wormley, W. M. (1990). Effects of race on organizational experiences, job performance evaluations, and career outcomes. *Academy of Management Journal*, *33*, 64–86.

Herzog, A. R., & Rodgers, W. L. (1981). Age and satisfaction: Data from several large surveys. *Research on Aging*, *3*(2), 142–165. doi:10.1177/016402758132002

Joshi, A., Liao, H., & Roh, H. (2011). Bridging domains in workplace demography research: A review and reconceptualization. *Journal of Management*, *37*, 521–552.

Judge, T. A., & Iles, R. (2004). Affect and job satisfaction: A study of the relationship at work and at home. *Journal of Applied Psychology*, *89*, 661–673.

Judge, T. A., Iles, R., & Scott, B. A. (2006). Work-family conflict and emotions: Effects at work and at home. *Personnel Psychology*, *59*, 779–814.

Judge, T. A., & Klinger, R. (2007). Job satisfaction: Subjective well-being at work. In M. Eid & R. Larsen (Eds.), *The science of subjective well-being* (pp. 393–413). New York, NY: Guilford Publications.

Judge, T. A., Parker, S., Colbert, A. E., Heller, D., & Ilies, R. (2001). Job satisfaction: A cross-cultural review. In N. Anderson, D. S. Ones, H. K. Sinangil, & C. Viswesvaran (Eds.), *Handbook of industrial, work, and organisational psychology*. London, UK: Sage.

Judge, T. A., & Watanabe, S. (1993). Another look at the job satisfaction-life satisfaction relationship. *Journal of Applied Psychology*, *78*, 939–948.

Kacmar, K. M., & Ferris, G. R. (1989). Theoretical and methodological considerations in the age-job satisfaction relationship. *Journal of Applied Psychology*, *74*, 201–207.

Kahneman, D., & Deaton, A. (2010). High income improves evaluation of life but not emotional well-being. *Proceedings of National Academy of Sciences*, *107*, 16489–16493.

Kalleberg, A. L., & Loscocco, K. A. (1983). Aging, values, and rewards: Explaining age differences in job satisfaction. *American Sociological Review*, *48*(1), 78–90. Retrieved from http://www.ncbi.nlm.nih.gov/pubmed/6838066

Kozlowski, S. W. J., & Klein, K. J. (2000). A multilevel approach to theory and research in organizations. In K. J. Klein & S. W. J. Kozlowski (Eds.), *Multilevel theory, research, and methods in organizations: Foundations, extensions, and new directions* (pp. 3–90). San Francisco, CA: Jossey-Bass.

Kunzmann, U., Kupperbusch, C. S., & Levenson, R. W. (2005). Behavioral inhibition and amplification during emotional arousal: A comparison of two age groups. *Psychology and Aging*, *20*, 144–158.

Lance, C. E., Lautenschlager, G. J., Sloan, C. E., & Varca, P. E. (1989). A comparison between bottom–up, top–down, and bidirectional models of relationships between global and life facet satisfaction. *Journal of Personality*, *57*(3), 601–624.

Lange, T. (2009). Attitudes, attributes and institutions: Determining job satisfaction in Central and Eastern Europe. *Employee Relations*, *31*(1), 81–97. doi:10.1108/01425450910916832

Lawrence, B. (1997). The black box of organizational demography. *Organization Science*, *8*, 1–22.

Lincoln, A. E., & Allen, M. P. (2004). Double jeopardy in Hollywood: Age and gender in the careers of film actors, 1926–1999. *Sociological Forum*, *19*, 611–631.

Lyness, K. S., & Thompson, D. E. (1997). Above the glass ceiling? A comparison of matched samples of female and male executives. *Journal of Applied Psychology*, *82*, 359–375.

Lyness, K. S., & Thompson, D. E. (2000). Climbing the corporate ladder: Do female and male executives follow the same route? *Journal of Applied Psychology*, *85*, 86–101.

McCain, B. E., O'Reilly, C. A., & Pfeffer, J. (1983). The effects of departmental demography on turnover: The case of a university. *Academy of Management Journal*, *26*, 626–641.

McKee-Ryan, F. M., Song, Z., Wanberg, C. R., & Kinicki, A. J. (2005). Psychological and physical well-being during unemployment: A meta-analytic study. *Journal of Applied Psychology*, *90*, 53–76.

Mookherjee, H. (1992). A comparative assessment of life satisfaction in the United States: 1978–1988. *The Journal of Social Psychology*, *132*(3), 407–409. Retrieved from http://www.tandfonline.com/doi/pdf/10.1080/00224545.1992.9924717

Mukerjee, S. (2013). Job satisfaction in the United States: Are blacks still more satisfied? *The Review of Black Political Economy*, *41*(1), 61–81. doi:10.1007/s12114-013-9174-6

Ng, T. W. H., & Feldman, D. C. (2010). The relationship of age with job attitudes: A meta-analysis. *Personnel Psychology*, *63*, 677–718.

Oishi, S., & Graham, J. (2010). Social ecology: Lost and found in psychological science. *Perspectives on Psychological Science*, *5*, 356–377.

Ostroff, C., & Atwater, L. E. (2003). Does whom you work with matter? Effects of referent group gender and age composition on managers' compensation. *Journal of Applied Psychology*, *88*, 725–740.

Peccei, R., & Lee, H.-J. (2005). The impact of gender similarity on employee satisfaction at work: A review and re-evaluation. *Journal of Management Studies*, *42*, 1571–1592.

Raudenbush, S. W., & Bryk, A. S. (2002). *Hierarchical linear models: Applications and data analysis methods* (2nd ed.). Thousand Oaks, CA: Sage.

Sacco, J. M., & Schmitt, N. (2005). A dynamic multilevel model of demographic diversity and misfit effects. *Journal of Applied Psychology*, *90*, 203–231. doi:0.1037/0021-9010.90.2.203

Schieman, S. (2002). Socioeconomic status, job conditions, and well-being: Self-concept explanations for gender-contingent effects. *The Sociological Quarterly*, *43*, 627–646.

Simons, T. (2002). Behavioral integrity: The perceived alignment between managers' words and deeds as a research focus. *Organization Science*, *13*(1), 18–35. Retrieved from http://pubsonline.informs.org/doi/abs/10.1287/orsc.13.1.18.543

Simons, T., Friedman, R., Liu, L. A., & McLean Parks, J. (2007). Racial differences in sensitivity to behavioral integrity: Attitudinal consequences, in-group effects, and "trickle down" among Black and non-Black employees. *Journal of Applied Psychology*, *92*(3), 650–665. doi:10.1037/0021-9010.92.3.650

Tay, L., Chan, D., & Diener, E. (2014). The metrics of societal happiness. *Social Indicators Research*, *117*, 577–600. doi:10.1007/s11205-013-0356-1

Tay, L., & Harter, J. K. (2013). Economic and labor market forces matter for worker well-being. *Applied Psychology: Health and Well-Being*, *5*, 193–208. doi:10.1111/aphw.12004

Tay, L., Morrison, M., & Diener, E. (2014). Living among the affluent: Boon or bane? *Psychological Science*. Advanced online publication. doi:10.1177/0956797614525786

Tay, L., Woo, S. E., & Vermunt, J. K. (2014). A conceptual and methodological framework for psychometric isomorphism: Validation of multilevel construct measures. *Organizational Research Methods*, *17*, 77–106. doi:10.1177/1094428113517008

Taylor, S. E., & Lobel, M. (1989). Social comparison activity under threat: Downward evaluation and upward contacts. *Psychological Review*, *96*, 569–575.

Thatcher, S. M. B., & Patel, P. C. (2011). Demographic faultlines: A meta-analysis of the literature. *Journal of Applied Psychology*, *96*, 1119–1139.

Thomas, M. E., & Hughes, M. (1986). The continuing significance of race: A study of race, class, and quality of life in America, 1972–1985. *American Sociological Review*, *51*(6), 830–841. Retrieved from http://www.ncbi.nlm.nih.gov/pubmed/11613887

Tsui, A. S., Egan, T. D., & O'Reilly, C. A. (1992). Being different: Relational demography and organizational attachment. *Administrative Science Quarterly*, *37*, 549–579.

Tuch, S. (1991). Race in the workplace: Black/White differences in the sources of job satisfaction. *Sociological Quarterly*, *32*(1), 103–116. Retrieved from http://scholar.google.com/scholar?hl=en&btnG=Search&q=intitle:Race+in+the+workplace+:+Black+/+White+differences+in+the+sources+of+job+satisfaction#9

van Knippenberg, D., & Schippers, M. C. (2007). Work group diversity. *Annual Review of Psychology*, *58*, 515–541.

Wanous, J. P. (1973). Effects of a realistic job preview on job acceptance, job attitudes, and job survival. *Journal of Applied Psychology*, *58*, 327–332.

Weaver, C. (1998). Black-white differences in job satisfaction: Evidence from 21 nationwide surveys. *Psychological Reports*, *83*, 1083–1088. Retrieved from http://www.amsciepub.com/doi/pdf/10.2466/pr0.1998.83.3.1083

Weaver, C. N. (1977). Relationships among pay, race, sex, occupational prestige, supervision, work autonomy, and job satisfaction in a national sample. *Personnel Psychology*, *30*(3), 437–445. doi:10.1111/j.1744-6570.1977.tb00436.x

Weaver, C. N. (1980). Job satisfaction in the United States in the 1970s. *Journal of Applied Psychology*, *65*(3), 364–367. doi:10.1037//0021-9010.65.3.364

Weaver, C. N. (2003). Happiness of Asian Americans. *Psychological Reports*, *93*(3 Pt 2), 1032–1034. Retrieved from http://www.ncbi.nlm.nih.gov/pubmed/14765565

Weaver, C. N., & Hinson, S. (2000). Job satisfaction of Asian Americans. *Psychological Reports*, *86*(2), 586–594. Retrieved from http://www.ncbi.nlm.nih.gov/pubmed/11729542

Weiss, H. M., & Rupp, D. (2011). Experiencing work: An essay on a person-centric work psychology. *Industrial Organizational Psychology*, *4*, 83–97.

Wright, T. A., & Cropanzano, R. (2000). Psychological well-being and job satisfaction as predictors of job performance. *Journal of Occupational Health Psychology*, *5*, 84–94.

Wunder, C., & Wiencierz, A. (2013). Well-being over the life span: Semiparametric evidence from British and German longitudinal data. *Review of Economics and Statistics*, *95*(March), 154–167. Retrieved from http://www.mitpressjournals.org/doi/abs/10.1162/REST_a_00222

Yap, M., Cukier, W., Holmes, M. R., & Hannan, C.-A. (2010). Career satisfaction: A look behind the races. *Relations Industrielles. [Industrial Relations.]*, *65*(4), 584–608. doi:10.7202/045587ar

APPENDIX: JOB SATISFACTION AND CURRENT LIFE SATISFACTION OF FULL-TIME WORKERS IN 2010

#	Country	Job Satisfaction	Life Satisfaction
1	Afghanistan	0.86	4.28
2	Albania	0.80	5.94
3	Algeria	0.70	5.60
4	Angola	0.70	5.59
5	Argentina	0.85	6.83
6	Armenia	0.60	4.69
7	Australia	0.88	7.42
8	Austria	0.94	7.56
9	Azerbaijan	0.75	4.97
10	Bahrain	0.83	5.65
11	Bangladesh	0.79	4.79
12	Belarus	0.73	5.65
13	Belgium	0.91	7.33
14	Benin	0.47	3.72
15	Bolivia	0.86	6.07
16	Bosnia and Herzegovina	0.80	5.58
17	Botswana	0.63	4.76
18	Brazil	0.87	7.14
19	Bulgaria	0.82	4.69
20	Burkina Faso	0.65	4.59
21	Burundi	0.54	4.31
22	Cambodia	0.76	4.12
23	Cameroon	0.56	4.42
24	Canada	0.92	7.68
25	Central African Republic	0.78	4.54
26	Chad	0.78	4.41
27	Chile	0.82	6.86
28	China	0.75	5.28
29	Colombia	0.86	6.74
30	Comoros	0.59	4.04
31	Congo (Kinshasa)	0.57	4.75
32	Congo Brazzaville	0.74	5.10
33	Costa Rica	0.91	7.45
34	Croatia	0.77	6.04
35	Cyprus	0.90	6.68
36	Czech Republic	0.82	6.50
37	Denmark	0.94	7.91
38	Djibouti	0.78	5.20
39	Dominican Republic	0.75	5.25
40	Ecuador	0.85	6.10
41	Egypt	0.77	4.60

(*Continued*)

#	Country	Job Satisfaction	Life Satisfaction
42	El Salvador	0.82	6.10
43	Estonia	0.80	5.60
44	Ethiopia	0.74	4.67
45	Finland	0.91	7.84
46	France	0.86	6.85
47	Gabon	0.58	4.57
48	Georgia	0.75	4.74
49	Germany	0.90	6.90
50	Ghana	0.65	5.80
51	Greece	0.83	5.99
52	Guatemala	0.89	6.31
53	Guinea	0.55	4.45
54	Haiti	0.45	4.43
55	Honduras	0.85	5.85
56	Hong Kong	0.81	5.69
57	Hungary	0.82	5.13
58	Iceland	0.96	7.78
59	India	0.74	4.94
60	Indonesia	0.79	5.44
61	Iran	0.73	4.80
62	Iraq	0.78	5.38
63	Ireland	0.90	7.10
64	Israel	0.85	7.58
65	Italy	0.85	6.42
66	Jamaica	0.75	5.97
67	Japan	0.76	6.11
68	Jordan	0.80	5.46
69	Kazakhstan	0.83	5.74
70	Kenya	0.53	4.60
71	Kosovo	0.87	5.50
72	Kuwait	0.87	6.52
73	Kyrgyzstan	0.82	5.10
74	Laos	0.84	4.85
75	Latvia	0.84	5.30
76	Lebanon	0.72	5.23
77	Lesotho	0.46	6.13
78	Liberia	0.80	5.13
79	Libya	0.79	5.21
80	Lithuania	0.82	5.74
81	Luxembourg	0.92	7.24
82	Macedonia	0.77	5.04
83	Madagascar	0.47	4.23
84	Malawi	0.55	4.93
85	Malaysia	0.85	5.83

(*Continued*)

#	Country	Job Satisfaction	Life Satisfaction
86	Mali	0.59	4.81
87	Malta	0.85	6.30
88	Mauritania	0.74	5.05
89	Mauritius	0.91	5.59
90	Mexico	0.85	7.49
91	Moldova	0.77	5.85
92	Mongolia	0.87	5.08
93	Montenegro	0.76	5.60
94	Morocco	0.67	5.12
95	Mozambique	0.69	5.30
96	Myanmar	0.59	3.57
97	Nepal	0.86	4.36
98	Netherlands	0.93	7.62
99	New Zealand	0.87	7.30
100	Nicaragua	0.82	5.88
101	Niger	0.85	4.58
102	Nigeria	0.66	5.67
103	North Cyprus	0.78	6.03
104	Norway	0.95	7.82
105	Oman	0.85	6.82
106	Pakistan	0.70	4.97
107	Palestinian Territories	0.76	5.11
108	Panama	0.91	7.50
109	Paraguay	0.90	6.02
110	Peru	0.82	5.94
111	Philippines	0.88	5.19
112	Poland	0.88	6.20
113	Portugal	0.87	5.74
114	Qatar	0.87	6.79
115	Romania	0.77	5.59
116	Russia	0.76	5.72
117	Rwanda	0.62	4.78
118	Saudi Arabia	0.84	6.56
119	Senegal	0.63	4.64
120	Serbia	0.71	5.03
121	Sierra Leone	0.74	5.40
122	Singapore	0.90	6.56
123	Slovakia	0.82	6.28
124	Slovenia	0.89	6.53
125	Somaliland region	0.88	5.82
126	South Africa	0.66	5.47
127	South Korea	0.73	6.17
128	Spain	0.90	6.77
129	Sri Lanka	0.88	4.35

(*Continued*)

#	Country	Job Satisfaction	Life Satisfaction
130	Sudan	0.63	4.83
131	Suriname	0.88	6.57
132	Swaziland	0.69	5.89
133	Sweden	0.93	7.57
134	Switzerland	0.93	7.69
135	Syria	0.57	3.96
136	Taiwan	0.80	6.46
137	Tajikistan	0.88	4.65
138	Tanzania	0.67	4.64
139	Thailand	0.95	6.43
140	Togo	0.48	3.16
141	Trinidad & Tobago	0.89	6.37
142	Tunisia	0.62	4.98
143	Turkey	0.77	5.51
144	Turkmenistan	0.94	5.90
145	Uganda	0.59	4.84
146	Ukraine	0.74	5.44
147	United Arab Emirates	0.89	7.16
148	United Kingdom	0.87	7.00
149	United States	0.87	7.35
150	Uruguay	0.83	6.47
151	Uzbekistan	0.91	5.54
152	Venezuela	0.91	7.31
153	Vietnam	0.84	5.82
154	Yemen	0.59	4.29
155	Zambia	0.68	5.79
156	Zimbabwe	0.64	5.29

ABOUT THE AUTHORS

Christopher J. L. Cunningham is a UC Foundation Associate Professor of Psychology and a graduate faculty member at The University of Tennessee at Chattanooga. He teaches multiple courses including organizational and occupational health psychology (OHP), organizational development and change management, statistics, and research methods. His research interests include stress and recovery, individual differences and health practices, and the management of multiple work and nonwork roles. Chris is an editorial board member for the *Journal of Occupational Health Psychology,* the *International Journal of Stress Management,* and *Stress & Health*, and a frequent reviewer for eight other applied psychology journals.

Shanna R. Daniels is an Assistant Professor of Management at Florida State University. Daniels received a Ph.D. in Management from Tulane University. Prior to her current position, she also served on the faculty at Southern University and A&M College as Assistant Professor of Management. Daniels is a member of the Academy of Management, Southern Management Association, and the Society for Industrial and Organizational Psychology. Her research focuses on workplace social experiences including interpersonal mistreatment, discrimination, and paternalism, and the ways in which those experiences affect employee well-being and organizational outcomes. Daniels is particularly interested in the intersection of race and gender when studying these relationships. In another line of work, Daniels investigates employee reciprocity, as a social exchange mechanism, with regard to positive and negative organizational phenomena. Her work has been published in the *Handbook of Industrial Organizational Psychology.*

Ed Diener was a Professor at the University of Illinois from 1974 until 2008 and is now professor emeritus, and a Senior Scientist for the Gallup Organization. He was the president of three scientific societies and the editor of *Journal of Personality and Social Psychology*. Diener was the founding editor of *Perspectives on Psychological Science* and *Journal of Happiness Studies*. He has over 325 publications and 84,000 citations of his work, and has been awarded many of the top scientific recognitions in psychology, as well as honorary doctorates. Diener explores the personality and cultural influences on subjective well-being (SWB) as well as the influences of income on well-being. He works on the development and validation of diverse measures of SWB. Diener spearheaded the drive to use national accounts of subjective well-being for policy purposes. He recently has been working to exploring the beneficial effects of subjective well-being on health, social relationships, productivity, and citizenship.

Emilija Djurdjevic is an Assistant Professor at the College of Business Administration at the University of Rhode Island. She received her Ph.D. in Business Administration from the Sam. M. Walton College of Business at the University of Arkansas. Her current research interests include performance appraisal, power, politics, and social influence processes, and work stress. Her publications have appeared in journals such as *Journal of Applied Psychology* and *Human Resource Management Review*.

Daniel C. Feldman is the Synovus Chair of Servant Leadership and the Associate Dean for Academic Affairs at the Terry College of Business at the University of Georgia. He received his Ph.D. in Organizational Behavior from Yale University. He is the author of seven books and over 150 articles on career development and career management in organizations. He served as Editor-in-Chief of *Journal of Management* and Chair of the Careers Division of the Academy of Management and was named a Fellow of the Society of Organizational Behavior in 2008.

Gerald R. Ferris is the Francis Eppes Professor of Management and Professor of Psychology at Florida State University. Ferris received a Ph.D. in Business Administration from the University of Illinois at Urbana-Champaign. Prior to his current position, he also served on the faculties at Texas A&M University, the University of Illinois at Urbana-Champaign, and the University of Mississippi. Ferris is a Fellow of the American Psychological Association, the Society for Industrial and Organizational Psychology, and the American Psychological Society. He has research interests in the areas of social and political influence in organizations. Ferris is the author of numerous articles published in a number of top-level journals. He founded, and served as editor of, the annual series, *Research in Personnel and Human Resources Management* from its origin in 1981 until 2003. Ferris has been the recipient of a number of distinctions and honors. In 2001, he was the recipient of the Heneman Career Achievement Award, and in 2010 he received the Thomas A. Mahoney

Mentoring Award, both from the Human Resources Division of the Academy of Management.

Steve Jex is currently Professor of Industrial/Organizational Psychology at Bowling Green State University. He has also held faculty appointments at Central Michigan University and University of Wisconsin Oshkosh. He received his Ph.D. in Industrial/Organizational Psychology from the University of South Florida in 1988. His primary research interests are occupational stress, employee health, and aging issues in the workplace. Dr. Jex is the author of five books, including *Stress and Job Performance: Theory, Research,* and *Implications for Managerial Practice* and *Organizational Psychology: A Scientist-Practitioner Approach (3rd Edition)* (with Tom Britt).

Eden King is an Associate Professor in the Industrial-Organizational Psychology program at George Mason University. She is pursuing a program of research that seeks to guide the equitable and effective management of diverse organizations. Her research integrates organizational and social psychological theories in conceptualizing social stigma and the work-life interface. This research addresses three primary themes: (1) current manifestations of discrimination and barriers to work-life balance in organizations, (2) consequences of such challenges for its targets and their workplaces, and (3) individual and organizational strategies for reducing discrimination and increasing support for families.

Rachel King, M.A. is currently a Ph.D. student in Industrial/Organizational Psychology at Bowling Green State University. She received her M.A. in Industrial/Organizational Psychology from Bowling Green State University in 2014. Her research interests are primarily in the areas of psychometrics, occupational health psychology, and the aging workforce.

Thomas Köllen, Ph.D., is an Assistant Professor at the Department of Management/Institute for Gender and Diversity in Organizations, Vienna University of Economics and Business (WU Wien). Dr. Köllen completed studies of Business Administration at Friedrich Schiller University in Jena, Germany; University of Turin, Italy; and WU Vienna, Austria. He was a Doc Team Fellow of the Austrian Academy of Sciences (2006–2009) and a Visiting Scholar at Goethe University Frankfurt, Germany (2007), and Fluminense Federal University (UFF) in Niteroi, Brazil (2012). Dr. Köllen's research focuses on issues related to bi- and homo-sexual employees and entrepreneurs, nationalities and nationalism in organizations, and intersectional approaches to diversity and diversity management. Dr. Köllen received several awards for his research and publications.

Lauren Kuykendall is a doctoral student in Industrial-Organizational Psychology at Purdue University. She received her bachelor's degree in psychology and philosophy from Wofford College and her master's degree in Industrial-Organizational Psychology from Purdue University. Her research interests include worker well-being, leisure, and virtues.

Alex Lindsey is a third year doctoral student in the Industrial/Organizational Psychology program at George Mason University. His research interests include diversity and inclusion as well as the promotion of employee well-being in the workplace. Specifically, Alex is interested in strategies that organizations, targets of prejudice, and allies can use to reduce workplace discrimination and promote the well-being of marginalized employees, with a special interest in lesbian, gay, and bisexual (LGB) populations. In the future, Alex hopes to obtain an academic position in which he can continue these streams of research while also pursuing his passions for teaching and service.

Vincent Ng is a graduate student in the Industrial-Organizational Psychology Ph.D. program at Purdue University. He received his B.A. in psychology from Vassar College and his M.S. in Industrial-Organizational Psychology from Salem State University. His current research interests include virtues, measurement, and ethical leadership.

Shannon L. Rawski is a Ph.D. Candidate at the University of Arkansas. She holds an M.A. in Business from the University of Nebraska – Lincoln and a B.S. in psychology from Bowling Green State University. Shannon's research interests include sexual harassment & workplace deviance, ethical decision-making & organizational punishment, and gender & identity issues in the workplace.

Isaac Sabat is a second year doctoral student in the Industrial/Psychology program at George Mason University. His research focuses on all aspects of diversity and discrimination in the workplace, with special focus on invisibly stigmatized identities. Most of his work deals with understanding the dynamics of stigma identity management within a workplace context, and identifying ways to improve the effectiveness of identity management strategies that stigmatized targets can engage in to remediate the discrimination that they experience. Isaac plans to pursue an academic career that will allow him to continue researching these very important topics.

Heiko Schulz is consultant for personnel and organizational development at Techniker Krankenkasse, one of the largest health insurance funds in Germany. Moreover, he has consulted various companies in different industries. His main interests are leadership behavior, managerial challenges related to the aging workforce, as well as evidence based human resource management.

Jennifer C. Sexton is an Assistant Professor of Management at West Virginia University. Sexton received a Ph.D. in Business Administration from Florida State University. Her research interests include organizational learning, knowledge-based and resource-based perspectives, innovation, top management teams, and mergers and acquisitions. She is especially interested in examining how firms develop, control, and change their innovation processes. While at Florida State University (FSU), Sexton was a 2008 BB&T Graduate Fellow and a 2011–2012 Leslie N. Wilson – Delores Auzenne Fellowship recipient. She has received the College of Business Doctoral Student Research Award, the College of Business Outstanding Teaching Assistant Award, and the FSU Outstanding Teaching Assistant Award. She has presented her research at the Strategic Management Society, the Babson College Entrepreneurship Research Conference, and the Southern Management Association, and her work has appeared in several scholarly journals and anthologies, including *Organizational Research Methods*.

Leah D. Sheppard received her Ph.D. from the University of British Columbia and is an Assistant Professor in the College of Business at Washington State University. She is researching issues related to gender stereotyping in organizations and female leadership. Leah is particularly interested in interpersonal workplace dynamics among women and how they are perceived and influenced by organizational observers. Her research on how female same-sex conflict at work is evaluated relative to male same-sex conflict has been featured in the Wall Street Journal and on the Canadian Broadcasting Company's Lang & O'Leary Exchange.

Louis Tay is an Assistant Professor in Industrial-Organizational Psychology at Purdue University. He received his Ph.D. in Industrial/Organizational Psychology from the University of Illinois in 2011. His research interests include subjective well-being, vocational interests, virtue, and methodology. He has published more than 40 papers and his work has appeared in multiple outlets including *Journal of Applied Psychology*, *Personnel Psychology*, *Organizational Research Methods*, *Psychological*

Science, and *Journal of Personality and Social Psychology*. He is currently serving on the editorial boards of *Organizational Research Methods* and *Journal of Management*.

Hannes Zacher is an Associate Professor in Organizational Psychology at the University of Groningen in the Netherlands. He received his Ph.D. in industrial and organizational psychology from the University of Giessen (Germany) in 2009. Subsequently, he was a postdoctoral fellow at Jacobs University (Germany) and lecturer at the University of Queensland (Australia). His research focuses on different forms of organizational sustainability, with emphases on successful aging and career development in the work context; proactivity, innovation, leadership, and entrepreneurship; and pro-environmental employee behaviors. He is consulting editor on the founding editorial board of *Work, Aging and Retirement* published by Oxford University Press.